PROGRESS IN SMOKING AND HEALTH RESEARCH

PROGRESS IN SMOKING AND HEALTH RESEARCH

THOMAS C. JEFFRIES
EDITOR

Nova Biomedical Books
New York

For permission to use material from this book please contact us:
Telephone 631-231-7269; Fax 631-231-8175
Web Site: http://www.novapublishers.com

Library of Congress Cataloging-in-Publication Data

Progress in smoking and health research / Thomas C. Jeffries (editor).
p. ; cm.
Includes bibliographical references and index.
ISBN-13: 978-1-60021-686-2 (hardcover)
ISBN-10: 1-60021-686-2 (hardcover)
1. Nicotine addiction--Treatment. 2. Smoking--Health aspects. 3. Smoking cessation. I. Jeffries, Thomas C.
[DNLM: 1. Tobacco Use Disorder--therapy. 2. Smoking--adverse effects. 3. Smoking Cessation.
WM 290 P9645 2007]RC567.P76 2007
616.86'50072--dc22 2007011127

Published by Nova Science Publishers, Inc. ✦ New York

Contents

Preface

Smoking is the most common risk factor for the development of lung cancer, which is the leading cause of cancer death. It is also associated with many other types of cancer, including cancers of the esophagus, larynx, kidney, pancreas, and cervix. Smoking also increases the risk of other health problems, such as chronic lung disease and heart disease. Smoking during pregnancy can have adverse effects on the unborn child, such as premature delivery and low birth weight.This new book presents cutting-edge research in this field.

Chapter I - Tobacco-use is a serious public health concern worldwide and remains the leading cause of preventable death in the United States, accounting for over 440,000 deaths annually. Healthcare providers have an obligation to their patients to provide the most current behavioral and pharmacotherapeutical tobacco cessation interventions available. Understanding the medications available for effective cessation interventions will do a great deal to help reduce the overwhelming disease burden caused by tobacco.

Chapter II - The purpose of this study was to examine risk and protective factors for the initiation and maintenance of cigarette smoking during varying developmental periods from childhood through late adolescence for African-American and white adolescents. The authors used data from a sample of 503 males who were first recruited in the first grade and followed annually for 14 years. Trajectory analyses identified three trajectory groups for African Americans and whites: nonsmokers, light smokers, and regular smokers. The following domains of risk and protective factors were included in the analyses: individual [hyperactivity/impulsivity/attention problem (HIA), depression, attitudes toward substance use, school performance, delinquency frequency, and religiosity], family (parental smoking and relationship with parents), peer (peer delinquency), and environmental [socioeconomic status (SES) and neighborhood quality]. First analyses were conducted separately by race to determine which factors represented risk and which represented protection. Then hierarchical logistic regression analyses were conducted to determine how these factors differentiated among the three trajectory groups and whether race interacted with these factors. Many of the variables were both risk and protective factors across different developmental periods. School performance and religiosity were only significantly related to smoking for African Americans and SES was only related for whites. For both races HIA, depression, delinquency, and peer delinquency were significantly related to smoking. In the multivariate analyses, race, SES, and delinquency were related to smoking at younger ages and delinquent peers was related to smoking at all ages. Only four interactions with race were significant for smoking. Good school performance was protective for African Americans at ages 7-9, but not whites. Having many delinquent peers was a stronger risk factor for African Americans at ages 13-16, but having many at ages 17-19 was a risk factor only for whites. Being low in delinquency was a stronger protective factor for whites at ages 13-16. Depression was related to regular smoking only for African Americans and attitudes toward substance use, parental smoking, and neighborhood quality were related only for whites. For both races HIA, school performance, delinquency, and peer delinquency were related to regular smoking. In the multivariate analyses, being African American protected against regular smoking at all ages. Only one interaction was significant; low depression was a protective factor for African American but not white regular smoking. Overall, the fact that there were few significant interactions of risk and protective factors with race suggests that the same factors can be targeted for both whites and African Americans in cigarette prevention programs.

Chapter III - Cigarette smoking is still considered a common habit in the Western world, even though it has come under increasing attack by numerous groups both within the United States and worldwide. Among smokers, increased plaque accumulation, higher incidence of gingivitis and periodontitis, higher rate of tooth loss, and increased resorption of the alveolar ridge, have been found in the oral cavity. The use of endosseous dental implants in various edentulous situations have increased over the past 10 years. Cigarette smoking may adversely affect wound healing, and thus jeopardize the success of bone grafting and dental implantation.

Bone grafts and sinus lift operations are both common and well documented procedures prior to dental implant placement. Autologous bone grafts for dental implants were originally described by Bränemark *et al.* in 1975, and is now a well-accepted procedure in oral and maxillofacial rehabilitation. A sinus lift operation has a predictable outcome with an implant survival rate of over 90% for 3 to 5 years. It is considered a safe treatment modality with only minor complications. Toxic by-products of cigarette smoking, such as nicotine, carbon monoxide and hydrogen cyanide, have been implicated as risk factors for impaired healing and thus may affect the success and complications of those surgical procedures.

Smoking also impairs wound healing in various surgical disciplines. It is the single most important risk factor for the development of post-operative complications in orthopedic surgery. In dermatology, smoking decreases the synthesis rate of collagen in skin, *in vivo,* and alters the balance of extracellular matrix turnover in skin. Tissue ischemia and wound-healing impairment, secondary to the influence of tobacco, are problematic for plastic surgeons.

An association between dental implants, grafting procedures (bone grafts, maxillary sinuses augmentation etc.), and history of smoking has been reported. A higher complication or failure rate was found in smokers with and without bone grafts.

The relationship between cigarette smoking and oral procedures with regard to dental implantations, i.e., sinus lift operations, onlay bone grafts and dental implantations, including the incidence of complications related to these procedures and long-term survival and success rates of dental implants among smokers and non-smokers will be described in this chapter.

This study was based on data from dental operations performed between the years 1995-2003, following accepted and well documented protocols. Criteria for patient inclusion in the study were: adequate information regarding age, gender, health status, pre- and post-operative radiographs, and follow-up for at least 6 months post-surgery.

All smoking habits were known at the time of operation. Current smokers were divided into two subgroups: number of cigarettes per day (less vs. more than 10) and duration of smoking (less vs. more than 10 years). Past smokers were defined as patients who stopped at least 6 months before the surgical procedure.

Chapter IV - In 2002, the New York City Department of Health and Mental Hygiene (DOHMH) launched an aggressive, comprehensive tobacco control program comprised of five components: taxation, legal action, cessation services, public education and evaluation. Smoking cessation has been delivered through two main approaches: the promotion of cessation behaviors, and the provision of specific population-based and targeted cessation services.

This chapter provides information on both the promotion of cessation behaviors and the provision of cessation services. It describes how cessation behaviors (e.g., making a quit attempt, adopting a smoke-free home policy) have been supported by the other four components of DOHMH's five-point tobacco control program (taxation, legal action, public education and evaluation) as well as provides details about the cessation services offered (giveaways of nicotine replacement therapy, face-to-face education of health care providers and their staff, and coordination of cessation services with the city's public hospital system).

By aggressively implementing a comprehensive tobacco control that includes the provision of cessation services and the promotion of cessation behaviors through taxation, legal action, public education and evaluation, New York City has been able to produce significant declines in smoking prevalence in less than 5 years.

Chapter V - Male smoking prevalence is considerably high in many Asian countries including Japan, but there have been few reports on effectiveness of smoking cessation measures. In this article, the authors examined the following four fundamental questions that public health professionals often face;

1) To what extent do smokers quit smoking? In many situations, the authors encourage smokers to quit smoking regardless of their intention to quit. In one of these situations, the authors implemented a smoking-cessation intervention in a workplace setting (263 male smokers, smoking prevalence: 62.9%) in a cross-over design, and ascertained that the cessation rate was 12.9% and 3.1% in the intervention and control groups, respectively.

2) To what extent do smokers maintain their cessation of smoking after having quit for more than four weeks? Many smokers successfully quit smoking, but later relapse. After the authors cross-over intervention study was completed, the authors then observed all ex-smokers who quit smoking at least once for more than four weeks, and ascertained that no relapse occurred after three years had passed since cessation and that 45% of them continued smoking cessation.

3) Is a small-scale intervention effective in reducing smoking prevalence? In smoking cessation programs, the authors are usually able to reach only a small portion of smokers, and most of them voluntarily participate in the program. The authors ascertained that small-scale annual interventions for smoking cessation repeated for ten years yielded lower smoking prevalence than doing no intervention at all.

4) Are comprehensive environmental changes as effective as direct intervention? It is usually hard to compare these two measures, because environmental changes affect all smokers, making concurrent comparison impossible. Smokers in Japan have experienced environmental changes since 2002, such as a price increase and implementation of laws. In the occupational setting described above, indoor smoking was banned in 2003. The authors compared the smoking abstinence rate in the intervention period and during the period of comprehensive environmental changes. The authors ascertained that the smoking abstinence rate was 8.9% and 7.1% in the periods of intervention and environmental changes, respectively, and revealed that comprehensive environmental changes are fairly effective in promoting smoking cessation.

Chapter VI - With 4.9 million people being killed each year due to smoking worldwide, tobacco is the only product that kills half its consumers. Across the E.U. countries, it is estimated that around 106.000 women die prematurely each year as a result of smoking. Women are affected by the main smoking-related diseases in the same way as men, but are also at risk of developing a number of gender-specific problems including cancer of cervix and problems related to reproductive health and osteoporosis.

An important question regarding quitting smoking is whether men and women should receive different cessation treatments. Although smoking cessation clinical trials reveal that the same pharmacotherapy treatments (Bupropion SR, Nicotine Replacement Therapies) benefit both men and women, there is strong evidence that the approach should be different towards female smokers. In fact, women may face different stressing parameters and barriers to quitting that may be useful to address in treatment decisions. These include greater likelihood of depression, greater weight control concerns, and hormonal cycle abnormalities. This suggests that women may benefit from tobacco dependence treatments that address these topics, although only few studies have examined programs targeted to one gender.

With regard to motivation in a smoking cessation program for females, one should underline benefits such as physical appearance and lower incidence of osteoporosis. In particular, women, who are candidates to become pregnant, may be more receptive to stop smoking because of the serious risks imposed on the fetus.

In conclusion, different smoking cessation treatment strategies with augmented psychosocial interventions and more intensive counseling about weight gain, osteoporosis, physical appearance, depression, and pregnancy may be needed for female smokers in order to achieve better abstinence rates.

Chapter VII - Overweight and obesity are the most common nutritional disorders in industrialized countries which continue to increase in their prevalences and, in particular, in the US. Childhood obesity predicts obesity in adulthood and later cardiovascular disease. Effective prevention strategies against childhood obesity are needed because therapeutic interventions are expensive and tend to have poor long term results. However, for primary prevention of childhood obesity potential modifiable risk factors have to be identified. Nowadays we know that more than energy intake alone regulates our body mass index. In fact, there are hormone-modulating risk factors that might promote obesity. A number of such new risk factors like intrauterine tobacco exposure were recently identified. The individual association of this risk factor to childhood obesity is estimated in a large population with respect to potential confounders and its impact on population level is estimated by using adjusted attributable risk fractions and preventable potentials.

Chapter VIII - Frequency: The prevalence of cigarette smoking is significantly higher among patients with schizophrenia (60-90%) than in the general population (23-30%). While tobacco smoking decreases in general population (from 45% in the 1960's to 23-30% in the 2000's), smoking in patients with schizophrenia remains high. Patients with schizophrenia smoke more deeply, thereby increasing their exposure to harmful elements in tobacco smoke.

Impact of smoking on patients with schizophrenia: As in the general population, smoking contributes to the reduced life expectancy in patients with schizophrenia. Patients with schizophrenia are at elevated risk for cardiovascular disease due to high rates of cigarette smoking. In the Department of Mental Health of the commonwealth of Massachussetts, cardiovascular disease was the factor that most strongly associated with excess mortality.

Improvement of cognitive deficits: Patients with schizophrenia may use nicotine to reduce cognitive deficits and negative symptoms or neuroleptic side effects. Smoking may transiently alleviate negative symptoms in patients with schizophrenia in increasing dopaminergic and glutamatergic neurotransmission in the prefrontal cortex. In patients with schizophrenia, nicotine improves some cognitive deficits : 1) Sensory gating deficits and abnormalities in smooth pursuit eye movements associated with schizophrenia are transiently normalized with the administration of nicotine 2) High-dose nicotine transiently normalizes the abnormality in P50 inhibition in schizophrenic patients and in their relatives 3) In tasks that tax working memory and selective attention, nicotine may improve performance in patients with schizophrenia by enhancing activation of and functional connectivity between brain regions that mediate task performance 4) Cigarette smoking may selectively enhance visuospatial working memory and attentional deficits in smokers with schizophrenia. However, Harris et al. found that nicotine affects only the attention without effects of nicotine on learning, memory or visuospatial/constructional abilities. In addition, smoking could facilitate disinhibition in patients with schizophrenia. Some authors stressed that nicotine does not appear to have a long-lasting therapeutic effect on schizophrenia's symptoms.

Impact of smoking on patients with schizophrenia who are on antipsychotic medications : Smoking increases the metabolism of the antipsychotic medications by inducing the cytochrome P450 1A2 isoform. Smoking lowers the blood levels of typical or atypical antipsychotic medications.

Treatment: Although patients with schizophrenia have low motivations to quit smoking, smoking cessation treatment can be effective for these patients. Atypical antipsychotic medications, in combination with the nicotine transdermal patch, or bupropion significantly enhanced the rate of smoking cessation.

Chapter IX - The aim of the study was the evaluation of the level of cotinine, socio-economic status of the patients and birth parameters of the newborn as an index for the behaviors of pregnant women in relation to smoking tobacco and ETS.

The research included 115 women delivering at the Gynecological-Obstetric Clinic University of Medical Sciences in Warsaw as well as 115 newborns. The patients were divided into three groups: smokers, exposed to ETS and the nonsmokers.

A questionnaire method concerning the socio-economic status, tobacco smoking/passive exposure and pregnancy was used in the research. Most often women smoking tobacco would have the secondary education and performed a white-collar work. 74.47% of women were inhabitants of Warsaw. Among the women who were inhaling the smoke passively, the highest percentage referred to women aged 25-29. 64% of patients had higher education. 72% of women performed the white-collar work. Among the women smoking tobacco, 46.05% were patients who smoked 1-5 cigarettes a day. In all the groups of the tested women, the consciousness of health consequences connected with tobacco smoking and ETS was almost 100%.

In the group of mothers smoking tobacco, there were 76.6% of newborns born at the right time, whereas 23.4% of newborns were born prematurely. The newborns of the smoking women were lighter by 610.9 g in comparison with the newborns of the nonsmoking mothers, and 280.3 g in relation to the newborn of women who were passively exposed to smoke.

The newborns of smoking mothers were 4.06 cm shorter in comparison to the children of non-smoking mothers and the ones who were not exposed to smoke. These newborns were also 1.72 cm smaller than the newborns of mothers passively exposed to smoke.

The concentration of cotinine in the urine and placenta of smoking mothers as well as the first urine of the newborns was respectively: 898 ng/mg of creatinine, 47 ng/g of placenta and 184 ng/mg of creatinine. For women exposed to ETS the concentrations were 53 ng/mg of creatinine, 19 ng/g and 26 ng/mg of creatinine respectively.

A statistically significant relation between the active and passive exposure to tobacco smoke during pregnancy and the risk of premature delivery, low birth body mass and body length was observed.

The presence of cotinine in the placenta and in the first urine of an newborn speaks volumes of the exposure of the fetus to toxic components of smoke.

Chapter X - Tobacco use is the number one cause of preventable death in the United States (U.S. Department of Health and Human Services, 2001). While there has been much research dedicated to adolescents and adolescent health risk activities, there remains a gap in knowledge surrounding parental awareness of these risk behaviors specifically as it relates to the decision to initiate tobacco use. The purpose of this current study is to examine parental awareness of adolescent tobacco use in a population of middle school students. Unique to this study is the dyadic approach to investigation. Twenty-two dyadic pairs of parents and adolescents were surveyed. The results of this study demonstrate that there is a gap in family communication around tobacco use. While parents were generally accurate when reporting that their own child did not smoke, they underestimated the behavior of their child's peers'. Adolescents report rarely having tobacco related conversations with mothers and sometimes talking with fathers about tobacco. There was also concordance between the parents' responses and the adolescents' response around collaborative decision making. The respondents felt that the adolescent within a family is being told exactly what to do by his or her parent; limiting their opportunity to make decisions. Parents must engage their children in conversation about their own behavior and that of their peers. During middle school and high school adolescents are faced with powerful peer influences and decisions about risk behaviors. If these teens are not able to make their own decisions in their home it can be assumed that they will have a difficult time with social decision making, which may lead to detrimental choices. Parents need to be aware of these facts so they can accurately monitor the behaviors of their child and child's peers and potentially health risk decision making.

Chapter XI - Adolescent behaviour is a dynamic process. Adolescent behaviour outcomes will be due to temporal dependencies, latent variables, feedback effect and other socio-economic and socio-environmental factors most of which are process outcomes themselves. Survey studies, cross-sectional and even some longitudinal studies show very little appreciation for the dynamic nature of the process and often concentrate on the socio-economic variables. Such an approach provides a flat snapshot view of a dynamic and multi dimension process which raises more questions than providing insight. The consequences of failing to account for the dynamic features of the process under study may be erroneous results and misleading conclusions with serious implications for the process of policy development. These issues are illustrated and discussed in this chapter using the behaviour outcome "teenage smoking".

In: Progress in Smoking and Health Research
Editor: T. C. Jeffries, pp. 1-3
ISBN: 978-1-60021-686-2

Expert Commentary

Tobacco Cessation or the Treatment of Tobacco Dependence?

Joan M. Davis[1] and Giuseppe Pizzo[2]

[1] Assistant Professor, Department of Dental Hygiene, College of Applied Sciences and Arts, Southern Illinois University, Carbondale, IL

[2] Senior Researcher and Assistant Professor, Department of Oral Sciences, University of Palermo, Italy

For many healthcare professionals, the educational goal when providing a health intervention to a tobacco-user is *tobacco cessation* – for the patient to set a quit date and then actually quit. The U.S. Public Health Service Guideline (2000) for tobacco cessation stresses the need to Ask if a patient uses tobacco, Advise them to quit, Assess their tobacco use, Assist in their quit attempt and finally Arrange follow-up after a cessation intervention [1]. Research has shown with just a brief intervention by a clinician, the chances of a successful quit attempt can double. Now considered a chronic, relapsing, progressive disease, tobacco-use represents behavioral, social and chemical dependent components where people often find themselves trapped in an addiction they did not see coming. Even with evidence-based interventions, pharmacotherapies, telephone quitlines, online resources and alternative quit methods, people still find it difficult to quit or stay quit. More than 70-90% of smokers who try to quit will relapse into regular tobacco use with the average smoker making five to seven quit attempts before actually succeeding long-term [1-3]. These 'failures' to succeed often lead a tobacco-user to give up all together and avoid another quit attempt for months or even years. The leveling off in the decline of smoking in the United States [4-5] may reflect, in part, this phenomenon of users who just are not able to quit. It could be argued that recommending a patient to quit over and over again at repeated office visits may discourage or alienate the very person needing help.

The question needs to be asked – *How do healthcare professionals/counselors effectively reach those patients who have tried to quit, failed, and are reluctant to try again?* One possible strategy would be for the healthcare field to change intervention paradigms and provide *tobacco dependence treatment* rather than tobacco cessation interventions [6]. The goal of both treatment approaches would be life-long discontinuance of all forms of tobacco-use but the *process* of ultimately quitting could look very different than from recommending immediate cessation.

For example, a 55 year old laborer who has been smoking two packs of cigarettes for 38 years states he is not interested in quitting. He is interested, though, in cutting back to help his health. Do we tell him he must quit – all or nothing - and tell him how to do it? Some patients may feel cornered and withdraw or become angry. A tobacco treatment strategy for this individual may be *reduction* from two packs to one pack then to a half of a pack. This would give the user a sense of success as well as an understanding on behavioral strategies on how to cut down use. In time, he may be much more receptive to information on pharmacotherapies to help overcome the remaining chemical dependence and quit.

Another approach with the treatment of tobacco dependence may include the off-label use of FDA approved pharmacotherapies. Rather than using the nicotine patch only or bupropion SR as isolated medications, a patient-tailored approach could be used according to the level of nicotine addition and reported withdrawal symptoms of the individual. For example, our two pack-a-day smoker could use the 4mg nicotine lozenge to replace cigarettes through out the day as he cuts down as he changes life habits connected to his smoking.

An open-ended approach is needed when treating tobacco dependence and involves building a trust relationship between clinician and patient. This is especially true for clinicians who see patients on an ongoing basis such as in the dental field. For the patient who is unwilling to quit, what do we say to encourage them to continue to seek preventive care but not make them feel they are going to get the 'tobacco talk' two or three times a year? We could ask 'Tell me how you are doing with your smoking." – then listen. If they are not ready to talk about cutting back or quitting, then a simple "I understand this is not a good time. When *you* are ready, we can talk about the several resources and medications available to help you. The decision is completely yours". This leaves an open door for reflection, ownership and self-determination.

Though the ultimate goal for any intervention is total abstinence, clinicians need to ask themselves what defines success when patients are treated for tobacco dependence. Have we failed if a quit date is not chosen at the first appointment? Have we succeeded if we get in the recommended 5A's? Have we failed if the patient has not quit by the next regular appointment? Do we quit treating the tobacco use if there is a hostile response to our recommendations to quit? Success may be opening communication lines and building trust with those who indicate an unwillingness to quit. Success may be a reduction from 20 cigarettes to ten. Success may be a patient stating that he has thought a lot about what was discussed at him last appointment and want to know more about the options to help him quit. Success may be a patient taking you by the arm in the waiting room and thanking you for respecting him enough to let him decide a system that worked for him – he has gone from two packs a day to two cigarettes a day.

The combination of increase taxes on tobacco products, indoor air standard as well as a change in social norms against tobacco-use, will likely drive more and more tobacco-users to want to cut-back or quit all together. More flexible tobacco treatment options need to be offered if we are going to be there for 'hard-core' users ready to do something.

References

[1] Fiore MC, Bailey WC, Cohen SJ, et al. Treating tobacco use and dependence. Clinical Practice Guideline. Rockville, MD: U.S. Department of Health and Human Services. Public Health Service. June 2000. Available at: URL: http://surgeongeneral.gov/tobacco/treating_tobacco_use.pdf. Accessed December 5, 2006.

[2] Tonnesen P, Paoletti P, Gustavsson MA, et al. Higher dosage nicotine patches increase on-year smoking cessation rates: results from the European CEASE trial. *Eur. Respir. J.* 1999;13:238-246.

[3] Hughes JR, Keely J, Naud S. Shape of the relapse curve and long-term abstinence among untreated smokers. *Addiction* 2003;99:29-38.

[4] Centers for Disease Control and Prevention. Tobacco use among adults—United States, 2005. *MMWR Morb. Mortal Wkly. Rep.* 2006;55:1145-1148.

[5] Centers for Disease Control and Prevention. Cigarette use among high school students—United States, 1991-2005. *MMWR Morb. Mortal Wkly. Rep.* 2006;55:724-726.

[6] Fagerstrom K, Groman E, Ruiz CA. Smoking cessation: problems and opportunities and future perspectives. *J. Smoking Cess.* 2006;1:1-2.

In: Progress in Smoking and Health Research
Editor: T. C. Jeffries, pp. 5-40
ISBN: 978-1-60021-686-2

Chapter I

Pharmacotherapies for Smoking Cessation

Giuseppe Pizzo [*,1], ***Maria E. Licata*** [1], ***Maria R. Piscopo*** [1] ***and Joan M. Davis*** [2]

[1] Department of Oral Sciences, University of Palermo, Italy
[2] Department of Dental Hygiene, College of Applied Sciences and Arts, Southern Illinois University, Carbondale, IL

Introduction

Tobacco-use is a serious public health concern worldwide and remains the leading cause of preventable death in the United States, accounting for over 440,000 deaths annually [1, 2, 3]. Healthcare providers have an obligation to their patients to provide the most current behavioral and pharmacotherapeutical tobacco cessation interventions available. Understanding the medications available for effective cessation interventions will do a great deal to help reduce the overwhelming disease burden caused by tobacco.

Smoking is the most common way to use tobacco. In the United States (U.S.), some 20.9% of all adults reported that they are currently smokers, while in the United Kingdom (U.K.) the adult smoking rates are currently around 27% and 38% of Australians have this habit. The highest reported rates of smoking are from China, where it has been estimated that 63% of males are current smokers [1, 4].

The cigarette is the most important risk factor for premature mortality. In the year 2000, an estimated 4.83 million premature deaths worldwide were a direct consequence of smoking. If smoking prevalence continues to increase in the developing world, the number of annual

* Corresponding Author: Giuseppe Pizzo, DDS; Dipartimento di Scienze Stomatologiche, Università di Palermo; Via del Vespro 129; 90127 Palermo, Italy; phone: +39-091-6552231 fax: +39-091-6552202; email: giuseppepizzo@unipa.it; secondary email: giuseppepizzo@odonto.unipa.it

deaths attributable to cigarette smoking will be 10 million by 2020 [1, 2, 5, 6]. Smoking mortality is a composite of the four leading causes of death: heart disease, cancer, cerebrovascular disease and chronic obstructive pulmonary disease. Tobacco use is estimated to cause 35% of all cancers, 33% of all heart attacks and strokes, and 90% of chronic obstructive pulmonary disease, including emphysema. Smokers who do not quit by age 35 have a 50% chance of dying from a tobacco-related disease. Their life expectancy is 8 years less than those who have never smoked [7, 8]. Other forms of tobacco-use include cigar smoking, reverse smoking and smokeless tobacco. These ways of tobacco consumption may pose a reduced risk to the general health because the tobacco smoke is not inhaled. Nevertheless, they represent important risk factors for other serious diseases, such as the oropharyngeal cancer and periodontitis [9, 10, 11].

There is some indication that an increasing number of users have stopped smoking with an estimated two-thirds of smokers making a quit attempt each year. In fact, in 1965, 42.4% of U.S. adults reported that they were currently smokers, and another 13.6% reported that they were former smokers. By 1997, 24.75 of adults were current smokers and 23% were former smokers. Among current smokers in 1997, 41% had stopped smoking for at least 1 day in the preceding year and 70% wanted to quit. However, during the 1990s evidence suggested the rate of decline in smoking had waned. Unfortunately, many smokers choose to make an unaided quit attempt, a method that has only a small chance of long-term success [1, 12, 13].

The primary reason why many tobacco users find difficult to quit is because of their dependence on nicotine. Tobacco-use (both smoked and smokeless) provides rapid delivery of nicotine to the central nervous system, where it facilitates the relapse of a number of neurotransmitters, such as dopamine and noradrenaline. In dependent users, nicotine deprivation precipitates a withdrawal syndrome, consisting of symptoms such as irritability, low mood, poor concentration, and urges to smoke. This physical dependence to nicotine is a key factor in continued tobacco-use and should be addressed when considering therapies for the treatment of cigarettes or other tobacco products.

Since the 1980s, several pharmacological agents have been introduced to treat this dependence. Current guidelines for tobacco cessation interventions include a pharmacotherapy program: nicotine replacement therapy (NRT), of which there are six different products, and the non-nicotine therapies [12]. NRT acts by replacing some of the nicotine users would have received from their cigarettes (or the other tobacco products), and in doing so relieves the severity of the withdrawal symptoms. Non-nicotine therapies use agents that mimic the reinforcing effects of nicotine or reduce the negative effects associated with abstinence. A large number of studies examining the efficacy of various pharmacological agents for smoking cessation have been published with positive evidence for their effectiveness [4, 12, 14]. Moreover, specific pharmacological approaches should be considered in unique groups of the population such as smokeless tobacco users, adolescents, women, cultural and ethnic minorities and users of multiple forms of tobacco. In these groups, pharmacological interventions have to be conducted in consideration of the patient's conditions (psychosocial, cognitive and cultural conditions, pregnancy) and habits [12, 15, 16].

Strategies being considered for future pharmacotherapies include using agents that block the reinforcing effects of nicotine, prevention of nicotine from crossing the blood-brain barrier, and altering the metabolism of nicotine. Moreover, pharmacogenetic studies are currently in progress to explore the use of genetic information to better tailor existing treatment agents to tobacco users [17].

Pharmacological interventions should be accompanied, whenever possible, by behavioral support (patient centered advice and assistance). The U.S. Public Health Service 2000 Guideline *Treating Tobacco Use and Dependence* demonstrated that even minimal support, combined with appropriate pharmacotherapies, would increase the chances of a sustained quit of smoking. The more intense intervention, the greater likelihood the patient would remain tobacco free [12].

Currently, pharmacological therapy is prescribed by physicians to support smokers making attempt to quit. Dentists and dental hygienists should be able to actively promote smoking cessation interventions in their dental practice [18, 19]. They need to provide patients with appropriate pharmacological agents used to treat nicotine dependence and, if needed, recommending the use of them. Every member of the dental team can play an effective role in tobacco cessation as they provide preventive and therapeutic services to a basically healthy population. Dentists and their staff, in fact, have the opportunity to see groups of patients not regularly seen by other healthcare professionals such as smokers who have not yet developed smoking-related diseases as well as young people experimenting with smoking or at risk of starting [20, 21, 22].

Nicotine Dependence

Dependence can be defined as a situation in which a drug controls behavior and is considered a chronic relapsing disease. The primary criteria for drug dependence are a highly controlled or compulsive use of a drug with psychoactive effects and the presence of drug-reinforced behavior. Additional criteria include stereotypic patterns of use, use despite harmful consequences, relapse following abstinence, and recurrent drug cravings or urges to use. Dependence-producing drugs are often associated with tolerance, physical dependence with withdrawal symptoms and pleasant subjective effects. Tolerance is the result of morphological changes in the brain, such as receptors desensitization and inactivation as well as upregulation of the density of receptors. As a result of this neuroadaptation, cessation of drug use results in withdrawal syndrome.

The signs and symptoms of tobacco withdrawal syndrome include cravings for tobacco, irritability, frustration or anger, anxiety, depressed mood, difficulty concentrating and insomnia. These symptoms generally begin in a minor form a few hours (4-6 h) after the last cigarette, as nicotine blood levels drop, and usually peak 2-3 days after quitting and gradually decrease over time. A study of 554 patients who were attempting to quit smoking without assistance observed that 87% (482 of 554) of the subjects reported withdrawal symptoms during the first week of the follow-up. Restlessness and an increased appetite or weight gain were the most common symptoms [23]. If tobacco abstinence is maintained, mood usually returns to baseline (pre-quitting) level after 3-6 weeks, although there is much individual variation. Anxiety, poor concentration, irritability, restlessness, and nocturnal awakening returned to pre-cessation levels by 30 days, however hunger symptoms and weigh gain remained increased at 30 days post-cessation. Although data are much more limited on the acute withdrawal effects from smokeless tobacco, the symptoms appear to be very similar though they may be less intense and fewer in number. Thus, nicotine dependence is maintained not only by the subjective positive effects that smokers experience, but also by the desire to avoid the negative symptoms associated with nicotine withdrawal [12, 24, 25].

The Fagerström Test for Nicotine Dependence (FTND) consists of six questions and has been widely used to determine the degree of nicotine dependence. Although the maximal score is 10, a score higher than 4 indicates probable nicotine dependence. This test emphasizes the "time to the first cigarette of the day"; in fact, nicotine has a relatively short half-life, and smokers may experience discomfort upon waking unless they smoke a cigarette [17, 26].

The addictive nature of nicotine makes tobacco cessation difficult and it was estimated that 30-40% of smokers attempt to quit annually, yet less than 5% do. Most smoking cessation attempts fail within the first two weeks; on average, four or more attempts are necessary before long-term cessation is achieved. Even in patients with tobacco-related diseases (cardiovascular disease, cancer, chronic obstructive pulmonary disease) where stopping tobacco use is critical to halt further deterioration of their medical condition, fewer than 50% quit [4, 16].

Mechanisms of Nicotine Dependence

The potential for abuse or dependence to a drug is generally determined by the magnitude of the positive reinforcing effects and the speed of drug delivery to the brain. Typically, the relationship between drug dose and the reinforcing effect of the drug is characterized by an inverted U-shaped curve. Generally, the more quickly the drug is delivered to the brain, the greater the potential for abuse. Nicotine from a smoked cigarette is fast-acting, arriving in the brain within 7 seconds of inhalation, with initial arterial nicotine concentration far surpassing venous concentration. Such rapid delivery contributes to its high abuse potential [15, 16].

There exists a greater body of research on smoked tobacco rather than smokeless tobacco, though with both there is a systemic absorption of pharmacologically significant amounts of nicotine. Although absorption of the nicotine via the buccal mucosa for smokeless, pipe and cigar smoking is slower than the pulmonary route, it gives rise to lower arterial levels. Similar venous nicotine levels are found in regular users of each product. Blood nicotine levels fall rapidly after each cigarette whereas levels plateau during and after smokeless tobacco use. With the latter, nicotine absorption continues after the tobacco is discarded from the mouth due to the release of nicotine from the mucous membranes and absorption of swallowed nicotine. The systematic absorption of nicotine per typical dose may be 3-4 fold greater for smokeless than for smoked tobacco. Due to the short half-life of nicotine (~ 2h) it accumulates throughout the day in regular smokeless tobacco users and persists overnight. Both routes give rise to physical and psychological dependence [4].

Nicotine has a number of neurobiological effects which can lead to dependence. These effects are complex and not entirely understood. Nicotine binds to nicotinic acetylcholine receptors located in the brain, autonomic ganglia, and neuromuscular junctions. Such binding leads to release of a number of neurotransmitters and hormones including dopamine, serotonin, norepinephrine (adrenaline), acetylcholine, vasopressin, glutamate and beta-endorphin. Nicotine also stimulates the release of growth hormones, adrenocorticotrophic hormone and prolactin [16, 17].

The rewarding properties of nicotine are believed to be mediated by dopamine release in the nucleus accumbens from ventral tegmental area neurons. The mechanism through which nicotine mediates the increase in nucleus accumbens synaptic dopamine may involve the μ-opioid receptors and its endogenous ligand, β-endorphin. Increasing synaptic dopamine in the nucleus accumbens is a mechanism of reward for many abused drugs and reinforces its self-administration. The release of this substance produces both arousing and relaxing effects modulating many of the subjective, cognitive and behavioral effects, such as increase in pleasure, improved mood, increased attention, enhanced cognition vigilance and motor performance, reduced anxiety and weight loss. For example, the rush of adrenaline causes a sudden release of glucose, an increase in blood pressure, and increased respiratory and heart rates. In the brain, the nicotine decreases the inhibitory response, associated with the levels of gamma amino butyric acid, in regions controlling pleasure and motivation. Even a brief exposure to nicotine results in the long-term excitation of the brain's reward areas. However, it is not clear to what extent these positive subjective effects reported by tobacco users are the result of primary intrinsic effects of nicotine and to what extent they simply reflect relief of withdrawal symptoms which can appear after only a couple of hours of abstinence [16, 17].

Tobacco smoking and nicotine have pronounced effects on endocrine function as well. Nicotinic acetylcholine receptors are found throughout the central nervous system and also in peripheral tissues. There are several binding sites for nicotine within the paraventricular nucleus of the hypothalamus, and the endocrine effects of nicotine appear to be the result of a combination of action at postsynaptic cholinergic sites that acutely regulate corticotrophin releasing factor (CRF), and presynaptic action on monoaminergic neurons. Acutely, smoking increase adrenocorticotrophic hormone (ACTH) and cortisol levels. This response appears to require quite intense intake, involving one than more cigarette, and has been attributed to nicotine exposure. It has recently been established that nitric oxide is an inhibitory mediator of nicotine-induced hypothalamic-pituitary-adrenocortical (HPA) activity, providing a direct link between inflammatory processes and the HPA activation stimulated by smoking. The relationship between smoking, cortisol, and nicotine is important because the HPA axis is implicated in addictive processes. Moreover, heightened levels of cortisol have a range of adverse effects on biological processes relevant to long-term health, including lipid profiles, immune function, central adiposity, bone mineral density, and reproductive function. Cortisol may therefore mediate some of the effects of smoking on health outcomes such as cardiovascular disease and the metabolic syndrome. It is also highly sensitive to psychological stress, and this can explain why smoking cessation is stressful for many smokers, and it may lead them to fail in quit attempts. It has been proposed that cortisol is directly involved in this process, and that changes in cortisol following smoking cessation may predict early relapse [27].

Nicotine Replacement Therapy (NRT)

Nicotine Replacement Therapy (NRT) is considered a first-line treatment for tobacco dependence. The rationale for NRT is to reduce the severity of nicotine withdrawal symptoms and cravings among tobacco users attempting to quit and to facilitate the cessation attempt by providing weaking doses of nicotine in a "clean" form to smokers. When smokers inhale cigarette smoke, they receive a bolus of nicotine that rapidly enters the brain and delivers immediate reinforcement to their drug-seeking behavior. NRTs are designed to provide a lower level and, in some cases, slower infusion of nicotine by slowing and reducing the arterial and venous concentration of the drug [4, 12, 28].

Currently, five dosage forms of NRT are marketed in the United States: nicotine gum, nicotine transdermal patch, nicotine inhaler, nicotine nasal spray, and nicotine lozenges. A nicotine sublingual tablet is marketed in some countries in Europe. All six products developed to date deliver pure nicotine (derived from tobacco) to the user's blood stream without the dangerous toxins and carcinogens that are present in tobacco or tobacco smoke which are very largely responsible for the damaging health effects. The products differ in terms of the speed of nicotine delivery, the frequency and ease of use, type of local sensory side effects, amount of "behavioral" substitution they provide, and the extent to which they enable the user to titrate their dose as and when needed.

Based on the rate of delivery NRTs can be divided into two main types: constant dose (transdermal patches) and more flexible, self-administered dosing (gum, inhalator, nasal spray, lozenges, sub-lingual tablets).

There is no evidence that any one product is more effective than another. A recent meta-analysis, that included data from more than 100 randomized trials that tested the effects of several forms of NRT, reported that all commercially available agents were effective for smoking cessation and showed no overall significant differences among products [29]. These agents increase the odds of quitting long-term as much as two fold. In fact, when trials of all forms of NRT were pooled, results showed that 17% of smokers undergoing NRT therapy were able to quit compared with 10% of those treated with placebo, representing a 74% increase in the odds of abstinence after at least 6 months. It is for this reason that clinicians should encourage patients committed to a quit date to use NRT and are advised to take the patients' preference and medical contraindications into account.

However, there are no sufficient trials with follow-up beyond one year to give a good estimate of the long-term benefit of NRT [30]. Although such treatment is still likely to be highly cost-effective in terms of life years gained, the substantial amount of relapse observed (more than 90% of those treated do not succeed) even after one year of abstinence question whether this therapeutic is the most appropriate. For this reason, nicotine addiction should be viewed as a chronic recurring disease of the brain, often requiring long-term treatment. This treatment should include the encouragement to make repeated quit attempts accompanied with multiple treatment episodes over many years [13]. Moreover, with all NRT products, the long-term abstinence rate is determined by the level behavioral support provided. Success rates will vary from about 5% or less for NRT used without any support and may increase up to 15-30% when used with intensive counseling [4].

Current guidelines recommended using NRT only after quitting smoking [12]. However, theoretical arguments and data support the hypothesis that pre-cessation use of NRT, and in particular skin patches, might be useful in reducing dependence on inhaled nicotine and serve as a helpful prelude to smoking cessation [31].

Nicotine Transdermal Patches

The nicotine patch was introduced in 1992. They are currently available in various shapes, sizes, and effects duration. There are three major brands: Harbitol (Novartis Consumer, East Hanover, NJ), Nicoderm CQ (SmithKline Beecham, Philadelphia, PA), and Nicotrol (McNeil Consumer, Fort Washington, PA). The patch is placed on waking up, on a relatively hair free site on the upper body typically between neck and waist.

With the application of all forms of nicotine patches, nicotine diffuses through the skin and with concentrations increasing gradually over four to eight hours, after which this level is maintained for approximately 15 and 24 hours, before gradually declining [4]. The Harbitol and Nicoderm CQ formulations are intended for 24 hour use and applied once daily. These patches are available in 21 mg, 14 mg, and 7 mg doses. The dose can be progressively weaned over 2 to 4 months. Depending on the brand and the level of nicotine dependence, users usually start on the highest strength (21 mg) for about 4-6 weeks and then move into the medium (14 mg) for 2-4 weeks, then low strength (7 mg) patches for about 2-4 weeks. It is very important to properly determining the level of nicotine dependence and current level of tobacco use. One cigarette delivers approximately 1-2 mg of nicotine to a smoker. Therefore, if a patient uses 14 cigarettes/day then a 14 mg patch would be a reasonable NRT to recommend [32]. The Nicotrol patch is intended for 16 hour daytime use. It should be applied in the morning and removed before bedtime. The patch is available at 15 mg dose. The recommended duration of treatment is 6 weeks without tapering. The duration of patch use can range from 6 to 12 weeks, depending on specific patient characteristic [15, 28, 33].

The optimum dosage is selected on the basis of frequency of smoking (20 or more; less than 20/day), and patient's characteristics (e.g., prior experience with the patch, amount of nicotine dependence). The Fagerström scale can be useful to guide initial dosing for heavy smokers with a high nicotine dependence score. The 24 hour patch has the advantage of controlling morning smoking urges by producing higher blood nicotine levels upon awakening. However, it may be associated with sleep disturbances or vivid dreams, where the 16 hour patch is not [4, 12, 25].

Adverse effects of patches are generally minimal and include (usually mild) local skin sensitivity and irritation characterized by erythema, pruritus, or burning under the patch. Rotating the patch site every day can minimize these effects. Up to 50% of patients have localized skin reaction with less than 5% requiring discontinuation of the patch therapy. Reactions are self-limited and most erythema will disappear spontaneously after 1 to 2 days. Rashes may be treated with steroid creams. Other adverse effects included generalized rash, headache, nausea, vertigo and dyspepsia [12, 15, 16, 28].

The patch 1) provides constant and therapeutic levels on nicotine from first day of use, 2) does not need any special technique, 3) has few local side effects, 4) has no social acceptability problems as it is worn out of sight, 5) it is extremely unlikely to give rise to problems of long-term use and dependence due to the very slow rate of nicotine delivery.

The efficacy of the nicotine patch has been assessed in numerous studies and summarized in several meta-analyses. The odds ratio versus placebo for 12 month sustained abstinence rates reported from meta-analysis of patch trials is 1.62 [34]. Moreover, evidence suggests that an 8 week course of therapy with the patch is an efficacious as longer courses (e.g., up to 28 weeks) and that no treatment difference exists between the 24 hour and 16 hour patches [29]. However, the results of meta-analysis and clinical trials provide little support for improved outcomes with treatment longer than 8 weeks in duration or with tapering versus abrupt cessation of treatment [17]. In a comparison of standard transdermal nicotine treatment and extended treatment (8 addictional weeks of "maintenance" therapy with the 21 mg dose, following by a tapering phase) in a group of 55 smokers with abstinence-induced depressed mood, significant differences in abstinence rates were not observed. However, when treatment dropouts were excluded, the extended treatment group had significantly lower rates of relapse [35]. This effect of extended therapy was observed only during the 21 mg dose phase and not during the tapering phase, suggesting that the benefits of extended high-dose treatment may be achieved only if individuals continue taking this dose [17].

Moreover, several studies suggest that a high-dose nicotine patch (until to double a standard dose) produces slightly higher abstinence rates in heavy smokers (i.e., those who smoke 30 or more cigarettes per day) and may be especially useful for heavy smokers who report persistent craving and other withdrawal symptoms during cessation [36]. Other studies, however, have not found better outcomes with the 44 mg dose of transdermal nicotine, even in short term [37].

Nicotine Gum

Nicotine gum (Nicorette [Glaxo Smith Kline Consumer Healthcare LP, Pittsburgh, PA]) has been available by prescription since 1985 and was approved for over the counter use (OCT) in 1996.

Absorption of nicotine from the gum is more rapid than with the patch and peak levels are obtained after about 20-30 minutes of use. Approximately 50% of the nicotine in the gum is released in the mouth and absorbed through the mucosa. The pharmacodynamics of the gum cause a gradual rising and falling of nicotine levels throughout the day. Repeated chewing of the nicotine gum delivers nicotine over time. Nicotine levels drop when the gum is not chewed and overnight during sleep. A daily cycle of neuroadaptation and abstinence develops, just like smoking cigarettes, but the amplitude of the cycles is blunted. Appropriate patient education is required for optimal use of the nicotine gum. Patients should be counseled that nicotine gum should not be chewed in the way one chews regular chewing gum. Nicotine gum should be intermittently chewed slowly until a "peppery" taste or tingling sensation occurs, and then placed between the cheek and buccal mucosa, to facilitate nicotine adsorption through the oral mucosa. This process should be repeated for about 30 minutes. Over-chewing and swallowing excess of nicotine can result in nicotine toxicity, in which the patient may experience nausea, vomiting, and/or upset stomach. Since an acidic environment impairs the buccal adsorption of nicotine, all food and beverages except water should be avoided for at least fifteen minutes before and during chewing [4, 25, 28, 33].

Currently, nicotine gum is available in 2 mg and 4 mg dosages. General guidelines suggest to use the 2 mg dosage for smokers who smoke fewer than 25 cigarettes per day, and the 4 mg dosage for heavy smokers who smoke at least 25 cigarette per day [12]. A meta-analysis in which the 2 mg and 4 mg doses of nicotine gum were compared found that among highly dependent smokers, those using the 4 mg gum had 21% greater success at cessation than those using the 2 mg gum [38]. Interestingly, for smokers low in nicotine dependence, the 2 mg gum may be more effective than the higher dosage. Over the counter gum labels recommended chewing 1 to 2 pieces per hour and average smokers use 10 to 15 pieces to achieve abstinence. It is recommended to instruct patients to chew the gum on a fixed schedule, instead of ad lib use, based on need [32]. The over the counter label recommends this treatment for 6 weeks followed by a 6 week taper. However, some studies suggest longer term use is more effective. It has been found that 10 to 25% of successful abstainers continue to use the gum for a year or longer [25]. Although patients should not be encouraged to use nicotine gum indefinitely, any risks associated with its long-term use are small relative to the risks associated with continued smoking.

Nicotine gum is a proven agent with smoking cessation. A meta-analysis estimated that 17.4% of smokers who used nicotine gum to treat tobacco dependence in clinical trials remained abstinent 12 months later [29]. Advantages of the gum include having a behavior to use with an urge to smoke that actively controls nicotine withdrawal mood changes [32]. Moreover, the gum has been shown, in dose-dependent manner, to be the only form of NRT which delay the weight gain normally associated with stopping smoking, though these results may not persist after the gum is discontinued [39].

Disadvantages include great effort to chew enough gum and adverse side effects that may include sore mouth, throat or temporomandibular joint problems, oral problems, hiccups, dysgeusia, dyspepsia, nausea, flatulence and gastrointestinal discomfort. Furthermore, the gum is not suitable for people with dentures or loose teeth. The jaw ache can be minimized by correct technique by simply compressing the gum with the teeth rather than chewing. Moreover, patient compliance is easier to achieve with the patch than with the gum, because use of the gum requires more behavior modification. Users may often underdose or neglect to follow the recommended dosing and chewing regimen, which could inhibit the agent's efficacy in reducing withdrawal symptoms [12].

Nicotine Inhaler

The nicotine inhaler (Nicotrol Inhaler, Pharmacia and Upjohn AB, Sweden) has been available in prescription since 1998. It comprises a small plastic mouthpiece about the size of a cigarette into which a replaceable nicotine cartridge is inserted. The cartridge contains 10 mg of nicotine and a 1 mg of menthol. The menthol is designed to decrease nicotine's irritant properties. Nicotine vapor is picked up from the cartridge by inhaling through the mouthpiece. The adsorption of nicotine occurs through the oral and pharyngeal mucosa and gastrointestinal tract secondary to swallowing, rather than through alveolar adsorption. The rate of nicotine is like the other oral products and it does not mimic the very rapid delivery of a cigarette. An acidic environment in the mouth may impair nicotine's absorption, therefore it is recommended that eating or drinking anything but water for at least fifteen minutes before and during inhalation be avoided. The blood nicotine levels are lower with the inhaler than with any other NRT [40].

A potential advantage of the nicotine inhaler is that it comes closest to mimicking the behavioral habit of smoking through puffing or handling the product. Thus, it may be the best choice for smokers that need a substitute for the mouth behavior, and the tactile/sensory stimulation the cigarette provides. Furthermore, the inhaler provides physiological replacement of nicotine and the smoker receives the reward of dopamine release in the brain [12, 40].

Each puff on the inhaler delivers at best $1/10^{th}$ of the nicotine from a puff (13 μg), much lower than from a cigarette, and users should aim to puff teadily for about 20 min per hour (equivalent of one cartridge) or two. Recommended minimum dosage is six cartridges per day up to a maximum of 12-16, for 6 to 12 weeks, with tapering over the subsequent 3 months. Each cartridge delivers 4 mg of nicotine over 80 inhalations, of which approximately 2 mg is absorbed. Delivery of nicotine from the inhaler declines significantly at temperatures below 40-59 F. In cold weather, the inhaler and cartridges should be kept in an inside pocket of warm area. Patients should be advised not to eat or drink 15 min prior to use as acidic drinks can change the absorption of nicotine [4, 12, 40].

Local irritation in the mouth and throat was observed in 40% of patients using nicotine inhaler. Coughing (32%) and rhinitis (23%) were also common. These local side effects could be avoided with shallow puffing versus deep inhalations, changing placement of the device, and not biting on the inhaler. Severity generally was rated as mild, and the frequency of such symptoms declined with continued use. Further side effects include headache, heartburn, hiccups, nausea, vomiting, sinusitis, nasal congestion, and aphthous ulcer. Less common side effects include sleep disturbances and dizziness. The use of a nicotine inhaler is contraindicated for patients with bronchospastic disease [24, 40].

Double-blind placebo-controlled trials found that the inhaler was useful for short-term smoking cessation with some potential for long-term cessation [41]. The efficacy of nicotine inhalers has been assessed in several studies, one of each found an odds ratio of 2.05 (95% CI:1.65 to 2.59) when using a nicotine inhaler relative to placebo [29]. The inhaler has been shown to be effective against other types of NRT for certain clients including those who smoke less than 10 cigarettes per day [42]. Critics of the nicotine inhaler cite the potential for its abuse. However, results from a study concluded that use for reasons other than cessation, abuse, and dependence were rare [43].

Nicotine Nasal Spray

Nicotine nasal spray (Nicotrol NS, Pharmacia and Upjohn Ab, Sweden) was introduced in 1996 and is currently available only by prescription. The medication is sprayed against lower nasal mucosa. It should not to be sniffed, swallowed, or inhaled. Adsorption of nicotine administered via the nasal spray is faster than that achieved with any of the other nicotine dosage forms (although slower than from smoking a cigarette) as the nasal mucosa is a very efficient delivery route, and mimics the nicotine bolus from cigarettes. Plasma nicotine levels are reached approximately in 5-10 minutes after administration and are about two-thirds those of cigarettes [4, 15].

The spray is available in a quantity of 10 ml. Each 0.05 ml spray delivers 0.5 mg of nicotine. Recommended dosage is 1-2 sprays per hour for 2 months and then gradual reduction to zero by 3 months. Patients should not exceed 5 doses per hour or 40 doses per day. The minimum recommended treatment is 8 doses per day for 3 to 6 months. Tapering of doses in the subsequent 4 to 6 week period is optimal to prevent withdrawal symptoms. As with the oral NRTs there is a technique to spraying effectively and is best delivered with the head tilted slightly back. Thus, smokers should to be instructed to use the nasal spray for up to 12 weeks, including a tapering period [4, 12].

Among the various NRT dosage forms, nicotine nasal spray is associated with the greatest frequency of adverse effects. Some 94% of users report moderate to severe nasal irritation in the first 2 days of use; 81% still reported nasal irritation after 3 weeks, although rated severity was mild to moderate [24]. Generally, the symptoms decrease with time although they may not dissipate entirely. Nasal congestion, runny eyes, coughing, throat irritation, headache and transient changes in sense of smell and taste were also reported. Users quickly develop tolerance to these irritant effects but may require some persuasion by a clinician to ensure users persist until tolerance is acquired. The quick absorption of nicotine raises questions about the addictive potential of this dosage form. Several studies have found that smokers continue to use nasal spray up to a year after initiating treatment, even if these concerns have not been shown in clinical trials. However, the health impact of ongoing use of the nicotine spray is small relative to continued smoking [12, 16].

Similar to nicotine gum, the nicotine nasal spray is particularly effective at rapidly relieving urges to smoke, thus it is used in place of smoking when the patient craves nicotine. Potential advantages of nicotine nasal spray, therefore, include a more rapid relief of craving than observed after administration of other NRTs, and an increased efficacy in highly dependent smokers. Some evidence suggests that the spray may delay though not prevent the weight gain normally associated with quitting smoking [12]. Nicotine nasal spray has been shown to be effective in improving smoking cessation rates. A recent meta-analysis showed an odds ratio of 2.35 (95% CI: 1.63 to 3.38) when compared to placebo [29].

Nicotine Lozenges

Lozenges are available in 3 doses (1, 2 and 4 mg nicotine). The 4 mg lozenge is for more dependent smokers normally smoking within 30 min of waking and the 2 mg for those who are awake for 30 min before smoking. The speed of nicotine delivery from lozenges is very similar to that from gum but completely dissolves thus delivering the full nicotine does as opposed to just 50% delivered by the gum. Another advantage of lozenges over gum would be the ease of use. The lozenge is place in the vestibule area and left there to melt. The lozenge should not be chewed or swallowed whole. Patient acceptance seems to be higher than the gum due to ease of use and newer flavors. Estimated odds ratio versus placebo from a recent meta-analysis is 2.05 (95% CI: 1.62 to 2.59) [29].

Nicotine Sub-Lingual Tablets

Similar to lozenge, the sub-lingual tablet, available in some countries of Europe only, is a small white tablet containing 2 mg of nicotine which is placed under the tongue and left to dissolve. Recommended dosage is one or two tablets every hour for about 3 months. Absorption rate is similar to the other oral NRTs. The number of doses used daily is determined by prior smoking levels. Users should be cautioned against sucking or chewing as this inhibits nicotine absorption. The sublingual tablets are as effective as the lozenges when compared to placebo [29].

Nicotine Containing Products

New forms of nicotine containing products are appealing to youth and can be found in the marketplace and on Internet. Physicians should remain vigilant for patients who use these products and advise them accordingly. The U.S. Food and Drug Administration has warned sellers of nicotine lollipops and lip balm that their products are illegal and that bottled nicotine water is an unapproved drug [44, 45].

Safety of NRT

Nicotine administered as a medication is always safer than actual tobacco use. While nicotine may be considered a neurotoxin, the currently available NRT products do not contain the thousands of hazardous chemicals in tobacco. The evidence clearly indicates that NRT products are safe when used in the doses recommended [12].

The active ingredient in NRT is nicotine which has no known risk in tobacco-related cancers and is not implicate in chronic obstructive lung disease. There are safety concerns relating to the use of NRT in people with pre-existing cardiovascular disease arising from clinical trials. Pharmacological data demonstrate nicotine is not associated with an increased risk of myocardial infarction (MI), stroke, or sudden death. Theoretical concerns over the safety of NRT in relation to potential adverse outcomes can therefore probably be discounted when the alternative for most smokers is continuing to use. Patients with pre-existing cardiovascular disease represent one of the groups most likely to benefit from smoking cessation interventions such as NRT. However, most NRT manufacturers recommended caution against the use of NRT in patients with acute disease such as unstable angina, recent MI, serious arrhythmia, and accelerated hypertension [46, 47, 48]. It has also been suggested the possibility of endogenous formation of carcinogenetic nitrosamines from nicotine metabolites, but lacks evidence.

Another concern of patients using NRT during smoking cessation is the sleep disruption. It has been hypothesized that nicotine can play a role in the sleep-wake cycle, due to neurotransmitter systems modified by nicotine are also involved in sleep-wake regulation. Preliminary evidence suggests that NRT can result in disrupted sleep, particularly in women. Different variables such as dosage, time and way of administration can change the way sleep is modified. However, pharmacological treatments designed to facilitate smoking cessation are ineffective for sustained abstinence in many smokers, which may be related to sleep disturbance [49].

While in theory all forms of NRT have some potential to sustain nicotine dependence, only a very small proportion of NRT users become long term-users. Furthermore, NRT can be used for a prolonged period even with concurrent use of cigarettes, with few adverse effects [12]. One concern with continued smoking is a theoretical increased risk of negative clinical outcomes. However, it has been found that some NRTs, such as nicotine patches, did not cause a significant increase in cardiovascular events among high risk outpatients with cardiac disease, even in the subgroup of patients who used the nicotine patch and continued to smoke [50].

Non-Nicotine Replacement Therapy

The various forms of NRT generally increase smoking quit rates as compared to placebo, but they usually do not result in quit rates of over 20% after one year [51]. To increase these rates, non-nicotine agents, such as antidepressant medications, have been employed. These medications, which include tricyclic inhibitors, selective serotonin reuptake inhibitors, and atypical antidepressants, have been widely studied as non-nicotine pharmacotherapy for smoking cessation.

Researchers have examined the effectiveness of antidepressant medication for use in smoking cessation for several reasons including the hypothesis that nicotine may have an antidepressant effect in humans. A strong association exists between smoking and depression: smokers are more likely than nonsmokers to report a history of depression. Quit attempts may also precipitate depression and several lines of clinical evidence suggest post-cessation depression can cause relapse [14]. Thus, the rationale for using antidepressants for smoking cessation is as follows: 1) abstinence increases depression 2) depression increases relapse and 3) depression can be prevented by antidepressants.

Bupropion

Bupropion was primarily developed as an antidepressant medication (Wellbutrin XL [GlaxoSmithKline, Research Triangle Park, NC]). However, clinical observers noted that patients treated with bupropion for depression spontaneously reduced or even quit smoking. Subsequent trials have shown bupropion to be efficacious in larger populations of non-depressed smokers, as well as in smokers with psychiatric (i.e., alcholism, depression, schizophrenia, post-traumatic stress disorders) and medical comorbidity (i.e., cardiovascular disease, chronic obstructive pulmonary disease) [14, 52, 53].

Bupropion sustained release (SR) (Zyban SR [GlaxoSmithKline]) is one of two non-nicotine medication approved by US Food and Drug Administration (FDA). In the U.K. and the European Union bupropion is the only non-nicotine pharmacotherapy used for smoking cessation treatment. It has been available for use since 1997. This agent is currently recommended as a first line pharmacotherapy by the U.S. FDA.

Mechanism of Action

Bupropion is an atypical antidepressant (aminoketone derivative antidepressant) which weakly inhibits the reuptake of dopamine and norepinephrine in the mesolimbic dopaminergic system, in the nucleus accumbens, and in the locus caeruleus of the brain, respectively. The nucleus accumbens is considered the pleasure reinforcing area of the brain for addictive drugs. Moreover, the locus caeruleus is the area which activates higher cortical function, such as alertness, concentration and memory [52].

Although the mechanism of action for smoking cessation is not known for certain, the increased levels of dopamine in the brain's areas may account for bupropion's stimulant-like effects, as well as a decrease in the activity of dopamine releasing neurons. Dopaminergic activation may also mediate craving in response to smoking cues. In a positron emission tomography (PET) study with smokers, bupropion treatment attenuated cue-induced craving and anterior cingulate cortex activation in smokers [52, 54, 55].

Moreover, bupropion increases synaptic norepinephrine levels by inhibiting the norepinephrine transporter, similar to its effects on the dopamine transporter. It was demonstrated that chronic nicotine exposure, as with smoking, may have long-term effects on noradrenergic activity. It was shown that clonidine, a substance similar to bupropion which inhibits noradrenergic activity by stimulating α_2-adrenergic receptors, attenuates craving for cigarettes and other nicotine withdrawal symptoms including anxiety, irritability, tension and hunger. These findings led to the hypothesis that tobacco withdrawal symptoms are mediated by noradrenergic system activation. Thus, the noradrenergic effect of bupropion may contribute to the ability of bupropion to attenuate symptoms of tobacco withdrawal [52, 55].

The dopaminergic and noradrenergic activities stimulate the reward achieved when tobacco is used and reduce withdrawal symptoms when tobacco-use is stopped, thereby preventing relapse. The principal action of bupropion is probably exerted during the withdrawal stage of smoking cessation, having little or no effect on the level of tobacco use until the smoker actually quits. Evidence also suggests that bupropion is a non-competitive nicotine receptor antagonist and block the reinforcing effect of nicotine. This feature might explain smokers' reports that bupropion makes smoking less enjoyable or satisfying and thus it may be useful in preventing relapse if one resumes smoking [52, 53, 55, 56].

Medication Dosing

The appropriate target dosage for bupropion SR is 300 mg/die (150 mg twice daily). The recommended course of treatment with bupropion for smoking cessation involves two phases. The first phase occurs in the 7-10 days prior to the targeted quit date, in order to achieve steady-state plasma levels of bupropion. The medication should be started at 150 mg/die for 3 days and then increased to 150 mg twice daily, with each dose taken 8-12 hours apart. In the second phase, smoking cessation begins; patients continue to take bupropion for a period of 7 to 12 weeks The treatment can be continued for as long as 6 months or up to 12 months to delay or prevent relapse [4, 12, 14]. The target quitting date for a smoker should be set between 8 and 14 days after starting the medication. The smokers continue to smoke as normal up to their quit date and then stop completely. If after 4 weeks of therapy an individual is still unable to maintain abstinence, continued therapy with bupropion SR may not be helpful and other treatment options should be offered [12].

The dosage of bupropion SR should be adjusted for some category of patients. The recommended dose in elderly patients or in smokers with renal or hepatic impairment is 150 mg once daily, as bupropion is metabolized in the liver and then the kidneys. For diabetic patients, the standard dose can be prescribed if 1) the diet is controlled 2) the diabetes is well controlled with insulin or 3) oral hypoglycaemics are used, 150 mg of bupropion SR once daily should be prescribed. Patients who have poorly controlled diabetes, the use of NRT should the tobacco cessation medication of choice. Smokers with a predisposition to seizures should not take bupropion unless the benefit of smoking cessation outweighs the risks associated with using the medication. Bupropion has been found safe to use in smokers with stable cardiovascular disease, and does not lead to adverse effects on the blood pressure or heart rate [4, 56]. Bupropion undergoes hepatic metabolism, primarly by isoenzyme CYP2B6. Therefore, other drugs that affect this enzyme (e.g., cimetidine, sodium valproate and cyclophosphamide) may affect bupropion metabolism. Bupropion inhibits the activity of CYP2D6, and may reduce the rate of metabolism of drugs such as betablockers, type 1C antiarrhythmics, antidepressants (MAOI) and antipsychotics. A dose reduction in these medications may be required. There are other contraindications and precautions with bupropion, including pregnancy, breast feeding, current or prior bipolar, eating disorders (anorexia nervosa, bulimia), withdrawal from alcohol or benzodiazepines, and tumor of the central nervous system [4, 14, 56]. Though this is an effective tobacco cessation pharmacotherapy, due consideration should be given to level of nicotine addiction as well as emotional, physical and pharmacologic issues of the patient prior to recommending bupropion.

Evidence for Efficacy

The efficacy of bupropion has been confirmed in several studies [14, 52]. In a meta-analysis based on 19 clinical trials it was found that smokers treated with bupropion alone were twice as likely as those treated with a placebo to achieve long-term abstinence at either 6 or 12 month follow-up visits (OR 2.06; CI 95%, 1.77-2.40) [57]. Furthermore, the efficacy of bupropion has been found comparable to that of NRT, but bupropion SR has been shown to produce significantly higher abstinence rates when combined with a transdermal nicotine patch [17, 52, 53].

Earlier studies examining the effectiveness of bupropion reported a dose-response relationship with a higher cessation rate at the end of treatment among smokers who received a higher dose. However, recent findings reported bupropion doses up to 300 mg/day had a significant effect on smoking cessation, but did not affect long-term (12 month) cessation rates [17, 53]. Moreover, the data on the efficacy of bupropion have been reported from highly controlled trials with multiple variables accounted for. Bupropion has been studied in real-world settings, where patients may have multiple diseases, imperfect adherence, and multiple medications. It appears that 12 month abstinence rates of patients using bupropion in real-world settings are similar to those found in the drug-treated groups of randomized, placebo-controlled trials [58].

The use of bupropion in relapse prevention has also been examined. Two studies asked smokers who successfully quit using bupropion to continue therapy for an additional 12 months. Both studies showed no significant benefit in preventing relapse with the extended treatment. Therefore, evidence currently available suggests that there is a little or no benefit for using bupropion long-term to prevent relapse. In fact, bupropion may delay the time to relapse but does not significantly increase long-term abstinence [55, 56, 59]. For smokers who failed to quit after initial NRT treatment, subsequent immediate treatment with bupropion has not been found to add any benefit, but for smokers with a past history of failure to quit with NRT, bupropion is more effective than placebo by the end of treatment. Moreover, for smokers who had failed in the past to quit after using bupropion, re-treatment with bupropion for 12 weeks does provide some benefit. For smokers wanting to reduce their amount of smoking rather than quit, bupropion may help sustain smoking reduction while on treatment, and reduce the time until the next cessation attempt [54, 55].

Bupropion showed to be particulary efficacious for smokers who may be more prone to relapse, such as women, African Americans, and smokers with higher levels of nicotine dependence [14, 17].

Bupropion for Postabstinence Weight Gain

Bupropion SR appears to provide an additional benefit of delaying weight gain that often follows smoking abstinence. In earlier clinical trials, a modest effect of bupropion SR on reducing weight gain during the drug treatment phase was observed, although a significant effect of reducing post-cessation weight gain in the active bupropion SR group was shown in a subsequent study [56, 60]. These findings may be important for people who want to quit but are concerned about gaining weight.

Common Adverse Effects of Bupropion

In all clinical trials of bupropion SR for smoking cessation, approximately 10% of subjects discontinued therapy due to an adverse drug-related reaction. The most common adverse effects reported with bupropion SR are insomnia and xerostomia or dry mouth. Insomnia may occur in 30% to 45% of individuals who take bupropion SR at the dosage of 300 mg/day. The adverse effect is often dose-related and is more common at higher doses. If patients experience insomnia, they should be instructed to take the first dose early in the morning and the second dose in the mid afternoon. Ultimately, the second dose may need to be eliminated, with the understanding that the clinical efficacy of bupropion SR also may be reduced at lower doses. Dry mouth occurs at rates of 5% to 15% may be dose-related, and has been correlated with lower body weight. These adverse effects are usually well tolerated and are not a cause for discontinuing of medication. The more common events leading to discontinuation of treatment include tremors and rashes [14, 56].

Other commonly reported minor adverse effects include headache, nausea, and anxiety. Headache and nausea have been reported to occur in clinical trials as frequently in the placebo as in the active treatment groups. Anxiety is commonly reported as an adverse effect, but the frequency of anxiety may be inversely proportional to the bupropion SR dose. This may indicate that anxiety symptoms are due to nicotine withdrawal and that withdrawal symptoms can be treated adequately with lower doses of bupropion SR. Active management of these minor adverse effects are usually not required since most improve over time [14, 56].

Bupropion SR has been associated with treatment-emergent hypertension in recent clinical trials. Treatment-emergent hypertension may be more common in patients receiving combination therapy with bupropion SR and NRT. No report exists of serious adverse effects resulting from uncontrolled hypertension due to bupropion SR treatment alone or in combination with NRT.

Serious Adverse Effects

In the U.K., the media reported a number of deaths in people using bupropion SR. However, none of the reported deaths have been causally associated to bupropion SR. In several cases, an underlying smoking-related disease was identified as the cause of death. In the U.S., no connection has been made between the use of bupropion SR and fatal outcomes [56, 61].

Seizures are a known risk factor associated with the use of many antidepressant medications. Bupropion is contraindicated in individuals who have a history of seizure disorder or eating disorder, are abruptly discontinuing alcohol or sedatives, are using another form of bupropion, or have used a monoamine oxidase inhibitor in the past 14 days. Studies of bupropion and seizures have suggested that the incidence rate of seizures is approximately 0.1% to 0.4%. The seizure risk with bupropion appears to be higher for the immediate-relase form of the drug when it is given at doses of 450 mg or more (experimental doses). All clinical trials using bupropion for smoking cessation have used the SR form of the drug. No seizures have been reported in clinical trials of bupropion SR for smoking cessation [52, 53, 56].

A recent study compared the death rate of smokers with cardiovascular diseases and admitted to the intensive care unit. The patients who were given NRT died more often than those who did not received NRT [62].

Varenicline

Varenicline (Chantix [Pfizer Inc., NY]) is a partial agonist at the subtype of neuronal nicotinic receptors composed of α4 and β2 subunits, located in the ventral tegmental area of the brain. Varenicline was recently tested and approved by the U.S. FDA as a first line smoking cessation aid and this is now available by prescription in the U.S. [63, 64, 65]. Varenicline is dosed at 10 mg once or twice day.

Recent research suggests that α4β2 nicotinic receptors play an important role in nicotinic dependence and craving. Furthermore, transgenic studies have shown that nicotinic receptors containing β2 subunits seem to play an essential role in nicotine self-administration and ensure normal sympathetic tone. Preclinical studies with another partial agonist at this nicotinic receptor (dianicline) suggest that these compounds, like nicotine, stimulate dopamine overflow in the shell of the accumbens. However, their effects are smaller than those evoked by nicotine injections and generalized to both nicotine and amphetamine in a drug discrimination paradigm [64, 66].

The ability of varenicline to desensitize neuronal nicotinic receptors has not been thoroughly explored. Test results suggest that the drug initially stimulates the $\alpha4\beta2$ receptors that mediate the effect of nicotinic agonist on dopamine release in the nucleus and behavioral responses (locomotor stimulation and reinforcement) that depend on this neural response. However, the receptors seem to desensitize rapidly on sustained exposure to the drug. Furthermore, the drug attenuates the effects of nicotine withdrawal and cravings. Smokers who have quit should experience diminished craving and withdrawal symptoms, thereby decreasing the chances to return to smoking. In most of the clinical trials, varenicline was used one week before quitting. With each cigarette, smokers may have experienced diminished positive reinforcement and, after attempted cessation, a lapse back to smoking may have been met with a lack of reinforcement. This could contribute both to ease of quitting upon quit day, as well as decreasing the likelihood of sustained relapse if a smoker returns to smoking. So, in part, varenicline's mechanism of action can be characterized as stabilizing perturbations in nicotine dependence motivational systems during the process of cessation [64, 66, 67].

Varenicline is the first smoking cessation treatment to demonstrate a significant long-term relapse prevention effect. Furthermore, the extended use of varenicline helps recent ex-smokers to maintain their abstinence and prevent relapse [67, 68]. The efficacy of varenicline has been demonstrated in a number of recent studies. Three phase III randomized trials reported that long-term (1 year) abstinence rates were more than twice those of the placebo group [63]. In one study, those who were quit at 12 weeks were more likely to remain abstinent at 24 weeks if they continued using varenicline [33]. The phase III placebo controlled trials included randomization to bupropion and showed that varenicline produced significantly higher short-term and long-term (1-year) abstinence rates than both placebo and bupropion SR groups [67, 69].

Varenicline appears to be safe and well tolerated for prolonged use with most adverse events being characterized as mild or moderate in intensity. Nausea was the only notable drug effect reported by trial participants but did not lead them to discontinue the use of the medication. Insomnia was reported less often among varenicline participants than among bupropion SR participants though some form of sleep disturbance is a common symptom of nicotine withdrawal and may not have been drug related [67, 68].

Nortriptyline

Nortriptyline (Aventyl, Ohm Laboratories, Gloverville, NY) is one of the two agents available as second-line medication for smoking cessation. A second-line agent should be used when a patient cannot use a first-line medication because of either contraindications, adverse events in response to, or lack of effectiveness. Furthermore, nortriptyline is not approved for smoking cessation by FDA [12, 14, 70].

This agent is an effective tricyclic antidepressant and is thought to exert therapeutic effects via the inhibition of the re-uptake of norepinephrine and serotonin with a greater effect on norepinephrine re-uptake. In smoking cessation, it is presumed to act through its noradrenergic mechanism, reducing the severity of withdrawal symptoms. Another possible mechanism may be as a nicotine receptor antagonist, even if this activity appears to be weak. Other hypothesis includes nortriptyline's anxiolitic effects and anticholinergic side-effects, such as dry mouth, which may make cigarettes less desiderable. Several studies also found that nortriptyline did not demonstrate superior efficacy for smokers with a past history of depression when compared to those lacking a history of depression. These findings suggest that the effectiveness of nortriptyline as a smoking cessation aids may be independent of the antidepressant properties [16, 70].

The treatment regimen involves a starting dose of 25 mg/day, increasing gradually over a period of 10 days to 5 weeks to a target dose of 75-100 mg/day which is generally needed to reach a therapeutic levels of 50 ng/ml. The quit date is usually set once therapeutic levels of the drug have been reached; this may take 10-28 days. The treatment period is tipically 12 weeks, after which the dose is tapered. There is limited evidence of benefit for extending treatment past 3 months though one study shows some decrease in relapse to smoking with extended medication treatment [57, 70].

The common side effects of nortriptyline are dry mouth, drowsiness, lightheadedness, blurred vision and constipation. Urinary retention, sexual difficulties and seizure risk are also reported. These side effects are related to the block of muscarinic cholinergic receptors (dry mouth, lightheadedness, blurred vision urinary retention and costipation), and H_1 histamine receptors (drowsiness). The use of nortriptyline is frequently associated with postural hypotension, which is related to the blocking of alpha adrenergic receptors. Several studies suggest that nortryptiline is as safe as existing smoking cessation medications, even if it has been tested in fewer smokers. Probably, a major reason for the relatively few adverse effects in these trials is the low nortryptiline level used [14, 16, 70].

Nortryptiline can also interact with several medications. The most common concern is sedation when it is combined with alcohol, antistamines, or sedating medications. As with other tryciclic antidepressants, nortriptyline can be fatal if taken in excessive amounts (overdose) especially when combined with alcohol or sedative drugs. Since some smokers become depressed after smoking cessation, this concern could be significant. Nortryptiline increases weight when used to treat depression. However, one smoking cessation study reported that, if anything, nortryptiline may have reduced weight gain [14, 70].

Nortryptiline has not been tested in several special populations, such as adolescents, the elderly, ethnic groups, pregnant women, or those with cardiovascular disease. However, this agent should be used with caution in the elderly and in patients with cardiovascular disease, or those who have experienced a recent MI or arrhythmia. The noradrenergic effects cause cardiac conduction delays leading to possible arrhythmias, thus in susceptible individuals or in overdose situations nortryptiline may not be the medication of choice. The possibility of significant adverse events might have warranted nortriptyline's classification as a second line medication by the U.S. FDA [12]. In addition, there are a number of precautions to note, such as use in people with a history of epilepsy or psychosis and severe liver disease, and women who are pregnant or breast-feeding [70].

Several clinical trials studying nortriptyline reported the odds doubled for long-term abstinence compared with the placebo (pooled OR 2.79; 95% CI, 1.70-4.59). The odds ratio for nortryptiline is resulted similar to that for NRT [28, 70]. In a study of Hall et al. [71] bupropion produced a numerically higher quit rate; however, it was not significant different from nortryptiline.

One possible advantage to nortryptiline is that, unlike with bupropion, therapeutic monitoring of blood levels is available, which can be used to ensure adequate medication exposure and avoidance of adverse effects. Another possible advantage is that, in most countries, it is a generic medication and thus less expensive [14, 28, 70].

Clonidine

Clonidine (Catapres, Boehringer Ingelheim Pharmacuticals, Rigefield, CT) is currently regarded as another second-line therapy, but it is not FDA approved for smoking cessation. It is an alpha-2 adrenoceptor agonist that reduces sympathetic activity by decreasing noradrenaline release. Clonidine is generally used as an antihypertensive and for prevention of recurrent migraines. It has also been used to treat opioid and alcohol dependence by decreasing sympathetic over-activity that characterizes their withdrawal syndromes [12, 16].

Treatment with clonidine should be started 2-3 days before quitting, allowing time to reach steady state concentration. Clonidine can be taken orally or through a transdermal patch. Oral doses typically start with 0.1 mg/day, and then are gradually increased, up to 0.4 mg/day. The transdermal doses are between 0.1 and 0.3 mg/day. The treatment period is usually short, given over the first 3-4 weeks after quitting when withdrawal symptoms are more intense. After this, the dose is reduced over several days, which is particularly important to avoid hypertensive crisis and hypoglycaemia in people with hypertension and diabetes, respectively [12].

The adverse or side effects associated with clonidine such as postural hypotension, dizziness and dry mouth, makes its use less desiderable. In addition, clonidine causes sedation, although this might be of some benefit to those who experience more intense symptoms of nicotine withdrawal. Depression, sleep disturbance and costipation are also reported, though these are also classic symptoms of nicotine withdrawal. Therefore it may be difficult to ascertain which of the two is the causal agent. Patients with a history of depression or occlusive peripheral vascular disease should avoid using clonidine. Furthermore, there is a possibility of sympathetic rebound resulting in a substantial increase in blood pressure, therefore clonidine must be tapered off slowly when discontinued [12, 72].

Clonidine has been shown to ameliorate the symptoms of tobacco withdrawal and, in some studies, increase abstinence rates [72]. Despite a number of published studies assessing its effect, the role of clonidine as a smoking cessation agent is still relatively unclear. One meta-analysis that looked at 12 double blind studies found a trend for increased smoking cessation with clonidine compared with the placebo [73]. However, a more recent meta-analysis looked at 6 studies that reported abstinence data at 3 months. At the completion of drug treatment, researchers found that clonidine was effective (pooled O.R. 1.89; 95% CI, 1.30-2.74) compared with placebo, despite only one of these studies reporting statistically significant findings [72]. Clonidine has also been found particularly useful for female smokers and for those who become agitated and anxious when quitting smoking [74].

Combination Therapy

Although few studies evaluated the effects of combining medications for nicotine dependence treatment, the use of combination therapy has been associated with higher odds of remaining abstinent. In fact, it has been shown that the use of combination therapy possibly offers some advantage compared with single or no medications. However, there remain many misperceptions among smokers and clinicians about this practice. This is due in part to the package labeling advising smokers not to combine these medications. For this reason, it is important to discuss with patients the concept of combining medications. Another advantage of utilizing multiple medications is the opportunity to offer flexible delivery options. In practice, the smokers using combination therapy are able to use different medications ad lib in various settings (e.g., lozenge during work, inhaler while driving, and nasal spray early in the morning). Longer duration of medications also seems to convey some benefit for abstinence. In fact, patients are encouraged to continue using short acting medications (gum, lozenge, inhaler, spray) as needed, usually at low doses for longer duration with the result of higher abstinence rates. There are several barriers to acceptance of combination therapy. A primary obstacle for individuals may be cost. In addition, availability and accessibility of treatments may also play a role in their use. Though some NRTs can be purchased over the counter (gum, lozenge, patch), other NRTs (nasal spray, nicotine inhaler) and oral medications (bupropion and varenicline) requires a prescription. Side effects, and perceptions of potential side effects of various medications, should be considered possible barriers to use of these agents in combination [75, 76].

Combination of NRTs

A growing body of evidence supports improved abstinence rates with NRT combination therapy, in which a fixed-dose formulation (patch) is combined with a flexible, self-administered dosage form (such as gum, inhaler or nasal spray). Most research has suggested that combining the patch with other flexible-dosage forms of NRT are both safe and effective. In a study comparing the use of nicotine inhalers with nicotine patches to inhalers with placebo patches for 18-26 weeks of treatment results showed that abstinence rates among the combination-treated group were consistently higher at the end of the year. Similar results were reported in a recent study reporting superiority of combined patch and nasal spray therapy at 6 weeks with no difference between groups at 6 months. However, a double-blind study found higher abstinence rates for subjects who received a nicotine patch and nicotine gum when compared with subjects who received a nicotine patch and placebo gum [33, 75].

Combination NRT therapy may be especially appropriate for highly dependent smokers, who have the greatest risk of developing tobacco-related illness. Combining the patch with an ad lib form of NRT is currently seen as more effective than monotherapy and should be encouraged if the smoker is unable to quit using only one medication. Nevertheless, the use of combinations of NRT therapy should be medically supervised [12, 48].

Combination of NRT with Bupropion

Bupropion may prove to be more effective in combination with NRTs therapy, even if research combining bupropion with the nicotine patch has shown mixed results. Studies comparing bupropion and nicotine patch monotherapy to a combination of both therapies found that the 4-week quit rates were higher in all treatment groups relative to the placebo, but only the bupropion and combined treatment groups were significantly superior to the placebo groups. The combination therapy resulted in 6- and 12- month quit rates higher than patch or the placebo group. However, another study failed to find significant incremental benefits in smoking abstinence by adding bupropion to nicotine patch use [16, 28, 65].

Combination of First-Line Pharmacotherapies with Behavioral Treatment

Numerous studies have evaluated the impact of both behavioral treatment components and first-line pharmacotherapy agents. These studies suggest that behavioral counseling using principles of effective brief therapies and cognitive behavioral therapy can enhance the gains achieved with first-line pharmacotherapies. The more time spent with the patients offering a tobacco cessation intervention, the greater the impact on a successful quit attempt. Thus, combination therapy that includes both a first-line pharmacotherapy and a well-specified behavioral treatment should be made available to every dependent tobacco user in order to provide the best chance of successful quit [12, 75].

Special Groups

While the above approach to tobacco cessation interventions provides a useful framework from which to begin, customized approaches and special considerations need to be given when treating special categories of tobacco users.

Age

Despite a recent decline in cigarette smoking among US adolescents, rates of tobacco-use remain quit high. Among middle school and high school students in the US, smoking averaged 10.1% and 22.9%, respectively. The mean age most teenagers start to smoke is about 14 years old. Among adolescents the order of tobacco usage is cigarettes, cigars, smokeless tobacco products and pipe smoking [77, 78].

Socio-demographic, environmental and personal factors put youth at an increased risk of initiating tobacco-use. Adolescent from families of low socioeconomic status are at increased risk of smoking. Environmental risk factors include: cigarette advertising, price, accessibility and availability of tobacco products, perceptions that tobacco-use is normal among peers and siblings, and lack of parental involvement and influence in adolescent daily life. Personal risk factors include the belief that tobacco-use provides a benefit, a low self-image and low self-esteem, and the lack of ability to refuse offers to use tobacco.

Following the onset of intermittent smoking, symptoms of nicotine dependence often develops rapidly in adolescent smokers. When adolescents try to quit, they experience withdrawal symptoms similar to those of adult smokers. However, relevant "adult" measures of dependence (i.e., cigarettes per day, time to first cigarette, smoking in spite of illness, avoiding places where smoking is prohibited) do not predict cessation outcome among daily adolescent smokers. In fact, no studies conclusively indicate either the reliability of exposure variables to measure dependence or predict successful cessation in dependent adolescent smokers [15, 79]. This complicates the clinician's ability to adequately assess nicotine dependence, and, subsequently, appropriate interventions for youth.

To date there are very few studies on the use of NRT by those under the age of 18 years old. These products appear to be safe for adolescents but have not yet been shown to be effective as a cessation aid for them. Experts from the United Kingdom and the United States, under the auspices of the Health Education Authority during a seminar in September 1999, concluded that NRT is less harmful than cigarettes and therefore should not be discouraged as a replacement for them and a cessation aid for this age group [48]. Additional recommendations included 1) specific cessation program should be developed for youth to use tobacco; 2) use of NRT by adolescents should be supervised by a health professional; 3) the level of dependence, motivation and readiness to quit should be assessed before recommending an appropriate form of NRT; 4) the implementation of any program should be monitored, records, kept, and the use of medications monitored with the outcomes noted [48].

Bupropion should not be prescribed in smokers under 18 years old. However, the US Public Health Service *Clinical Practice Guideline* recommends that, although there is little evidence of efficacy, clinicians may consider prescribing bupropion SR for youth when they are motivated to quit and there is clinical evidence of nicotine dependence. Furthermore, quit rates should be enhanced with adjunctive psychosocial or cognitive behavioral therapies [12].

Gender

The sex of an individual is an important variable in relation to the extent of nicotine addiction, the tobacco related pathologies and the susceptibility to the pharmacological therapies for smoking cessation. In the United States, over 23% of men and 18% of women smoke cigarettes. Women who smoke have twice the risk of MI and lung cancer than men. The risk of MI and stroke is further exacerbated in women when taking oral contraceptives. Other effects of tobacco-use particular to women include an increased risk of breast cancer, increased menstrual bleeding and duration of dysmenorrhea, greater variability of menstrual cycle length, difficulty in getting pregnant, and reaching menopause one to two years earlier [80].

Quitting smoking has been reported to be more difficult for women than men, partially because of the concern of the perceived potential risk of gaining weight if they do quit. Other reasons that women may have a more difficult time in quitting include greater susceptibility to environmental cues (such as friends and moods) and the feeling of control associated with the smoking. Furthermore, in women the menstrual cycle affects nicotine withdrawal symptoms as well as their response to cessation drugs which vary by cycle phase. Finally, during the quit attempt, men may provide less support to women than women give to men, while women were less compliant with treatment protocols and reported more depression symptoms as a result of quitting [15, 80].

A recent meta-analysis showed that NRTs (especially gum and patches) may not be as effective in women and that men benefited from NRT at all follow-up points, irrespective of the intensity of the support, while women benefited more from combining NRT with high-intensity psychosocial support [81].Women may use cigarettes to provide sensorimotor and social reinforcement and therefore nicotine replacement is not a central factor in quitting. Furthermore, it has been demonstrated that, at higher doses, the side effects rates associated with NRT, in particular with transdermal nicotine patches, were significantly higher for women than men [50, 80]. Research is currently being conducted to explore hormonal influences on nicotine dependence. These results show that women tend to experience greater withdrawal symptoms during the luteal or late luteal phases of the menstrual cycle. Nicotine patches appear to equally reduce the extent of withdrawal whether the woman quits smoking during the fullicular or late luteal phase of her menstrual cycle [16].

Gender differences may include the presence of postmenopausal periods in women, which may influence smoking cessation outcomes. Postmenopausal women represent approximately 30% of the female smoking population in U.S. Postmenopausal women are at greater risk than their non-smoker female counterparts to develop cancer, cardiovascular and pulmonary disease, and osteoporosis. Unfortunately, older women are less interested in quitting and are less likely to make a quit attempt within a given year. Weight gain and menopausal symptoms may be additional barriers to smoking cessation. Moreover, women with a history of depression were less likely to quit smoking, irrespective to the treatment they received [82].

The use of hormone replacement therapy (HRT) could influence the smoking treatment outcomes. One study reported that depressive symptoms increase during short-term smoking abstinence among women using HRT compared to those not using these hormones. This finding suggests that HRT may adversely impact cessation treatment outcomes [82]. Another study, however, found that HRT alleviates mood disturbances which can occur after smoking cessation [83]. There is also some evidence that HRT facilitates the improvement of clinical depression and the efficacy of antidepressants, so it is impossible that women on HRT could experience improved smoking outcomes than women not on hormonal therapy [84]. A recent study reported that transdermal nicotine patch use (at the dosage of 21 mg/day) helped to increase short-term smoking cessation rates in postmenopausal smokers. Unfortunately, the beneficial effect of the patch did not persist at a 1-year follow-up visit [82].

Pregnancy

Women who are pregnant should be strongly encouraged to stop for their health and health of their unborn child [12]. There is direct relationship between smoking and numerous adverse effects such as miscarriage, neonatal death and low birth weight. Pregnant smokers should receive clear and accurate information on the risks of smoking to the fetus. First, they should be provided special behavioral counseling to stop. If counseling is not sufficient, then use of pharmacological agents should be considered, especially if the risk of smoking outweighs the risk of using nicotine products with and without concomitant smoking. In fact, for women who continue to smoke during pregnancy, NRT may be considered safer than smoking, although there is potential danger nicotine may be a fetal teratogen and may contribute to obstetric complications as well as sudden infant death syndrome. The use of NRT is likely to be less hazardous than continued smoking, which exposes the fetus and mother to many other toxins, such as carbon monoxide and nicotine. NRT also generally provides lower doses of nicotine than does smoking.

A placebo-controlled trial has been published on the use of nicotine patches in pregnant smokers. This study reported that although no significant differences were observed for quit rates between the placebo and active nicotine patch group, the birth weights of babies born to mothers assigned to the active nicotine patch were higher than babies of mothers assigned to the placebo patch [85]. Because nicotine replacement products are not without risk to the fetus, such products should be used with caution by pregnant women for whom non-pharmaceutical interventions have failed. This assessment should be made by physicians in the early stage of pregnancy or, if possible, before. Moreover, pregnant women treated with NRTs should be given the lowest effective dose and monitored for nicotine and cotinine (a nicotine metabolite) levels. Nicotine products with intermittent rather continuous delivery are recommended [48].

There are limited data on the effects of bupropion on pregnant women, though animal studies have revealed no evidence of harm. Of note, bupropion and its metabolites cross the placenta and are secreted in breast milk [52, 53].

Smokers with Cardiovascular Disease

Smoking cessation is probably the most important risk factor modification for the primary and secondary prevention of cardiovascular disease. Stopping smoking reduces morbidity and mortality rates even among people who do not quit until after cardiovascular disease is diagnosed. Unfortunately, recent European data indicate that more than one-fifth of the people hospitalized for coronary heart disease (coronary artery bypass graft, coronary angioplasty or acute MI) continue to smoke [86].

The safety of NRT use by people with stable cardiovascular disease has been widely documented. Current research indicates that withholding NRT from smokers with cardiovascular disease is not warranted. There is evidence that it is more dangerous for patients with heart disease to continue to smoke than to use NRT. Given to the seriousness of their medical condition, cardiac patients who cannot quit should be among those first considered for NRT [87, 88]

Although little data are available on the safety of NRT for people with cardiovascular disease, current warnings range from careful use for people with stable cardiovascular disease to absolute contraindications in acute or instable cases. NRT should be recommended for smokers with stable cardiovascular disease who have tried and failed to quit without the use of appropriate medication. In addition, the patient's doctor should be notified of the cessation treatment plan and pharmacotherapy recommendation. For those patients who have experienced a serious cardiovascular event, or been hospitalized for a cardiovascular complaint in the previous four weeks (e.g., stroke, MI, unstable angina, cardiac arrhythmia, coronary heart bypass graft and angioplasty) or have uncontrolled hypertension, the patient's consulting physicians should be involved in the decision to recommend NRT [48, 87, 88].

Bupropion has been associated with hypertension, although it is virtually free of cardiovascular adverse effects. People with stable cardiovascular disease treated with bupropion, compared with placebo, achieved higher than 1-year continuous abstinence rates [14].

Patients with Chronic Obstructive Pulmonary Disease (COPD)

Cigarette smoking is the primary cause of COPD accounting for greater than 75% of all reported cases. Patients suffering from this disease are more likely to seek treatment due to disabling symptoms such as dyspnoea which impact on their quality of life. The positive effect of smoking cessation on COPD symptoms provides clinicians with a powerful "teachable moment" for smokers to move them to consider a quit attempt. Sharing information on potential improvements in lung function and symptoms could potentially "prime" COPD smokers for receiving and benefiting from smoking cessation treatment by enhancing their motivation to quit prior to a quit attempt.

However, despite the fact that smoking cessation is the only evidence-based intervention for treating COPD, little is known about the effectiveness of the interventions in COPD patients. Although reviews of the literature from the past few years concluded that a combination of pharmacotherapy with intensive individual counseling appears to be effective for treating patients with COPD, many gaps exists in cessation interventions that would best assist them [12, 89, 90]. Smokers with COPD may have a different pattern of smoking than those without COPD (e.g., greater nicotine dependence, heavier smoking, and higher CO concentrations in expired air). Moreover, it is not exactly known how quit rates compare in patients with varying degrees of COPD severity. Finally, no conclusions could be drawn regarding the effectiveness of behavioral intervention alone due to the lack of studies comparing such interventions with placebo or no treatment control conditions [89].

Tonnesen et al. [91] addressed some of these gaps by evaluating the efficacy of both pharmacologic and behavioral interventions in COPD smokers with a wide range of severity levels. In this study, point prevalence cessation rates were significantly greater with sublingual nicotine therapy compared to placebo at both 6-month and the 12-month follow-up, which is consistent with the results of prior studies of the sublingual nicotine tablet in a general population of smokers. The efficacy of bupropion used in smokers with mild to moderate COPD was associated with significantly higher abstinence rates at six months, but not at one year [14, 90].

Smokeless Tobacco Users

Smokeless tobacco or spit tobacco (ST) is cured, cut and often flavored tobacco that is not burned when used. The plug or chaw of ST is usually placed in the oral cavity against the mucosal sites permitting the absorption of nicotine into the blood stream. The tobacco juice generated by the combination of tobacco and saliva is either spit (thus spit tobacco) or swallowed. There are two main types or forms of ST: chewing tobacco and snuff. It may be used alone or in combination with other substances. Chewing tobacco comes in loose leaf, plug or block of cut tobacco or twist; snuff can be dry or moist though snuff is the most common type used.

Smokeless tobacco is a well-recognized risk factor for oral cancer due to the presence of tobacco specific N-nitrosamines [9, 10]. Moist snuff and chewing tobacco present a cancer risk also for upper respiratory and gastrointestinal sites, respectively, with dry snuff usage presenting an even higher risk. Continual use of ST can lead to localized gingival recession and snuff dippers' pouch. Senses of taste and smell are reduced so users generally eat more salt and sweet food [10, 78].

The amounts of nicotine absorbed, and the distribution and elimination are the same when using NRT as with smoked tobacco. Nicotine absorbed from smokeless tobacco is still euphoriant and reinforcer, and causes neuroadaptation that leads to tolerance and physiological dependence. Thus, there remains good reason to promote cessation programs for smokeless tobacco users [10].

Studies to date suggest tobacco cessation interventions for smokers are moderately effective when used with ST users. Smokeless tobacco users should be considered in a different category of patients. Therefore, prevention and cessation programs should be specific and distinct from smoking programs. Smokeless tobacco users may find an oral NRT a particularly helpful treatment approach. For patients who use ST cessation techniques could include alternatives such as bubble gum and sugarless candy. These oral alternatives can be combined with NRTs [4, 15].

Currently, there are few large-scale methodologically rigorous trials examining the efficacy of NRT for cessation of smokeless tobacco. A systematic review of treatment for spit-tobacco cessation found NRT (patch or gum) significantly increased six month point prevalence tobacco abstinence and that bupropion SR is probably effective for increasing smokeless tobacco abstinence at three months [92]. A number of studies also provided evidence of a positive treatment effect with behavioral interventions for ST users [4].

Cultural and Ethnic Minorities

Cultural and ethnic minorities deserve special consideration due to the increase of disease risk directly related to differences in patterns of smoking. Serum cotinine levels have been found to be higher among African American smokers than among white or Mexican American smokers. This may help explain why African American find it harder to quit and are more likely to experience higher rates of lung cancer than white smokers [93].

Chinese Americans exhibit a lower nicotine intake per cigarette, smoke fewer cigarettes per day, and exhibit a slower clearance of nicotine. Latinos exhibit similar nicotine intake per cigarette to whites, but smoke fewer cigarettes. The implication is that Chinese Americans, and perhaps other Asian, may require lower doses of NRTs [94]. The use of bupropion to aid in cessation has been shown to be effective in African Americans and New Zealand Maori smokers [53].

Individuals with Psychiatric Illness

Individuals with psychiatric illness have a disproportionate disease burden from cigarette smoking and tobacco-related mortality. Individuals with a current psychiatric illness are likely to be regular smokers and are less likely to quit smoking. Ninety-two percent of persons with schizophrenia have smoked compared to 20% of the general population. Rates of current smoking are also elevated among person with bipolar disorder (69%), major depression (37%), and generalized anxiety disorder (46%). There is some evidence for a common genetic etiology for smoking and psychiatric illness which supports the role of the α_7 neuronal nicotinic receptor in both schizophrenia and bipolar disorder [17].

Although smoking cessation treatments have not been extensively studied in persons with psychiatric illness, some pharmacotherapies have shown promise. In two randomized clinical trials of smoking cessation intervention for persons with schizophrenia or schizoaffective disorder, bupropion was found to be safe and significantly more effective than a placebo. Unfortunately, relapse rates were high. Evidence for the safety and efficacy of transdermal NRT, especially in conjunction with atypical antipsychotic agents, has been also reported [17, 53].

Pharmacogenetic Approaches to Nicotine Dependence Treatment

Despite the progress made in the pharmacological treatment of nicotine dependence, the efficacy of available treatment may be limited. Although transdermal nicotine is currently recommended as a first-line treatment for nicotine dependence, the vast majority of smokers receiving transdermal nicotine relapse to their former smoking practice [95, 96]. Bupropion has been shown to produce higher quit rates than NRT, yet it is effective for only a minority of smokers [97].

Several studies have attempted to identify pretreatment variables that can be used to individualize pharmacotherapies for nicotine dependence, but with limited success. Measures of nicotine dependence, such as smoking rate, level of dependence and cotinine level have predicted outcome in some NRT studies, but not in others [98, 99, 100]. Smokers with low to moderate nicotine dependence levels, nonobese smokers, and Caucasian smokers may benefit more from transdermal nicotine, while smokers who are highly dependent, obese, or members of minority groups may benefit more from nasal spray [101]. Bupropion may be a more effective treatment for women and smokers with higher levels of nicotine dependence [102, 103]. These data do not provide an empirical basis on which to tailor the choice of treatment to individual smokers, but pharmacogenetic research may identify smokers for whom bupropion and NRT will have the strongest benefit [17].

Smoking behaviors and the different response to pharmacotherapy for nicotine dependence is likely due to genetic variations in multiple genes and candidate genes may be involved in the central or peripheral mechanism of smoking. Candidate genes involved in the central mechanism include genes encoding for the nicotinic acetylcholine receptors, dopamine receptors, dopamine transporters and opiod receptors. For example, the dopamine D2 receptor (DRD2) is associated with an increases likelihood of nicotine abstinence symptoms, a reduced likelihood of sustained abstinence and greater efficacy of transdermal nicotine treatment relative to placebo [104, 105, 106]. Candidate genes involved in peripheral mechanisms include drug-metabolizing enzymes which metabolize nicotine and bupropion. Genetic variation in these targets may contribute to the genetic risk for smoking behaviors.

A recent pharmacogenetic study investigated the effect of genetic variations in the mechanism of slow metabolism of nicotine, mediated by cotinine. Approximately 70-80% of nicotine consumed during smoking is metabolically inactivated to cotinine, and roughly 90% of this conversion is mediated by CYP2A6. It was demonstrated that variability in the rate of nicotine metabolism owing to CYP2A6 genetic polymorphisms may influence nicotine plasma levels and that the variation of this gene, causing reduced or absent enzyme activity, is associated with a reduced risk of being a smoker, lower amount smoked, altered smoking intensity, and increased quitting. Moreover, it may influence pretreatment smoking behavior and affect plasma levels obtained from, and usage of, NRT [107].

Genetic information can lead to new treatments by identifying novel drug targets based on natural pharamacogenetic advantages in cessation. It can also lead to improvements in current treatments by enabling individualization of treatment based on the smoker's genetic background. The use of genetic information can lead to new drugs that augment our current smoking cessation therapies and the incorporation of genetic information into current treatment strategies can improve abstinence rates and help maximize the chances for long-term smoking cessation success. However, due to the complexity of the nicotine dependence phenotype, it seems that no one medication will show efficacy and safety for a majority of nicotine dependent individuals [17, 104].

References

[1] Centers for Disease Control and Prevention (CDC). Cigarette smoking among adults-United States, 2003. *MMWR Morb. Mortal Wkly. Rep.* 2005;54:509-513.

[2] World Health Organization (WHO). Why is tobacco a public health priority? Geneva: WHO, 2005. Available at: *http://www.who.int/tobacco/health_priority/en/ index.html.* Accessed December 4, 2006.

[3] Centers for Disease Control and Prevention (CDC). Annual smoking-attributable mortality, years of potential life lost, and economic costs-United States: 1997-2001. *MMWR Morb. Mortal Wkly. Rep.* 2005;54:625-628.

[4] Warnakulasuriya S, Sutherland G, Scully C. Tobacco, oral cancer, and treatment of dependence. *Oral Oncol.* 2005;41:244-260.

[5] Centers for Disease Control and Prevention (CDC). Youth tabacco surveillance-United States, 2000. *MMWR CDC Surveill. Summ.* 2001;50:1-84. Erratum in: *MMWR CDC Surveill. Summ.* 2001;50:1036.

[6] Ezzati M, Lopez AD. Regional, disease specific patterns of smoking-attributable mortality in 2000. *Tob. Control* 2004;13:3888-395.

[7] Shields PG. Tobacco smoking, harm reduction, and biomarkers. *J. Natl. Cancer Inst.* 2002;94:1435-1444.

[8] Lightwood JM, Phibbs CS, Glantz SA. Short-term health and economic benefits of smoking cessation: low-birth weight. *Pediatrics.* 1999;104:1312-1320.

[9] Warnakulsuriya S. Smokeless tobacco and oral cancer. *Oral Dis.* 2004;10:1-4.

[10] Rodu B, Jansson C. Smokeless tobacco and oral cancer: a review of the risks and determinants. *Crit. Rev. Oral Biol. Med.* 2004;15:252-263.

[11] Fisher MA, Taylor GW, Tilashalski KR. Smokeless tobacco and severe active periodontal disease, NHANES III. *J. Dent. Res.* 2005;84:705-710.

[12] Fiore MC, Bailey WC, Cohen Sj, Dorfman SF, Goldstein MG, Gritz ER, et al. Treating tobacco use and dependence. Clinical Practice Guideline. Rockville, MD: U.S. Department of Health And Human Service. June 2000. Available at: *http://surgeongeneral.gov/tobacco/treating_tobacco_use.pdf.* Accessed December 4, 2006.

[13] Centers for Disease Control and Prevention (CDC). Cigarette smoking among adults-United States, 2000. *MMWR Morb. Mortal. Wkly Rep.* 2002;51:642-645.

[14] McRobbie H, Lee M, Juniper Z. Non-nicotine pharmacotherapies for smoking cessation. *Respir. Med.* 2005;99:1203-1212.

[15] Anczak JD, Nogler RA. Tobacco cessation in primary care: maximizing intervention strategies. *Clin. Med. Res.* 2003;1:201-216.

[16] Kotlyar M, Hatsukami DK. Managing nicotine addiction. *J. Dent. Educ.* 2002;66:1061-1073.

[17] Berrettini WH, Lerman CE. Pharmacotherapy and pharmacogenetics of nicotine dependence. *Am. J. Psychiatry.* 2005;162:1441-1451.

[18] Brothwell DJ. Should the use of smoking cessation products be promoted by dental offices? An evidence-based report. *J. Can. Dent. Assoc.* 2001;67:149-154.

[19] Warnakulasuriya S. Effectiveness of tobacco counseling in the dental office. *J. Dent. Educ.* 2002;66:1079-1087.

[20] Shelley D, Cantrell J, Faulkner D, Haviland L Healton C, Messeri P. Physician and dentist tobacco use counseling and adolescent smoking behavior: results from the 2000 National Youth Tabacco Survey. *Pediatrics* 2005;115:719-725.

[21] Gorin SS, Heck JK. Meta-analysis of the efficacy of tobacco counseling by health care providers. *Cancer Epidemiol. Biomarkers Prev.* 2004;13:2012-2022.

[22] Tomar SL. Dentistry's role in tobacco control. *J. Am. Dent. Assoc.* 2001;132:30-35.

[23] Ritz ER, Carr CR, Marcus AC. The tobacco withdrawal syndrome in unaided quitters. *Br. J. Addict.* 1991;86:57-59.

[24] Mecklenburg RE, Backinger CL. Tobacco and chemical dependencies. In: Daniel SJ, Harfst SA, Eds. Mosby's Dental Hygiene. *Concepts, Cases, And Competencies*. St. Louis: Mosby, Inc., 2002:228-244.

[25] Fried J. Tobacco cessation. In: Darby ML, Walsh MM, Eds. Dental Hygiene. *Theory and Practice.* 2nd ed. St. Louis: Saunders, 2003:589-603.

[26] Heatherton TF, Kozlowshi LT, Frecker RC, Fagerström KO. The Fagerström test for nicotine dependence: a revision of the Fagerström tolerance questionnaire. *Br. J. Addict.* 1991;86:1119-1127.

[27] Steptoe A, Ussher M. Smoking, cortisol and nicotine. *Int. J. Psycophysiol.* 2006;59:228-235.

[28] Lam CY, Minnix JA, Robinson JD, Cinciripini PM. A brief review of pharmacotherapies for smoking cessation. *J. Ntl. Compr. Canc. Netw.* 2006;4:583-589.

[29] Silagy C, Lancaster T, Stead L, Mant D, Fowler G. Nicotine replacement therapy for smoking cessation. *Cochrane Database Syst. Rev.* 2004; 3:CD0000146.

[30] Etter J, Stapleton JA. Nicotine replacement therapy for long-term smoking cessation: a meta-analysis. *Tob. Control* 2006;15:280-285.

[31] Rose JE, Behm FM, Westman EC, Kukovich P. Precessation treatment with nicotine skin patch facilitates smoking cessation. *Nicotine Tob. Res.* 2006;1:89-101.

[32] Henningfield JE, Fant RV, Buchhalter AR, Stitzer ML. Pharmacotherapy for nicotine dependence. *CA Cancer J. Clin.* 2005;55:281-299.

[33] Karnath B. Smoking cessation. *Am. J. Med.* 2002;112:399-405.

[34] National Institute for Clinical Excellence (NICE). Technology Appraisal Guidance - No. 39. Guidance on the use of nicotine replacement therapy (NRT) and bupropion for smoking cessation. March 2002. Available at: *http://www.nice.org.uk/pdf/Nice NRT39GUIDANCE.pdf*. Accessed December 4, 2006.

[35] Pomerlau OF, Pomerlau CS, Marks JL, Snedecor SM, Mehringer AM, Namenek Brouwer RJ, et al. Prolonged nicotine patch use in quitters with past abstinence-induced depressed mood. *J. Sust. Abuse Treat.* 2004;24:13-18.

[36] Dale LC, Hurt RD, Offort KP, Lawson GM, Croghan IT, Schroeder DR. High-dose nicotine patch therapy: percentage of replacement and smoking cessation. *J. Am. Med. Assoc.* 1995;274:1353-1358.

[37] Jorenby DE, Smith SS, Fiore MC, Hurt RD, Oddford KP, Kroghan IT, et al. Varying nicotine patch dose and type of smoking cessation of smoking cessation counseling. *J. Am. Med. Assoc.* 1995;274:1347-1352.

[38] Tang JL, Law M, Wald N. How effective is nicotine replacement therapy in helping people to stop smoking? *Br. Med. J.* 1994;308:21-26.

[39] Doherty K, Militello FS, Kinnunen T, Garvey AJ. Nicotine gum dose and weight gain after smoking cessation. *J. Consult. Clin. Psychol.* 1996;64:799-807

[40] Burkett JS. The use of the nicotine inhaler in smoking cessation. *J. Am. Acad. Nurse Pract.* 2006;18:83-91.

[41] Schneider NG, Olmstead RE, Steinberg C, Sloan K, Daims RM, Brown HV. Efficacy of a nicotine inhaler in smoking cessation: a double-blind, placebo-controlled trial. *Addiction* 1996;91:1293-1306.

[42] Hjalmarson A, Nilsson F, Sjostrom L, Wiklund O. The nicotine inhaler in smoking cessation. *Arch. Int. Med.* 1997;157:1721-1728.

[43] Hughes JR, Adams EH, Franzon MA, Maguire MK, Guary J. A prospective study of off-label use of, abuse of, and dependence on the nicotine inhaler. *Tob. Control* 2005;14:49-54.

[44] U.S. Food and Drug Administration (FDA). FDA warns sellers of nicotine lollipops and li pbalm that their products are illegal. FDA Talk Paper (T02-17), April 10, 2002. Available at: http://www.fda.gov/bbs/topics/ANSWERS/2002/ANS01144.html. Accessed December 4, 2006

[45] "Nicotine water" is unapproved drug. *FDA Consum.* 2002;36:5

[46] Dacosta A, Guy JM, Tardy B, Gonthier R, Denis L, Lamaud M, et al. Myocardial infarction and nicotine patch; a contributing or a causative factor? *Eur. Heart J.* 1993;14:1709-1711.

[47] Hubbard R, Lewis S, Godfrey C, Smeeth L, Farrington P and Britton J. Use of nicotine replacement therapy and the risk of acute miocardial infarction, stroke, and death. *Tob. Control* 2005;14:416-421.

[48] World Health Organization European Partnership Project to Reduce Tobacco Dependence. Regulation of nicotine replacement therapies: an expert consensus. World Health Organization Regional Office for Europe. Copenhagen, 2001. Available at: *http://www.euro.who.int/document/e74522.pdf*. Accessed December 4, 2006.

[49] Salin-Pascual RJ. Effects of nicotine replacement therapies on sleep. *Sleep Med.* 2006;7:105-106.

[50] Stein MD, Anderson BJ, Niaura R. Nicotine replacement therapy. Patterns of use after a quit attempt among methadone-manteined smokers. *J. Gen. Intern. Med.* 2006;21:753-757.

[51] Kotlyar M, Golding M, Hatsukami DK, Jamerson BD. Effect of nonnicotine pharmacotherapy on smoking behavior. *Pharmacother.* 2001;21:1530-1548.

[52] Mooney ME, Sofuoglu M. Bupropion for the treatment of nicotine withdrawal and craving. *Expert Rev. Neurotherapeutics* 2006;6:965-981.

[53] Tong EK, Carmody TP, Simon JA. Bupropion for smoking cessation. A review. *Compr. Ther.* 2006;32:26-33.

[54] Learned-Coughlin SM, Bergstrom M, Savitcheva I, Ascher J, Schmith VD, Langstrom B. In vivo activity of bupropion at the human dopamine transporter as measured by positron emission tomography. *Biol. Psychiatry* 2003;54:800-805.

[55] Warner C, Shoaib M. How does bupropion work as a smoking cessation aid? *Addict. Biol.* 2005;10:219-231.

[56] Hays JT, Ebbert JO. Bupropion sustained release for treatment of tobacco dependence. *Mayo Clin. Proc.* 2003;78:1020-1024.

[57] Hughes JR, Stead LF, Lancaster T. Antidepressants for smoking cessation. *Cochrane Database Syst. Rev.* 2003;4:CD000031.

[58] Paluck EC, McCormack JP, Ensom MH, Levine M, Soon JA, Fielding DW. Outcomes of bupropion therapy for smoking cessation during routine clinical use. *Ann. Pharmacother.* 2006;40:185-190.

[59] Killen JD, Fortmann SP, Murphy GM, Hayward C, Arredondo C, Cromp D, et al. Extended treatment with bupropion SR for cigarette smoking cessation. *J. Consult. Clin. Psychol.* 2006;74:286-294.

[60] Hays JT, Hurt RD, Rigotti NA, Niaura R, Gonzales D, Durcan MJ, et al. Sustained-release bupropion for pharmacologic relapse prevention after smoking cessation: a randomized, controlled trial. *Ann. Intern. Med.* 2001;135:423-433.

[61] Dobson R. Antismoking drugs comes under scrutiny after deaths. *Br. Med. J.* 2001;322:452.

[62] American College of Chest Physicians (ACCP). Smoking Cessation Therapy May Be Harmful For ICU Patients. Available at: http://www.medicalnewstoday.com/medicalnews.php?newsid=55405. Accessed December 5, 2006

[63] Foulds J. The neurobiological basis for partial agonist treatment of nicotine dependence: varenicline. *Int. J. Clin. Pract.* 2006;60:571-576.

[64] Niaura R, Jones C, Kirkpatrick P. Varenicline. *Nat. Rev. Drug Discov.* 2006;5:537-538

[65] U.S. Food and Drug Administration. FDA approves novel medication for smoking cessation. *FDA News May* 11 2006. Available at: *www.fda.gov/bbs/topics/NEWS/* 2006. Accessed November 30, 2006.

[66] Fagerström K, Balfour DJK. Neuropharmacology and potential efficacy of new treatments for tobacco dependence. *Expert Opin. Investig. Drugs* 2005;15:107-116.

[67] Jorenby DE, Hays JT, Rigotti NA, Azoulay S, Watsky EJ, Williams KE, et al. Efficacy of varenicline, an α2β4 nicotinic acetylcoline receptor partial agonist, vs placebo or sustained-release bupropion for smoking cessation. *J. Am. Med. Assoc.* 2006;296:56-63.

[68] Tonstad S, Tonnesen P, Hajek P, Williams KE, Billing CB, Reeves KR, et al. Effect of manteinance therapy with varenicline on smoking cessation: a randomized controlled trial. *J. Am. Med. Assoc.* 2006;296:64-71.

[69] Gonzales D, Rennard SI, Nides M, Oncken C, Azoulay S, Billing CB et al. Varenicline, an alpha4beta2 nicotinic acetylcholine, receptor partial agonist, vs sustained-release buproprion and placebo for smoking cessation. A randomized controlled trial. *J. Am. Med. Assoc.* 2006;296:47-55.

[70] Huges JR, Lindsay FS, Lancaster T. Nortryptiline for smoking cessation: a review. *Nicotine Tob. Res.* 2005;4:491-499.

[71] Hall SM, Humfleet GL, Reus VI, Munoz RF, Hartz DT, Maude-Griffin R. Psychological intervention and antidepressant treatment in smoking cessation. *Arch. Gen Psychiatry* 2002;59:930-936.

[72] Gourlay SG, Stead LF, Benowitz NL. Clonidine for smoking cessation. *Cochrane Database Syst. Rev.* 2004;3:CD000058.

[73] Covey NS, Glassman AH, A meta-analysis of double-blind placebo controlled trials of clonidine for smoking cessation. *Br. J. Addict.* 1991;86:991-998.

[74] Gourlay SG, Benowitz NL. Is clonidine an effective smoking cessation therapy? *Drugs* 1995;50:197-207.

[75] Ingersoll KS, Cohen J. Combination tratment for nicotine dependence: state of science. *Subst. Use Misuse* 2005;40:1923-1943.

[76] Steinberg MB, Foulds J, Richardson DL, Burke MV, Shah P. Pharmacotherapy and smoking cessation at tobacco dependence clinic. *Prev. Med.* 2006;42:114-119.

[77] Centers for Disease Control and Prevention (CDC). Middle school youth risk behavior survey, 2003. U.S. Department of Health and Human Services 2005. Available at *www.cdc.gov/healthyyouth/yrb/middleschool2003/pdf.* Accessed November 30, 2006.

[78] Centers for Disease Control and Prevention (CDC). Cigarette use among high school students-United States, 1991-2005. *MMWR Morb. Mortal Wkly. Rep.* 2006;55:724-726.

[79] Franken FH, Pickworth WB, Epstein DH, Moolchan ET. Smoking rates and topography predict adolescent smoking cessation following treatment with nicotine replacement therapy. *Cancer Epidemiol. Biomarkers Prev.* 2006;15:154-157.

[80] Evans SE, Blank M, Sams C, Weaver MF, Eissenberg T. Transdermal nicotine-induced tobacco abstinence symptom suppression: nicotine dose and smokers' gender. *Exp. Clin. Psychopharmacol.* 2006; 14:121-135.

[81] Cepeda Benito A, Renoso JT, Erath S. Meta-analysis of the efficacy of nicotine replacement therapy for smoking cessation: differences between men and women. *J Consul. Clin. Psychol.* 2004;72:712-722.

[82] Onchen C, Cooney J, Feinn R, Lando H, Kranzler R. Transdermal nicotine for smoking cessation in postmenopausal women. *Addict. Behav.* 2007;32:296-309.

[83] Allen SS, Hatsukami DK, Bade T, Center B. Transdermal nicotine use in postmenopausal women: does the treatment efficacy differ in women using and not using nicotine replacement therapy? *Nicotine Tob. Res.* 2003;6:777-788.

[84] Miller KJ. The other side of estrogen replacement therapy: outcome study results of mood improvement in estrogen users and nonusers. *Curr. Psychiatry Rep.* 2003;5:439-444.

[85] Wisborg K, Henriksen TB, Jespersen LB, Secher NJ. Nicotine patches for pregnant smokers: a randomized controlled study. *Obstet. Gynecol.* 2000;96:967-971.

[86] Euroaspire II Study Group. Lifestyle and risk factor management and use of drug therapies in coronary patients from 15 countries: principal results from EUROASPIRE II Euro Hearth Survey Programme. *Eur. Hearth J.* 2001;7:554-572.

[87] Ford CL, Zlabek JA. Nicotine replacement therapy and cardiovascular disease. *Mayo Clin. Proc.* 2005;80:652-656.

[88] McRobbie H, Hajek P. Nicotine replacement therapy in patients with cardiovascular disease: guidelines for health professionals. *Addiction* 2001;96:1547-1551.

[89] van der Meer RM, Wagena EJ, Ostelo RW, Jacobs JE, van Schayck CP. Smoking cessation for chronic obstructive pulmonary disease. *Cochrane Database Syst. Rev.* 2003;2:CD002999

[90] Wagena EJ, van der Meer RM, Ostelo RW, Jacobs JE, van Schayck CP. The efficacy of smoking cessation strategies in people with chronic obstructive pulmonary disease: results from a systematic review. *Respir. Med.* 2004;98:805-815.

[91] Tonnesen P, Mikkelsen K, Bremann L. Nurse-conducted smoking cessation in patients with COPD, using nicotine sublingual tablets and behavioral support. *Chest* 2006;130:334-342.

[92] Ebbert JO, Rowland LC, Montori VM, Vickers KS, Erwin P, Dale LC. Treatments for spit tobacco use: a quantitative systematic review. *Addiction* 2003;98:569-583.

[93] Caraballo RS, Giovino GA, Pechacek TF, Mowery PD, Richter PA, Strauss WG, et al. Racial and ethnic differences in serum cotonine levels of sigarette smokers: Third National Health and Nutrition Examination Survey, 1988-1991. *J. Am. Med. Assoc.* 1998;280:135-139.

[94] Benowitz NL, Perez-Stable EJ, Herrera B, Jacob P 3rd. Slower metabolism and reduced intake of nicotine from cigarette smoking in Chinese-Americans. *J. Natl. Cancer Inst.* 2002;94:108-115.

[95] Fiore MC. Treating tobacco use and dependence: an introduction to the US Public Health Service Clinical Practice Guideline. *Respir. Care.* 2000;45:1196-1199.

[96] Fiore MC, Smith SS, Jorenby DE, Baker TB.The effectiveness of the nicotine patch for smoking cessation: a meta-analysis. *J. Am. Med. Assoc.* 1994;27:1940-1947.

[97] Gold PB, Rubey RN, Harvey RT. Naturalistic, self-assignment comparative trial of bupropion SR, a nicotine patch, or both for smoking cessation treatment in primary care. *Am. J. Addict.* 2002;11:315-331.

[98] Paoletti P, Fornai E, Maggiorelli F, Puntoni R, Viegi G, Carozzi L et al. Importance of baseline cotinine plasma values in smoking cessation: results from a double-blind study with nicotine patch. *Eur. Respir. J.* 1996;9:643-651.

[99] Norregaard J, Tonnesen P, Petersen L. Predictors and reasons for relapse in smoking cessation with nicotine and placebo patches. *Prev. Med.* 1993;22:261-271.

[100] Kenford SL, Fiore MC, Jorenby DE, Smith SS, Wetter D, Baker TB. Predicting smoking cessation: who will quit with and without the nicotine patch. *J. Am. Med. Assoc.* 1994;271:589-594.

[101] Lerman C, Kaufmann V, Rukstalis M, Patterson F, Perkins K, Audrain-McGovern J, Benowitz N. Individualizing nicotine replacement therapy for the treatment of tobacco dependence: a randomozed trial. *Ann. Intern. Med.* 2004;140:426-433.

[102] Collins BN, Wileyto EP, Patterson F, Rukstalis M, Audrain-McGovern J, Kaufmann V, et al. Gender difference in smoking cessation in a placebo-controlled trial of bupropion with behavioral counselling. *Nicotine Tob. Res.* 2004;6:27-37.

[103] Dale LC, Glover ED, Sachs DP, Schroeder DR, Offord KP, Croghan IT, et al. Bupropion for smoking cessation: predictors of successful outcome. *Chest* 2001;119:1357-1364.

[104] Lee Am, Tyndale RF. Drugs and genotypes: how pharmacogenetic information could improve smoking cessation treatment. *J. Psycopharmacol.* 2006;20:7-14.

[105] Lerman C, Jepson C, Wileyto EP, Epstein LH, Rukstalis M, et al. Role of functional genetic variation in the dopamine D2 receptor (DRD2) in response to bupropion and

nicotine replacement therapy for tobacco dependence: results of two randomized clinical trials. *Neuropsycopharmacology* 2006;31:231-242.

[106] Dahl JP, Jepson C, Levenson R, Wileyto EP, Patterson F, Berrettini WH, et al. Interaction between variation in the D2 dopamine receptor (DRD2) and the neuronal calcium sensor-1 (FREQ) genes in predicting response to nicotine replacement therapy for tobacco dependence. *Pharmacogenomics J.* 2006;6:194-199.

[107] Malaiyandi V, Lerman C, Benowitz NL, Jepson C, Patterson F, Tyndale RF. Impact of CYP2A6 genotype on pretreatment smoking behaviour and nicotine levels from and usage of nicotine replacement therapy. *Mol. Psychiatry* 2006;11:400-409.

In: Progress in Smoking and Health Research
Editor: T. C. Jeffries, pp. 41-70
ISBN: 978-1-60021-686-2

Chapter II

Developmental Risk and Protective Factors for Cigarette Smoking among African-American and White Adolescent Males

Helene Raskin White*[1], Lisa Metzger[2], Magda Stouthamer-Loeber[3], Nancy Violette[4] and Daniel Nagin[5]

[1] Center of Alcohol Studies, Rutgers University, New Jersey, United States
[2] University of Washington, Washington, United States
[3] Western Psychiatric Institute and Clinic, University of Pittsburgh, Pennsylvania, United States
[4] Center of Alcohol Studies, Rutgers University, New Jersey, United States
[5] H. J. Heinz III School of Public Policy and Management, Carnegie Mellon University, Pennsylvania, United States

Abstract

The purpose of this study was to examine risk and protective factors for the initiation and maintenance of cigarette smoking during varying developmental periods from childhood through late adolescence for African-American and white adolescents. We used data from a sample of 503 males who were first recruited in the first grade and followed annually for 14 years. Trajectory analyses identified three trajectory groups for African Americans and whites: nonsmokers, light smokers, and regular smokers. The following domains of risk and protective factors were included in the analyses: individual [hyperactivity/impulsivity/attention problem (HIA), depression, attitudes toward substance use, school performance, delinquency frequency, and religiosity], family (parental smoking and relationship with parents), peer (peer delinquency), and

* Correspondence to: Helene Raskin White, Rutgers Center of Alcohol Studies, 607 Allison Road, Piscataway, New Jersey, 08854-8001; hewhite@rci.rutgers.edu

environmental [socioeconomic status (SES) and neighborhood quality]. First analyses were conducted separately by race to determine which factors represented risk and which represented protection. Then hierarchical logistic regression analyses were conducted to determine how these factors differentiated among the three trajectory groups and whether race interacted with these factors. Many of the variables were both risk and protective factors across different developmental periods. School performance and religiosity were only significantly related to smoking for African Americans and SES was only related for whites. For both races HIA, depression, delinquency, and peer delinquency were significantly related to smoking. In the multivariate analyses, race, SES, and delinquency were related to smoking at younger ages and delinquent peers was related to smoking at all ages. Only four interactions with race were significant for smoking. Good school performance was protective for African Americans at ages 7-9, but not whites. Having many delinquent peers was a stronger risk factor for African Americans at ages 13-16, but having many at ages 17-19 was a risk factor only for whites. Being low in delinquency was a stronger protective factor for whites at ages 13-16. Depression was related to regular smoking only for African Americans and attitudes toward substance use, parental smoking, and neighborhood quality were related only for whites. For both races HIA, school performance, delinquency, and peer delinquency were related to regular smoking. In the multivariate analyses, being African American protected against regular smoking at all ages. Only one interaction was significant; low depression was a protective factor for African American but not white regular smoking. Overall, the fact that there were few significant interactions of risk and protective factors with race suggests that the same factors can be targeted for both whites and African Americans in cigarette prevention programs.

Keywords: race, African Americans, cigarettes, smoking, risk factors, protective factors.

Introduction

Smoking initiation and maintenance are serious public health concerns. In fact, smoking is the number one preventable cause of death in developed countries (Baker, Brandon, and Chassin, 2004). Despite the known health risks, large proportions of young people establish regular smoking habits (Johnston, O'Malley, and Bachman, 2003). Although there have been declines in smoking among adolescents since the mid-1990s, the rate of decline has been decelerating during the past several years. Data from the 2005 Monitoring the Future Study indicate that 50% of high school seniors had tried cigarette smoking, 23% had smoked within the last 30 days, and 14% had smoked daily (www.monitoringthefuture.org).

Racial differences in developmental patterns of cigarette smoking have been identified in numerous studies. Whites compared to African Americans begin smoking earlier and reach higher levels of use into their mid 20s (Griesler and Kandel, 1998; Williams and Covington, 1997). Racial differences in adolescent smoking hold across community and school samples even when bioassays are used to validate self report (Baker et al., 2004). At some point during early adulthood the prevalence of smoking for African Americans increases dramatically (Kandel, Chen, Warner, Kessler, and Grant, 1997; US Department of Health and Human Services, 1998; Williams and Covington, 1997). In fact, recent data indicate that current smoking prevalence rates are similar for white (24%) and African American (22%)

adults (National Center for Chronic Disease Prevention and Health Promotion, 2004). White, Nagin, Repologle, and Stouthamer-Loeber (2004) examined racial differences in developmental trajectories of smoking from late childhood into young adulthood. They identified the same three trajectory groups for African Americans and whites: nonsmokers, light smokers, and regular smokers. For each group, the African American and white trajectories followed similar shapes over time, but for the two smoker groups (light and regular), white trajectory levels were higher than African-American levels. That is, white regular smokers smoked more cigarettes per day than African American regular smokers at each assessment and the same was true for light smokers. In addition, there were differences in the timing and rapidity of development of for regular smokers with whites starting earlier and increasing more rapidly (see below).

Given that the development and patterns of smoking vary by race, it would be expected that the precursors of smoking would also vary by race and, in fact, some studies have found different predictors of smoking for whites and African Americans (e.g., Flint, Yamanda, and Novotny, 1998; Landrine, Richardson, Klonoff, and Flay, 1994; Robinson, Klesges, Zbikowski, and Glaser, 1997). However, other studies have found that similar variables predict smoking for both African Americans and whites (e.g., Gritz, Prokhorov, Hudmon, Chamberlain, Taylor, DiClemente et al., 1998; Kandel, Kiros, Schaffran, and Mei-Chen, 2004). Furthermore, it is possible that risk factors vary at different ages, although few studies have examined this possibility in a single sample. Thus, more research is needed to delineate the common and unique risk and protective factors for transitional stages in smoking behavior in order to develop racially appropriate prevention programs (Flint et al, 1998; Gritz et al., 1998; Gottfredson and Koper, 1996; Landrine et al. 1994). Studying these differences at different age periods can help inform the development of more effective prevention programs, which target adolescents when they are most vulnerable to specific risks. This study examines both risk and protective factors for the initiation of smoking and regular smoking among African Americans and whites at various developmental periods from childhood through late adolescence.

Risk and Protective Factors

Over the last few decades, studies of protective (or promotive) and risk (or vulnerability) factors have used alternative conceptualizations to define positive and negative predictors of problem and adaptive behaviors (for a review, see Stouthamer-Loeber, Wei, Loeber, and Masten, 2004). Some researchers view risk and protective factors as opposite ends of a continuum. Others conceptualize protective factors as moderators that buffer the effects of risk factors or as factors that reduce the likelihood that risk factors will occur (Schulenberg and Maggs, 2002, p. 57). In many cases it is not clear whether negative conditions should be viewed as risk factors or whether the absence of such conditions should be viewed as protective factors. Stouthamer-Loeber and colleagues (Stouthamer-Loeber, Loeber, Farrington, Zhang, van Kammen, and Maguin, 1993; Stouthamer-Loeber, Loeber, Wei, Farrington, and Wilkstrom, 2002) have argued that the positive and negative ends of protective/risk factors may have differential significance for varying dependent variables. In other words, they argue that there may be a nonlinear association between protective/risk ends of variables and subsequent outcomes. Furthermore, the positive or negative end of a variable may have differential effects during different developmental periods. In this paper, we examine both the positive and negative end of factors presumed to influence cigarette smoking among youth. We use the term protective factor to refer to the positive end and the term risk factor to refer to the negative end. We examine whether risk and protective factors differ by race across different developmental periods from childhood to late adolescence. We do not, however, examine racial differences in the magnitude of risk and protection (see Wallace and Muroff, 2002).

Current theories of substance use emphasize multiple risk and protective factors across several domains including individual factors and social contexts (Schulenberg, Wadsworth, O'Malley, Bachman, and Johnston, 1996). Multiple factors affect smoking, and their relative impacts vary across the developmental phases of smoking (Baker et al., 2004). In a recent review, Mayhew, Flay, and Mott (2000) identified numerous risk factors, including male gender, white race, positive attitudes and belief about smoking, concerns with body weight, affect regulation, perception of smoking as a relaxation tool, perceptions of cigarette accessibility, number of cigarette offers, intentions to smoke in the future, other drug use, minimization of smoking risks, tolerance for deviance, anti-social behaviors, low academic expectations, less educational achievement, lower expectations for school achievement, and working part time, tobacco use among parents and siblings, parental approval of smoking, adolescent perception of parents' permissiveness toward smoking, parental involvement, and having friends who smoke (for an additional review, see also Baker et al., 2004). After reviewing the literature, Mayhew et al. (2000) and Baker et al. (2004) both concluded that there were more common than unique predictors of smoking among African Americans and whites.

On the other hand, Gardiner (2001) suggested that there were factors related to smoking that were unique for African Americans. He enumerated several protective factors for African Americans that may account for their lower rates of cigarette smoking, including: 1) the cost of cigarettes, 2) sports participation, 3) body-type preferences (i.e., African Americans are less likely to smoke for weight loss); 4) peer and parental smoking status (i.e., having fewer peers and parents who smoke), 5) marijuana use (which often takes the place of tobacco as a gateway drug), and 6) ethical and religious concerns. He also noted several factors that may increase risk for cigarette smoking among African Americans, including: 1) tobacco industry marketing directly to African American teens and sponsorship of African American events, 2) adoption of smoking by segments of the hip-hop culture, 3) greater access to tobacco, and 4) racial discrimination and poverty.

We have selected a set of risk and protective factors across multiple domains, which have been demonstrated to influence the initiation and / or the maintenance of cigarette smoking for whites, African Americans, or both and were available within our data set (Baker et al., 2004; Mayhew et al., 2004). The risk and protective factors that we selected come from four domains: 1) individual (hyperactivity/impulsivity/attention problems, depression, attitudes toward substance use, school performance, delinquency frequency, and religiosity), 2) family (parental smoking and relationship with parents), 3) peer (peer delinquency), and 4) environmental (SES and neighborhood quality). Below, we briefly summarize the literature that supports our choice of these factors and whether racial differences have previously been found.

Negative affect and temperament have been associated with smoking behavior in several studies. There is a relatively strong link between impulsivity, hyperactivity, and attention problems and cigarette use, although studies have not examined racial differences (Baker et al., 2004; Burke, Loeber, and Lahey, 2001). In community samples, higher levels of depression have been found to predict smoking behavior (Glassman, Helzer, Covey, Cottler, Stetner, Tipp et al., 1990; Kandel and Davies, 1986; Newcomb McCarthy, and Bentler, 1989; Patton, Hibbert, Rosier, Carlin, Caust, and Bowes, 1996), although the findings have been inconsistent across studies (e.g., Breslau, Kilbey, and Andreski, 1991; White, Pandina, and Chen, 2002; Winefield, Winefield, and Tiggemann, 1992). In some studies, depression has not been linked to smoking among African Americans (e.g., Juon, Ensminger, and Sydnor, 2002; Lloyd-Richardson, Papandonatos, Kazura, Stanton, and Niaura, 2002).

Beliefs and attitudes concerning substance use have also been shown to be important determinants of smoking behavior (Baker et al., 2004; Chassin, Presson, Rose and Sherman, 1996; Flay, Hu, Siddiqui, Day, Hedeker, Petraitis et al., 1994). African Americans hold less positive attitudes about smoking than whites (Robinson et al., 1997), which might account for African Americans' lower rates of use. Positive attitudes towards smoking are also significant predictors of smoking behavior for whites (Flay et al., 1994). In our analysis, we used attitudes toward substance use (i.e., alcohol and illicit drugs) as a proxy measure because we did not have a measure of attitudes toward tobacco use.

Religiosity is another factor that may differentially protect against smoking initiation for African Americans and whites (Wallace, Brown, Bachman, and Laveist, 2003). Wallace and colleagues (2003) contend that the protective aspects of religiosity for African American youth may be due to the important cultural and social functions offered by church life. Juon and colleagues (2002) found that familial religiosity, as well as church attendance, was a significant protective factor for African American smoking. Other studies have shown that only attitudes towards religion are related to smoking behavior among whites (Griesler and Kandel, 1998).

Studies have consistently found that smoking is related to other deviant behaviors and inversely related to conventional behaviors (Baker et al., 2004; Newcomb et al., 1989). High academic achievement and school attachment appear to be protective factors for both races (Hestick, Perrino, Rhodes, and Sydnor, 2001; Kandel et al., 2004; Lloyd-Richardson et al., 2002). However, Griesler and Kandel (1998) reported that positive attitudes toward school were associated with less smoking for whites, but were not related to smoking for African Americans. In a recent study, Kandel and colleagues (2004) found that a positive scholastic attitude reduced the risk for smoking initiation for whites but not for African Americans. In contrast, they found that a positive scholastic attitude reduced the risk of daily smoking for African Americans but not for whites. Delinquency has been strongly associated with cigarette use (Breslau, Kilbey and Andreski, 1993; Chassin, Presson, Sherman, Montello, and McGrew, 1986; Diem, McKay, and Jamieson, 1994) and this association appears to hold for both races (Derzon and Lipsey, 1999; Kandel et al., 2004; Griesler and Kandel, 1998).

The effects of family smoking are differentially related to smoking by whites and African Americans. Having a parent who currently smokes has a strong predictive effect on adolescent regular smoking behavior and on lower cessation rates for whites (Chassin et al., 1996; Griesler and Kandel, 1998), but has only been shown to be significant for African American cigarette experimentation (Robinson et al., 1997; Hestick et al., 2001). Flay and colleagues (1994) found that parental smoking only had indirect effects on smoking initiation and escalation for both African Americans and whites. Furthermore, for both races, the effects of peer smoking were much stronger than the effects of parent smoking. High quality of parent-child interaction (e.g., closeness and monitoring) has been demonstrated to reduce the likelihood of lifetime smoking among African Americans, but has not had as strong an effect for whites (Griesler and Kandel, 1998). Kandel and colleagues (2004) found that stronger parent-child connectedness protected against daily smoking for both African Americans and whites. In addition, African American parents more closely monitor their children, which can reduce smoking, as well as influence peer group selection (Wallace and Muroff, 2002).

Peer cigarette use has been shown to be one of the strongest predictors of adolescent smoking initiation and maintenance for both whites and African Americans (Botvin, Baker, Botvin, Dusenbury, Cardwell, and Diaz, 1993; Gardiner, 2001; Grtiz et al., 1998; Kandel et al., 2004). We did not have a measure of peer smoking, so we used a measure of peer delinquency as a proxy. Affiliation with delinquent peers has also been shown to predict cigarette use (Baker et al., 2004).

Socioeconomic and neighborhood differences between African Americans and whites may account for differential access to cigarettes. Chaloupka (2003) argued that the high price of cigarettes serves as a deterrent for some youths by limiting access. On the other hand, Wallace and Muroff (2002) have noted that, regardless of race, youngsters of lower SES are more likely to smoke. Yet, family SES appears to have a stronger influence for whites than for African Americans (Griesler and Kandel, 1998). Wallace and Muroff (2002) argued that, because African American teens are more likely to live in poorer neighborhoods with greater availability of both licit and illicit drugs, they are at greater overall risk.

Current Study

Although several studies have examined racial differences in the predictors of cigarette use, these studies have had limitations, which weaken their ability to inform and improve prevention programs. Some studies have been cross-sectional, which limits their ability to establish directionality and examine patterns of smoking over time. Many of the longitudinal studies have had high attrition rates, posing generalization and validity issues, especially because dropouts tend to exhibit higher rates of smoking (Chassin, Presson, Sherman, and Kim, 2002). Many studies have not differentiated between different types of smoking (i.e., experimentation and regular use), which prevents them from addressing differences in transitions between levels of use. When smoking levels are taken into account, studies have used different operational definitions, which lead to contradictory findings across studies, as well as the inability to compare results (for greater detail see White et al., 2002). Most studies contain either racially homogeneous samples or heterogeneous samples that tend to have a much greater numbers of whites than African Americans. Furthermore, most studies of racial differences in predictors of smoking have included limited numbers of variables and have not examined multiple domains and predictors at varying age periods. Finally, few studies have empirically differentiated between risk and protection.

The present study attempts to fill a gap in the literature by examining racial differences in risk and protective factors for smoking at different developmental periods from childhood to late adolescence. We address the limitations of previous research by using a community sample with a large proportion of both African Americans and whites, using annually-collected, longitudinal data spanning childhood until late adolescence with low attrition, empirically defining smoking trajectory groups, and including multiple domains of variables and multiple sources of data. In addition, we examine both risk and protective factors for smoking and use a new empirical method for determining risk and protection. We examine these risk and protective factors at various developmental periods marking childhood (ages 7-9), early adolescence (ages 10-12), middle adolescence (ages 13-16) and late adolescence (ages 17-19). Although we have continuous annual data from approximate age 7 to age 19, we divided the ages into these developmental periods to determine if there were developmentally distinct risk and protective factors. Because the risk and protective factors were measured at various developmental periods from ages 7 to 19 and the outcome variable was based on smoking trajectories from ages 10 through 19, only the childhood risk and protective factors precede the trajectory group measurement and represent potential predictors of trajectory group membership. The other risk and protective factors were measured concurrently with smoking behavior and, thus, causal inferences cannot be assumed. Nevertheless, we believe that it is important to examine those variables that are associated with risk and protection of smoking behavior over time. This study will contribute to the literature by exploring risk and protective factors for smoking initiation and regular smoking in the context of specified age ranges. The results should have implications for the design of culturally and age appropriate prevention programs for cigarette smoking.

Method

Design and Sample

The data come from the Pittsburgh Youth Study (PYS), a prospective, multiple cohort, longitudinal study of the development of delinquency, substance use, and mental health problems (Loeber, Farrington, Stouthamer-Loeber, and Van Kammen, 1998). In 1987-88, random samples of first, fourth, and seventh grade boys enrolled in the City of Pittsburgh public schools were selected. Approximately 850 boys in each grade (85% of the target sample) were screened. Families were paid for their participation, and informed written consent was obtained from both the participants and their legal guardians. The 15% nonparticipation rate did not result in sample bias, at least in regard to achievement test results and racial distribution, which were the only two variables that could be compared from school records (Loeber et al., 1998).

About 500 boys in each grade (the 30% who scored highest on a risk assessment for later antisocial behavior and another 30% randomly selected from the remainder) were selected for the first follow up 6 months later; therefore, approximately half of each cohort was selected for potential high risk and half was not. There was no significant difference in the percent high risk by race. The present analyses will focus on the youngest cohort (from approximately age 7 through age 19).[1] After the first follow up, the members of the youngest cohort were subsequently followed up at 6-month intervals for six additional assessments and then at yearly intervals for a total of 14 years. Attrition has remained relatively low and the completion rate has averaged above 90% across 14 years of data collection (for more information about recruitment and retention see Stouthamer-Loeber and Van Kammen, 1995). The youngest cohort is 56% African American, 42% white and 2% other or mixed. Over one third of the boys' families received public assistance or food stamps. (For greater detail on design and sample see Loeber et al., 1998.)

Measures

The data come from self reports from the youth, their primary caretaker (usually a mother), and their teacher. The youth and his primary caretaker were interviewed separately, usually in their own home. Teachers completed mailed questionnaires. We combined the early 6-month assessments to create annual measures for each year. The measures were assessed in the same manner at each assessment, unless stated so below.

Race. Youths reported on their *race/ethnicity* at screening. For these analyses, we eliminated the other and mixed groups and included only the African Americans (N=281; coded 2) and whites (N=208; coded 1).

Cigarette use. At screening the respondents were asked if they had ever used tobacco (cigarettes, cigars/pipes and smokeless tobacco) and, if yes, at what age they first used. Subsequent to that, they were asked whether or not they smoked in the last year (last 6-months in the first few assessments). The response to this question was used to indicate annual *prevalence* each year. The first time the respondent reported using tobacco was coded as their *age of onset*. Those who smoked were asked how many cigarettes they smoke per day, which provided a *quantity* measure. Smoking trajectories were based on the number of cigarettes smoked per day.

Risk and protective factors. For the present analyses, we divided the risk and protective factors into four developmental periods representing childhood (ages 7-9), early adolescence (10-12), middle adolescence (ages 13-16), and late adolescence (ages 17-19). Developmental period scores were derived by calculating the mean of all the ages within the period for which data were available.

Hyperactivity/impulsivity/attention (HIA) problems represented 14 descriptors (e.g., "can't concentrate," "can't sit still," "is impulsive") related to hyperactivity, impulsivity, and attention problems. The descriptors were measured by 12 items from the primary caretaker on

[1] We chose to focus on the youngest cohort because they had data spanning childhood through late adolescence. There were no data on childhood precursors for the oldest cohort because they were first sampled at approximately age 12. Follow up of the middle sample stopped after age 13 not allowing for the investigation of the development of subsequent smoking behavior.

the Child Behavior Checklist (Extended CBCL; Achenbach and Edelbrock, 1979) and 13 items from the teacher on the Teacher Report Form (Extended TRF; Edelbrock and Achenbach, 1984). If either informant said that a descriptor was true for the boy sometimes or often, the youth received a positive score for that descriptor. The descriptors were then counted to create the final construct. This variable was assessed at all age periods except 17-19 (average alpha across developmental periods = .89).

Depression was the sum of 13 items on the Recent Mood and Feelings Questionnaire (Costello and Angold, 1988) responded to by the youth. The 13 questions covered the symptoms (during the previous 2 weeks) necessary for making a diagnosis of major depression according to the DSM-III-R criteria (American Psychiatric Association, 1987). This variable was assessed at all age periods (average alpha = .84).

Attitude toward substance use was based on the youth's judgment, on a 5-point scale, of the acceptability of behaviors related to drug use. At ages 7-10, it was made from three items about attitudes toward drinking alcohol, smoking marijuana, and sniffing glue. For the later ages, it was made from four items including attitudes about drinking alcohol, smoking marijuana, using hard drugs, and selling hard drugs (average alpha = 80).

Religiosity was measured by two questions asked of the youth: "Do you like going to religious services?" and "If you had to choose between going to a religious service or doing something else, which would you do?" Scores ranged from 0 to 2 with 2 being the least religious (did not attend services) (average alpha = .74). It was measured at all ages except 17-19.

Delinquency was the frequency of youth self-reported delinquency covering theft, violence, vandalism, and fraud but not status offenses (e.g., truancy or running away). It was measured at all ages.

School performance was the sum of the standardized scores for the Academic Achievement and School Motivation scales (average alpha = .86). Academic Achievement combined the caretakers', teachers', and youths' evaluations of the youth's performance in reading, math, writing, and spelling; caretakers and youths also evaluated up to three other academic subjects. Performance was rated on a 4-point scale, ranging from failing (highest score) to above average (lowest score). The ratings of all academic subjects by all informants were averaged to create the construct. School Motivation was based on the teachers' rating, on a 7-point scale, of how hard the youth was working in school. This measure was available at all ages except 17-19.

Parental smoking was a dichotomous measure of whether the male or female caretaker smoked as reported by the primary caretaker when the youth was approximately age 13 and reported by the youth when he was age 17. If either caretaker smoked, then it was coded as 1 and if neither smoked, then it was coded as 0.

Relationship with parents was the sum of the standardized scores for three constructs: Caretaker Positive Parenting, Caretaker/Child Communication, and Relationship with Primary Caretaker (average alpha = .83). Caretaker Positive Parenting combined 9 items from the caretakers' and 7 items from the youths' reports of the frequency of the caretaker's positive behaviors toward the youth (e.g., giving special privileges or compliments). Relationship with Primary Caretaker combined 13 items from the youths' and 16 items from the caretakers' perceptions of the quality of their relationship (e.g., how often the caretaker bugs the youth and how often the caretaker thinks that the youth is a good child). Caretaker/Child Communication summarized 30 items from the caretaker and 28 from the youth regarding everyday communication between caretaker and youth in terms of emotions, disagreements, and problems (e.g., how often they discuss the youth's personal problems together, whether the caretaker could interpret the youth's emotional state without asking). This scale was measured at all ages except 17-19.

Peer delinquency was a construct that summarized the proportion of friends who engaged in various delinquent activities, such as stealing and vandalism, based on the self report of the youth. It was measured at all age periods (average alpha = .83).

Socioeconomic status (SES) was measured using the Hollingshead (1975) index of social status based on data collected from the primary caretaker. It was equal to the highest score attained between the two caretakers or to the score attained by the single caretaker. Scores were reverse coded so that a higher score equals lower SES. It was measured at all age periods except 17-19.

Neighborhood quality was the caretaker's assessment of the neighborhood in which the family lived at the time of the interview. It included 17 items reflecting level of neighborhood safety/stability (e.g., the prevalence of abandoned buildings, unemployment, racial tension, and various criminal activities) (*alpha* = .95). It was measured at all age periods except 17-19.

Analyses

Smoking trajectories. In a previous study (White et al., 2004), we developed smoking trajectories based on the number of cigarettes smoked per day using group-based trajectory modeling (Jones, Nagin, and Roeder, 2001; Nagin, 1999, 2005). This method identifies groups of individuals following distinctive developmental trajectories. As described in Nagin and Tremblay (1999, 2001) and Nagin and Land (1993), the trajectory groups are designed to trace out complex forms of population heterogeneity in developmental patterns using a statistical technique called finite mixture modeling. These unique trajectories not only reveal differences in the level of behavior at a given time, but also identify differences in the development of the particular behavior over time (Nagin and Tremblay, 1999). Model estimation used a SAS-based procedure, called Proc Traj, described in Jones et al. (2001). For the trajectory analyses, the youngest and oldest cohorts were combined and separate trajectory analyses were conducted by race from age 10 through age 25 years.

A key issue in the application of a group-based model is making a determination of how many groups define the best fitting model. We followed the lead of D'Unger, Land, McCall, and Nagin (1998) and used the Bayesian Information Criterion (BIC) as a basis for selecting the optimal model (see Raftery, 1995). They recommend selection of the model with the maximum BIC. We tested four sequential models each adding another group. Based on the BIC criteria, a three-group model fit the data best for each race. These three trajectories groups were: nonsmokers, light smokers, and regular smokers (see results below for greater detail). Individuals in the estimation sample were then assigned to the group to which they most likely belonged based on a statistic called the posterior probability of group membership

(PPGM) (see Nagin, 1999, 2005). The PPGM measures the probability that the individual belongs to that trajectory group. Ideally, the PPGM for an individual for his/her assigned group is 1; when the mean classification probability for individuals assigned to each of the respective trajectory groups exceeds .7, conventional normal-based hypothesis tests of differences across trajectory groups are little affected by classification error (Roeder, Lynch, and Nagin, 1999; Nagin, 2005). For these models the average PPGM for all individuals assigned to each group was .97 and above for both whites and African Americans (for greater details on the analytic technique and the creation of the trajectory groups see White et al., 2004). For some of the analyses below, the trajectory groups were dichotomized to reflect smoking (nonsmokers vs. light and regular smokers) and regular smoking (light vs. regular smokers).

Risk and protective factors. We used an empirical method developed by Stouthamer-Loeber et al. (2004) to identify whether a variable's relation to cigarette smoking was determined by the protective and / or the risk end. All variables were coded so that the higher score reflected potentially greater risk for cigarette smoking. We first tested each variable to see whether it had a significant protective association, a significant risk association, or both. To do this, each variable was trichotomized separately for whites and African Americans into the bottom 25%, the middle 50%, and the top 25%, which served to isolate the 25% of the youth at the potentially protective end, the 50% neutral, and the 25% at the potentially risk end, respectively. We then cross-tabulated the protective end (bottom 25%) with the 50% neutral (excluding those at the risk end) and cross-tabulated the risk end (top 25%) with the 50% neutral (excluding those at the protective end) by the smoking (nonsmokers vs. light and regular smoker) and regular smoking (light vs. regular smokers) dichotomies to determine whether the independent variable had a risk or protective association for each race.

After determining the protective and / or risk association of each variable for each race, the variable was then dichotomized 25%/75% (either the 25% protective vs. the rest or the 25% risk vs. the rest) so that all youth were included in the analyses. Chi-square analyses (2 X 2) and odds ratios were calculated for each protective and / or risk factor by the two dichotomized measures of smoking trajectory group membership described above separately by race. Parental smoking was treated as a dichotomy throughout the analyses to reflect the presence or absence of the risk factor.

Those protective and risk factors that were significantly associated ($p<.05$) with smoking initiation or regular smoking in the second set of cross-tabulations were then included in hierarchical logistic regression analyses for the age period and trajectory dichotomy for which they were significant. None of the independent variables were multicollinear within models. For the present analyses we conducted two sets of logistic regressions as suggested by Cohen, Cohen, West, and Aiken (2003). In the first set examining risk and protective factors for smoking initiation, we compared nonsmokers to light and regular smokers. In the second set examining risk and protective factors for regular smoking, we compared light to regular smokers. In the first step of the hierarchical logistic regression analyses, we entered each of the significant risk and protective factors and race; in the second step, we added the interactions between race and each of the risk and protective factors simultaneously. The models were tested separately at four points in time: childhood (ages 7-9), early adolescence (ages 10-12), middle adolescence (ages 13-16), and late adolescence (ages 17-19).

Results

Descriptive Results

Whites (mean=12.6 years) began smoking significantly earlier than African Americans (mean=13.6 years) by about one year (t= -2.20, p=.029). By age 19 significantly more whites (67.0%) than African Americans (47.6%) had ever smoked a cigarette (chi square= 27.56, df=1, p<.001).

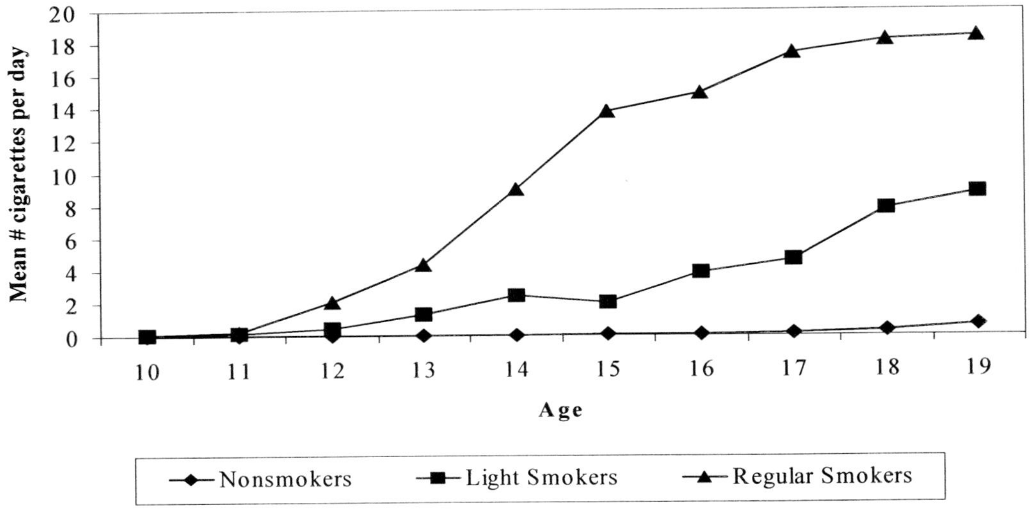

Figure 1. Observed Mean Number of Cigarettes Smoked for White Trajectory Groups.

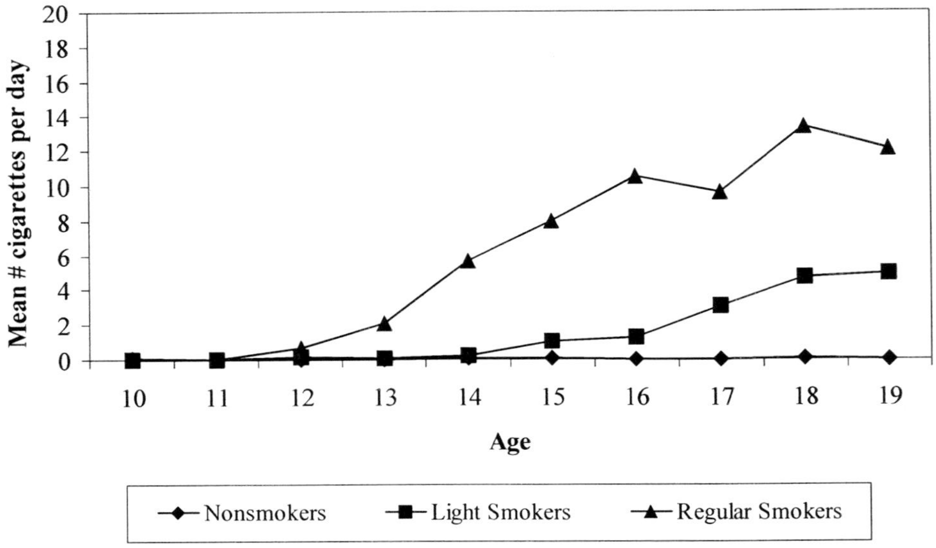

Figure 2. Observed Mean Number of Cigarettes Smoked for African American Trajectory Groups.

The average number of cigarettes smoked per day over time for each trajectory group is shown in Figure 1 for whites and Figure 2 for African Americans. Group membership differed significantly by race (chi square = 7.23, df=2, p<.03). There were more African Americans (56.6%) than whites (48.6%) in the nonsmoker group and more whites (28.4%) than African Americans (18.1%) in the regular smoker group. There were similar proportions of whites (23.1%) and African Americans (25.3%) in the light smoker group. Within both the light and regular smoker groups, whites began smoking earlier and smoked more cigarettes per day than African Americans at all ages (for greater detail see White et al., 2004).

Racial Differences in Risk and Protective Factors for Smoking

Table 1 shows the risk and protective factors significantly related to smoking based on the chi square analyses for the total sample conducted separately for whites and African Americans. We did not control for the number of chi square analyses that were conducted because we were first trying to classify all variables into risk or protection. The later multivariate analyses helped to isolate those variables that were most strongly related to smoking. Depression, delinquency, school performance, peer delinquency, and attitude toward substance use acted as both risk and protective factors for smoking either at the same age period or at different age periods. In other words, these variables had both positive and negative ends. Within each age period, those variables that had only a risk effect are listed first, followed by those that had only a protective effect, and then those that had both protective and risk effects. Only variables that were significant in the chi square analyses are listed.

For whites at ages 7-9, having many delinquent peers was a risk factor and having few was a protective factor. As an example of how to read table 1, 39% of the nonsmokers compared to 16.8% of the smokers had few delinquent peers and having few delinquent peers reduced the risk of smoking by about one-third [Odds Ratio (OR) = .32]. Also, 35.5% of the smokers compared to 13% of the nonsmokers had many delinquent peers and having many delinquent peers increased the risk of smoking almost four-fold [Odds Ratio (OR) = 3.69]. In addition, being high in delinquency was a risk factor and being low in depression and coming from a high SES family were protective factors. At ages 10-12, being high in HIA was a risk factor and having few delinquent peers and coming from a high SES family were protective factors. At ages 13-16, school performance, delinquent peers, and attitudes toward substance use had both protective and risk associations with smoking. In addition, low depression, low delinquency, and good relationships with parents were protective factors. At ages 17-19 having a parent who smoked and many delinquent peers were risk factors, whereas having negative attitudes toward substance use was a protective factor.

Many of the same risk and protective factors for smoking were identified for African Americans, although not necessarily at the same ages as whites. At ages 7-9, high HIA, depression, and delinquency were risk factors for African Americans, whereas doing well in school, good relationships with parents, and having few delinquent peers were protective factors. At ages 10-12 high HIA and poor school performance were risk factors and low delinquency and few delinquent peers were protective factors for smoking among African

Americans. At ages 13-16, having many delinquent peers was a risk factor and having few was a protective factor for smoking. In addition, having high HIA, positive attitudes toward substance use, and a parent who smoked were risk factors and being high in religiosity and doing well in school were protective factors. At ages 17-19, none of the variables were risk factors, but having negative attitudes toward substance use and low depression were protective factors.

In summary, all of the factors except neighborhood quality were significantly related to smoking for at least one race at one or more developmental period. School performance (as a risk and protective factor) and religiosity (as a protective factor) were significant only for African Americans. SES (as a protective factor) was related only for whites. The variables most frequently related to smoking for both races were HIA (only as a risk factor), depression (mostly as a protective factor), delinquency (as both a risk and protective factor), and peer delinquency (more often as a protective factor than a risk factor).

We selected all of the risk and protective factors that were significant at each developmental age period for either race and included them in multivariate hierarchical logistic regression analyses with smoking trajectory group as the dependent variable (light or regular smokers versus nonsmokers). In the previous analysis, we found that high SES was a protective factor in the two younger age periods (7-9 and 10-12) for whites. We decided to include SES as a protective factor in all of the models because of the need to control for SES when examining race differences (Rose, Chassin, Presson, and Sherman, 1996). In the 17-19 age period, we used the SES measure from ages 13-16 because family SES was not available at ages 17-19. If a variable had both a risk and protective effect for one race, but a clear risk or protective effect for the other race, then we went with the clear effect. Otherwise, if a variable had both a risk and a protective effect, then we included the effect with the best odds ratio from the cross-tabular analyses reported above. The analyses were conducted separately for each developmental period. We first tested the main effects of the risk and protective factors and race. Then we added the interactions of race with each of the risk factors simultaneously. The results are presented in table 2.

In the main effects model, at ages 7-9, depression, delinquency, peer delinquency, and race were all significant predictors of smoking. Being low in depression, having few delinquent peers, and being African American protected against smoking; frequently engaging in delinquent activities increased the risk for smoking. In the second model that included the interactions, only the interaction between race and school performance was significant. A probe of that interaction showed that high school performance protected against smoking for African Americans (OR = .32, CI = .18-.60, $p<.001$), but was not a protective factor for whites (OR= .82, CI= .44-1.55, $p>.05$).

At ages 10-12 delinquency, peer delinquency, family SES, and race were significantly related to smoking. Being non-delinquent, having few delinquent peers, coming from a high SES family, and being African American were protective factors for smoking. None of the interactions was significant.

Table 1. Significant Risk and Protective Factors for Cigarette Smoking by Race and Developmental Period

	White			*African American*		
	Nonsmoker %	**Smoker %**	**OR (95% CI)**	**Nonsmoker %**	**Smoker %**	**OR (95% CI)**
Ages 7-9						
Risk Factors						
High HIA				18.9	32.0	2.02 (1.17-3.50)
High Delinquency	11.0	38.3	5.03 (2.40-10.51)	15.1	32.0	2.64 (1.48-4.71)
Protective Factors						
Good School Performance				34.0	13.9	.32(.17-.58)
Good Relationship with Parents				30.2	19.7	.57 (.32-.99)
High SES	33.3	16.8	.40 (.21-.78)			
Both Risk and Protective Factors						
High Depression				18.2	31.2	2.03 (1.16-3.54)
Low Depression	38.0	13.1	.25 (.12-.49)			
Many Delinquent Peers	13.0	35.5	3.69 (1.82-7.46)			
Few Delinquent Peers	39.0	16.8	.32 (.17-.60)	33.3	13.9	.32 (.18-.60)
Ages 10-12						
Risk Factors						
High HIA	17.5	29.5	1.97 (1.01-3.86)	18.4	33.3	2.21 (1.27-3.87)
Poor School Performance				17.8	34.2	2.40 (1.37-4.21)
Protective Factors						
Low Delinquency				47.0	30.0	.48 (.29-.80)
Few Delinquent Peers	35.1	13.3	.29 (.14-.57)	28.8	14.2	.41 (.22-.76)
High SES	34.0	16.2	.37 (.19-.73)			
Ages 13-16						
Risk Factors						
High HIA				17.8	33.9	2.37 (1.34-4.19)
Parental Smoking				54.6	69.8	1.93 (1.15-3.23)
Protective Factors						
Low Depression	31.9	16.4	.42 (.21-.82)			
High Religiosity				30.8	17.0	.46 (.25-.83)
Low Delinquency	68.1	30.8	.21 (.11-.38)			
Good Relationship with Parents	34.7	16.4	.37 (.19-.72)			
Both Risk and Protective Factors						
Positive Attitude to Substance Use	16.0	34.6	2.79 (1.41-5.53)	16.4	36.4	2.91(1.64-5.19)
Negative Attitude to Substance Use	28.7	12.5	.36 (.17-.74)			
Many Delinquent Peers	12.8	34.6	3.62 (1.75-7.49)	11.0	39.0	5.19 (2.74-9.82)
Few Delinquent Peers	37.2	14.4	.28 (.14-.57)	34.9	14.4	.31 (.17-.58)
Poor School Performance	11.6	37.5	4.58 (2.18-9.64)			
Good School Performance	37.9	13.5	.26 (.13-.51)	37.7	9.3	.17 (.08-.34)
Ages 17-19						
Risk Factors						
Parental Smoking	35.6	55.3	2.24 (1.24-4.06)			
Many Delinquent Peers	12.4	35.6	3.92 (1.85-8.27)			
Protective Factors						
Low Depression				33.1	20.4	.52 (.29-.93)
Negative Attitude To Substance Use	33.7	14.4	.33 (.16-.67)	34.6	15.0	.34 (.18-.63)

Table 2. Hierarchical Logistic Regression Results for Smoking[a]

	Model I	Model II
Ages 7-9 (N= 487)		
High HIA	1.15 (0.72-1.84)	0.89 (0.17-4.76)
Low Depression	0.55 (0.34-0.88)*	0.13 (0.03-0.67)
High Delinquency	2.46 (1.53-3.96)*	6.21 (1.10-35.15)
Good School Performance	0.64 (0.40-1.03)	3.93 (0.75-20.66)
Good Relationship with Parents	0.79 (0.50-1.24)	0.84 (0.18-3.97)
Few Delinquent Peers	0.47 (0.29-0.75)*	0.51 (0.11-2.40)
High SES	0.66 (0.42-1.04)	0.21 (0.04-1.05)
Race	0.66 (0.45-0.98)*	0.66 (0.32-1.37)
Race x HIA		1.20 (0.45-3.25)
Race x Depression		2.52 (0.95-6.70)
Race x Delinquency		0.57 (0.21-1.57)
Race x School Performance		0.32 (0.12-0.89)*
Race x Relationship with Parents		0.96 (0.37-2.46)
Race x Delinquent Peers		0.96 (0.36-2.51)
Race x SES		2.04 (0.78-5.34)
Likelihood Ratio χ^2	68.87***	80.33***
Ages 10 – 12 (N=466)		
High HIA	1.59 (0.97-2.60)	2.20 (0.32-15.28)
Low Delinquency	0.59 (0.39-0.91)*	0.39 (0.10-1.59)
Poor School Performance	1.53 (0.94-2.48)	0.38 (0.06-2.39)
Few Delinquent Peers	0.49 (0.29-0.82)*	0.28 (0.05-1.47)
High SES	0.52 (0.32-0.83)*	0.22 (0.05-1.08)
Race	0.64 (0.43-0.96)*	0.39 (0.19-0.78)
Race x HIA		0.87 (0.29-2.63)
Race x Delinquency		1.30 (0.55-3.10)
Race x School Performance		2.32 (0.80-6.69)
Race x Delinquent Peers		1.42 (0.50-4.00)
Race x SES		1.71 (0.66-4.47)
Likelihood Ratio χ^2	49.76***	54.59***
Ages 13 – 16 (N=414)		
High HIA	1.61 (0.95-2.72)	2.63 (0.42-16.61)
Low Depression	1.03 (0.60-1.76)	0.69 (0.11-4.43)
Positive Attitude to Substance Use	1.65 (0.97-2.83)	2.07 (0.32-13.52)
High Religiosity	0.77 (0.45-1.33)	2.13 (0.30-15.27)
Low Delinquency	0.73 (0.44-1.20)	0.07 (0.01-0.38)
Good School Performance	0.34 (0.19-0.60)*	1.66 (0.25-10.93)
Parental Smoking	1.64 (1.04-2.58)*	0.83 (0.17-4.01)
Good Relationship with Parents	0.88 (0.51-1.52)	0.61 (0.09-4.31)
Many Delinquent Peers	2.48 (1.36-4.51)*	0.30 (0.04-2.39)

Table 2. (Continued).

	Model I	Model II
High SES	0.74 (0.43-1.27)	0.40 (0.06-2.56)
Race	0.68 (0.44-1.06)	0.26 (0.08-0.81)
Race x HIA		0.75 (0.25-2.25)
Race x Depression		1.33 (0.43-4.08)
Race x Attitude to Substance Use		0.86 (0.28-2.66)
Race x Religiosity		0.56 (0.18-1.81)
Race x Delinquency		4.53 (1.59-12.87)*
Race x School Performance		0.35 (0.11-1.16)
Race x Parental Smoking		1.61 (0.62-4.23)
Race x Relationship with Parents		1.15 (0.36-3.68)
Race x Delinquent Peers		3.76 (1.06-13.27)*
Race x SES		1.40 (0.44-4.41)
Likelihood Ratio χ^2	84.07***	97.62***
Ages 17 – 19 (N=405)		
Low Depression	0.92 (0.57-1.49)	2.12 (0.43-10.37)
Negative Attitude to Substance Use	0.30 (0.18-0.51)*	0.20 (0.03-1.21)
Parental Smoking	1.74 (1.14-2.66)*	2.91 (0.67-12.62)
Many Delinquent Peers	1.80 (1.09-2.97)*	13.93 (2.33-83.19)
High SES	0.51 (0.30-0.86)*	0.91 (0.16-5.17)
Race	0.75 (0.49-1.13)	1.37 (0.62-3.03)
Race x Depression		0.59 (0.22-1.56)
Race x Attitude to Substance Use		1.30 (0.44-3.85)
Race x Parental Smoking		0.73 (0.30-1.75)
Race x Delinquent Peers		0.28 (0.10-0.80)*
Race x SES		0.71 (0.24-2.09)
Likelihood Ratio χ^2	50.12***	57.23***

[a] Odds Ratio presented; 95% Confidence Intervals in parentheses.
* p < .05; ** p < .01; *** p < .001.

In middle adolescence (ages 13-16), school performance, parental smoking, and peer delinquency were significantly related to smoking. Having a parent who smoked and having many delinquent peers increased the risk of smoking, whereas good school performance decreased the risk. In the second model, low delinquency and many delinquent peers interacted with race. Probes of these interactions indicated that being low in delinquency was a stronger protective factor for whites (OR = .21, CI = .11-.38, p<.001) than for African Americans (OR = .48, CI = .29-.81, p<.01). On the other hand, having many delinquent peers was a somewhat stronger risk factor for African Americans (OR = 5.19, CI = 2.74-9.82, p<.001) than whites (OR = 3.62, CI = 1.75-7.49, p<.001).

There were several factors in late adolescence (ages 17-19) that were significantly related to smoking in the multivariate analyses, including attitude toward substance use, parental smoking, peer delinquency, and family SES. At ages 17-19, those young men who had a parent who smoked and many delinquent peers were at increased risk for smoking. On the other hand, those who came from a higher SES family and held negative attitudes toward substance use were less likely to smoke. The interaction between race and delinquent peers was significant. Having many delinquent peers at ages 17-19 was a risk factor for whites (OR = 3.92, CI = 1.85-8.27, p<.001), but not for African Americans (OR = 1.76, CI = .99-3.15, p>.05).

In the main effects model, at ages 7-9, depression, delinquency, peer delinquency, and race were all significant predictors of smoking. Being low in depression, having few delinquent peers, and being African American protected against smoking; frequently engaging in delinquent activities increased the risk for smoking. In the second model that included the interactions, only the interaction between race and school performance was significant. A probe of that interaction showed that high school performance protected against smoking for African Americans (OR = .32, CI = .18-.60, p<.001), but was not a protective factor for whites (OR= .82, CI= .44-1.55, p>.05).

At ages 10-12 delinquency, peer delinquency, family SES, and race were significantly related to smoking. Being non-delinquent, having few delinquent peers, coming from a high SES family, and being African American were protective factors for smoking. None of the interactions was significant.

In middle adolescence (ages 13-16), school performance, parental smoking, and peer delinquency were significantly related to smoking. Having a parent who smoked and having many delinquent peers increased the risk of smoking, whereas good school performance decreased the risk. In the second model, low delinquency and many delinquent peers interacted with race. Probes of these interactions indicated that being low in delinquency was a stronger protective factor for whites (OR = .21, CI = .11-.38, p<.001) than for African Americans (OR = .48, CI = .29-.81, p<.01). On the other hand, having many delinquent peers was a somewhat stronger risk factor for African Americans (OR = 5.19, CI = 2.74-9.82, p<.001) than whites (OR = 3.62, CI = 1.75-7.49, p<.001).

There were several factors in late adolescence (ages 17-19) that were significantly related to smoking in the multivariate analyses, including attitude toward substance use, parental smoking, peer delinquency, and family SES. At ages 17-19, those young men who had a parent who smoked and many delinquent peers were at increased risk for smoking. On the other hand, those who came from a higher SES family and held negative attitudes toward substance use were less likely to smoke. The interaction between race and delinquent peers was significant. Having many delinquent peers at ages 17-19 was a risk factor for whites (OR = 3.92, CI = 1.85-8.27, p<.001), but not for African Americans (OR = 1.76, CI = .99-3.15, p>.05)

Racial Differences in Risk and Protective Factors for Regular Smoking

Table 3 shows the significant risk and protective factors for regular smoking for whites and African Americans. At each age period, fewer significant risk and protective factors were identified for regular smoking than for smoking, possibly due to less power (i.e., eliminating the nonsmokers from the analyses).

Table 3. Significant Risk and Protective Factors for Regular Cigarette Smoking by Race and Developmental Period

	White			*African American*		
	Light Smoker %	**Regular Smoker %**	**OR (95%CI)**	**Light Smoker %**	**Regular Smoker %**	**OR (95%CI)**
Ages 7-9 Risk and Factors						
Poor School Performance	16.7	37.3	2.97(1.18-7.49)			
Protective Factors						
Low HIA				29.6	11.8	.32 (.12-.86)
Good Neighborhood	14.6	35.7	3.24 (1.16-9.02)			
Ages 10-12 Protective Factors						
Low Depression				25.7	6.0	.18 (.05-.67)
Low Delinquency				38.6	18.0	.35 (.15-.83)
Good School Performance	36.2	13.8	.28 (.11-.73)			
Ages 13-16 Risk Factors						
Positive Attitude to Substance Use	21.7	44.8	2.93 (1.20-6.99)			
High Delinquency	21.7	50.0	3.60 (1.51-8.59)	19.1	52.0	4.58 (2.02-0.41)
Parental Smoking	46.7	72.2	2.97 (1.29-6.85)			
Many Delinquent Peers	19.6	46.6	3.58 (1.47-8.74)			
Protective Factors						
Low HIA	30.4	8.8	.22 (.07-.67)	26.5	6.0	.18 (.05-.64)
Risk and Protective Factors						
Poor School Performance				23.5	48.0	3.0 (1.36-6.60)
Good School Performance	28.3	1.7	.04 (.01-.36)			
Ages 17-19 Risk Factors						
Parental Smoking	39.0	67.9	3.3 (1.41-7.76)			
Protective Factors						
Few Delinquent Peers				11.6	27.3	2.86 (1.05-7.71)

For whites at ages 7-9, poor school performance was a risk factor for regular smoking and living in a good neighborhood was a protective factor. At ages 10-12, no risk factors were identified, but good school performance was a protective factor. At ages 13-16, positive attitudes towards substance use, high delinquency, having many delinquent peers, and having a parent who smoked were risk factors, whereas low HIA and doing well in school were protective factors. At ages 17-19, having a parent who smoked was the only factor related to regular smoking for whites.

For African Americans, low HIA protected against regular smoking at ages 7-9 and low depression and low delinquency protected at ages 10-12. At ages 13-16, high delinquency and poor school performance were risk factors, and low HIA was a protective factor. Having few delinquent peers at ages 17-19 was a risk factor for regular smoking rather than a protective factor as would be expected.

Table 4. Hierarchical Logistic Regression Results for Regular Smoking[a]

	Model I	Model II
Ages 7-9 (N=208)		
Low HIA	0.53 (0.24-1.17)	2.34 (0.18-30.97)
Poor School Performance	1.36 (0.72-2.58)	11.99 (1.15-125.06)
High SES	0.63 (0.29-1.34)	0.26 (0.02-3.51)
Good Neighborhood	1.90 (1.00-3.61)	6.54 (0.66-64.69)
Race	0.49 (0.28-0.87)*	0.97 (0.40-2.38)
Race x HIA		0.39 (0.08-2.01)
Race x School Performance		0.25 (0.06-1.01)
Race x SES		1.68 (0.35-8.15)
Race x Neighborhood		0.44 (0.11-1.71)
Likelihood Ratio χ^2	16.16***	22.45***
Ages 10-12 (N=224)		
Low Depression	0.60 (0.28-1.26)	10.81 (0.78-150.18)
Low Delinquency	0.73 (0.40-1.32)	3.31 (0.47-23.57)
Good School Performance	0.42 (0.20-0.89)*	0.13 (0.01-1.39)
High SES	0.81 (0.39-1.72)	0.74 (0.06-8.66)
Race	0.49 (0.28-0.87)*	0.86 (0.40-1.88)
Race x Depression		0.14 (0.02-0.77)*
Race x Delinquency		0.35 (0.10-1.22)
Race x School Performance		1.97 (0.41-9.30)
Race x SES		0.99 (0.21-4.60)
Likelihood Ratio χ^2	15.75***	26.53***
Ages 13-16 (N=193)		
Low HIA	0.30 (0.11-0.78)*	0.19 (0.01-4.49)
Positive Attitude to Substance Use	1.13 (0.56-2.28)	3.69 (0.27-50.44)
High Delinquency	2.58 (1.21-5.53)*	0.88 (0.06-13.08)
Good School Performance	0.19 (0.05-0.74)*	0.01 (<0.01-1.00)
Parental Smoking	2.13 (1.04-4.36)*	4.17 (0.37-47.07)
Many Delinquent Peers	1.32 (0.61-2.85)	1.31 (0.09-18.57)
High SES	1.38 (0.56-3.42)	0.12 (0.01-2.86)
Race	0.44 (0.23-0.84)*	0.38 (0.09-1.66)
Race x HIA		1.23 (0.17-9.18)
Race x Attitude to Substance Use		0.55 (0.12-2.59)
Race x Delinquency		2.05 (0.41-10.33)
Race x School Performance		9.38 (0.55-160.10)
Race x Parental Smoking		0.64 (0.14-2.89)
Race x Delinquent Peers		0.95 (0.19-4.73)
Race x SES		4.98 (0.75-33.28)
Likelihood Ratio χ^2	45.67***	53.48***
Ages 17-19 (N=193)		
Parental Smoking	1.57 (0.87-2.83)	8.77 (1.23-62.76)
Few Delinquent Peers	1.26 (0.57-2.81)	0.25 (0.02-3.66)
High SES	0.74 (0.33-1.69)	0.16 (0.01-2.21)
Race	0.48 (0.27-0.86)*	0.62 (0.24-1.65)
Race x Parental Smoking		0.31 (0.09-1.04)
Race x Delinquent Peers		2.95 (0.58-15.10)
Race x SES		3.03 (0.58-15.99)
Likelihood Ratio χ^2	9.71*	17.88*

[a] Odds Ratio presented; 95% Confidence Intervals in parentheses

* $p < .05$; ** $p < .01$; *** $p < .001$.

In sum, all of the variables except religiosity and SES were related to regular smoking across developmental periods for at least one race. Depression (as a protective factor) was related to regular smoking for African Americans only and attitudes toward substance use (protective), parental smoking (risk), and neighborhood quality (protective) were related for whites only. The variables related to smoking for both races were HIA (only protective), school performance (both risk and protective), delinquency (risk and protective), and peer delinquency (only protective).

As was done before for the smoking analyses, for each developmental period, the significant risk and protective factors were included in hierarchical logistic regression analyses. Now regular smoking was the dependent variable (i.e., the regular smoker group vs. the light smoker group). (Nonsmokers were not included in these analyses.) The same criteria as above were used to determine whether the risk or protective end would be used in the regression analyses. For these analyses, we also controlled for high SES. The results are presented in table 4.

None of the predictors at ages 7-9, except race, was significantly related to regular smoking. African Americans were less likely to become regular smokers than whites. None of the interactions was significant.

At ages 10-12, school performance and race were significantly related to regular smoking. Those who did well in school compared to those who did worse were less likely to be regular smokers and African Americans were less likely to be regular smokers than whites. In the second model, there was a significant interaction of race with depression. Being low on depression protected against regular smoking for African Americans (OR = .18, CI= .05-.67, $p<.01$), but not for whites (OR = .99, CI= .37-2.63, $p>.05$).

In middle adolescence (ages 13-16), HIA, delinquency, school performance, parental smoking, and race were significantly related to regular smoking. Those who had a parent who smoked and were high in delinquency had an increased risk for regular smoking. Being low in HIA, having good school performance, and being African American protected against regular smoking. None of the interactions was significant.

Finally, in late adolescence (ages 17-19) only race was related to regular smoking. African Americans were more likely to be regular smokers than whites. None of the interactions with race was significant.

Conclusion

In this chapter we examined risk and protective factors for smoking and regular smoking among African Americans and whites across multiple domains. We had expected to find differential risk and protective factors for African Americans and whites. Instead we found that, for the most part, similar variables were related to smoking and regular smoking for both races. Our findings are consistent with those of Kandel and colleagues (2004), who also found that the same variables predicted smoking initiation and regular smoking for whites and African American youth. In addition, some variables acted as protective factors, others acted as risk factors, and many acted as both. We also found that similar variables acted as risk and / or protective factors across different development periods.

In accord with other research (Baker et al., 2004; Griesler and Kandel, 1998; Hestick et al., 2001; Lloyd-Richardson et al., 2002), we found that school performance was related to smoking; however it appears to be more consistently related to regular smoking than to smoking initiation. It was significantly associated (as a protective factor) with smoking only for African Americans and with regular smoking (as both a risk and protective factor) for both races. Regardless of its risk or protective association, the implications for prevention are clear. Smoking prevention programs should be targeted to students doing poorly in school and those with low school motivation (see also Kandel et al., 2004). Helping such students to improve their academic skills and motivation may also reduce smoking (see Storr, Ialongo, Kellam, and Anthony, 2002). Targeting students with poor school performance could also be preventative for other substance use, as well as problem behaviors such as delinquency, given the reciprocal nature of these relationships (Baker et al., 2004). Because the temporal order between smoking and school performance was not assessed at each developmental period, it is also possible that smoking may have led to declines in academic achievement and motivation over time (e.g., through associations with deviant peers). Nevertheless, childhood good school performance protected against smoking for African Americans highlighting the importance of early school performance as a target for smoking prevention.

Having or not having delinquent peers and being high or low on delinquency were also consistently related to smoking and regular smoking for both races. Deviant adolescents are more likely to affiliate with deviant and substance using peers due both to socialization and selection effects (Baker et al., 2004; Gorman and White, 1995). In this study, we did not have a measure of peer cigarette smoking and we used delinquent peers as a proxy measure. The findings indicate that affiliation with delinquent peers is related to cigarette smoking regardless of peer cigarette use. However, given the association between delinquency and cigarette smoking (Baker et al., 2004), it is reasonable to assume that many of the delinquent peers were also cigarette smokers, who could have influenced smoking by modeling smoking behavior, increasing perceptions that smoking is normative, and / or providing opportunities for use (Baker et al., 2004). Previous research examining the association between an adolescent's cigarette use and his or her friends' use has found that the effect of peers is stronger for whites than African Americans (Baker et al., 2004; Unger, Rohrbach, Cruz, Baezconde-Garbanati, Palmer, and Johnson, 2001). Our results suggest that when other types of deviance are included in the peer measure, the associations between smoking and peer behaviors in childhood and adolescence are equally strong for both races, although the effects varied at different periods of development. In late adolescence, having few compared to many delinquent peers was a risk rather than protective factor for regular smoking among African Americans. The reasons for this finding are unclear, but perhaps the negative influence of peers diminishes over time for African Americans. Nevertheless, the overall results suggest that smoking prevention programs need to target delinquent youth. It should be noted that peer delinquency was reported by the youth and thus reflects perceptions of peer behavior rather than peer actual behavior. Other studies have shown that the effects of peers may be overestimated because youth are likely to attribute their own behavior to those of peers (e.g., Bauman and Ennett, 1994).

As found in previous research, parental smoking was a risk factor for smoking (Chassin et al., 1996; Griesler and Kandel, 1998; Hestick et al., 2001; Robinson et al., 1997). Among

African Americans it was related to smoking and for whites it was related to regular smoking. These findings are consistent with those of other studies that found that parental smoking was related to initiation for African Americans, but not to regular use (Hestick et al., 2001; Robinson et al., 1997). Parental smoking retained its significance in three of the four multivariate analyses in which it was included. This strong association between a youth's smoking and his parent's smoking may reflect modeling or effects or heredity (i.e., heritable individual differences in the pharmacological effects of tobacco or personality characteristics) (Baker et al., 2004, p. 470). In this study we could not disentangle such effects.

High HIA was consistently a risk factor for smoking over time, especially for African Americans. In contrast low HIA was a protective factor for regular smoking for both races. However, HIA was only significant in one of the multivariate models (age 13-16 for regular smoking). It is possible that the inclusion of other variables, such as delinquency, in the models may have mediated the effects of HIA. That is, attention deficit/hyperactivity disorder has not been found to predict adolescent substance use when co-occurring conduct disorder is included in the model (Baker et al., 2004). Our measure of HIA did not separate out the effects of attention problems from hyperactivity problems, and some studies have found that these differential components have varying effects on tobacco use (Burke et al., 2001). Nevertheless, the results suggest that boys high in HIA during childhood may be an important risk group for early cigarette prevention.

Low depression was primarily a protective factor for smoking for both races, however, it did not maintain significance in the multivariate analyses. There was one significant interaction with depression indicating that low depression was protective for African Americans, but not whites (at ages 10-12). Our failure to find a stronger association between depression and cigarette smoking is consistent with some of the previous research (Baker et al., 2004; White et al., 2002) and may reflect the fact that we did not have a diagnostic measure of depression nor of cigarette dependence. We expected that depression would be especially important for regular smoking inasmuch as cigarettes are often used for negative affect regulation (Baker et al., 2004). Overall, our findings are consistent with the literature in that externalizing factors were more strongly related to smoking than were internalizing factors (see Baker et al., 2004).

In middle and late adolescence, attitudes toward substance use were related to smoking for both races and, in middle adolescence, attitudes were related to regular smoking by whites. However, attitudes were only significant in one multivariate model. Our measure did not include attitudes towards cigarettes, which might explain the absence of a stronger effect. Nevertheless, the fact that the attitude variable was significant at all suggests that negative attitudes about substance use generalize across substances. Therefore, prevention programs need to reinforce negative attitudes and counter positive attitudes toward substance use among youth.

High religiosity was protective only at one age period (13-16) for smoking for African Americans and at no age periods for regular smoking for either race. Furthermore, in the multivariate models, religiosity did not emerge as a protective factor in contrast to what has been found in other studies, especially of African Americans (e.g., Juon et al., 2002).

However, our measure was quite weak and may not have captured religiosity as used in other research.

High SES was protective against smoking in childhood and early adolescence for whites, but not for African Americans at any age and SES was not related to regular smoking for either race. Similarly, neighborhood quality was not related to smoking for either race and was only related to regular smoking at one age period for whites. These findings are in contrast to claims that low SES and disadvantaged neighborhoods increase the risk of smoking for African Americans (Gardiner, 2001). In the presence of behavioral variables (i.e., delinquency and school performance), SES and neighborhood may not be important. It is possible, however, that SES has an indirect impact on smoking behavior through its impact on school performance, delinquency, and peer delinquency. Future research should test such mediation models.

The fact that we found mostly similar risk and protective factors for both races may have had to do with the way we defined our factors. That is, we identified the risk and protective end cutoffs separately by race. Therefore, African Americans and whites may have differed in terms of absolute levels of risk and protective factors but not in terms of relative effects (see Wallace and Muroff, 2002). For example, the means for delinquency frequency were higher for African Americans than whites (not shown), however, for both races being in the highest 25% in terms of delinquency frequency for one's race was a significant risk factor for smoking. In contrast, Griesler and Kandel (1998) found that although African Americans experienced a disproportionate number of risk factors for smoking compared to whites, these factors were more often associated with smoking for whites than for African Americans. They found few consistent predictors across race except for behavior problems. Most of our common risk factors were also related to behavior (i.e., school performance, delinquency, peer delinquency, and HIA). In the presence of other risk and protective factors, being African American was a protective factor for smoking in childhood and early adolescence and for regular smoking from childhood through late adolescence.

The results of the present study should be considered within the limitations of the data. The present study was limited to one geographical location. However, lifetime prevalence rates for the whites and African-Americans at age 17 were very close to their racial counterparts of male (and female) high school seniors in the 2000 and 2001 Monitoring the Future studies (Johnston et al., 2003). We only included males, and the findings may not be generalizable to females. Because the PYS study oversampled boys who were at risk for antisocial behavior, it is possible that the significant associations may not generalize to other samples. However, the association between race and whether the boy was originally in the high antisocial risk group was not statistically significant and, therefore, racial differences identified in this study do not appear to be influenced by the high-risk nature of the sample.

For the present study, we relied on self reports and did not confirm our smoking measures with bioassays. However, other studies have found that self-reports of smoking behavior are valid (e.g., Chassin, Presson, Rose, and Sherman, 1990; Patrick, Cheadle, Thompson, Diehr, Koepsell, and Kinne, 1994). In addition, not all independent variables were measured at each age period. Therefore, analyses within age periods relied on different sets of risk and protective factors, which could have influenced the number of significant associations found. In addition, the meaning of certain variables may differ over time, and certain measures may have better validity in childhood than adolescence or vice versa. Also, we did not measure the pharmacological effects of nicotine nor individual's motivations for smoking. These types of measures are especially important for understanding why individuals transition from experimental to regular smoking (Baker et al., 2004). In addition, we did not have a measure of nicotine dependence within the data set and our group of regular smokers was based solely on their quantity of cigarettes over time. Therefore, we could not address potential racial differences in the use of cigarettes for negative affect control or in the development of dependence.

Many of the risk and protective factors were measured at the same time as the smoking behaviors. Therefore, as discussed in the Introduction, we were not able to assess the temporal associations between the adolescent risk and protective factors and smoking behavior. We could, however, identify those factors that were significantly associated with different smoking trajectories during adolescence. In addition, we could identify those childhood risk and protective factors that predicted later smoking trajectory group membership.

In addition, there are contextual influences, which we did not measure, that can play an important role in the onset of smoking. It is important to consider the influence of the community, racial discrimination, pricing, media access, school policies, and smoke-free air laws, and how these differentially affect African Americans compared to other ethnic/racial groups (Chaloupka, 2003; Gardiner, 2001; Wilcox, 2003). Kandel and colleagues (2004) found that individual factors were better predictors of smoking initiation and daily smoking than were contextual factors. In their multivariate analyses, the only significant contextual predictor of smoking initiation was state-level bans on cigarette vending machines. Given that our sample all came from the same state, and, in fact, the same city, this variable would not have had any variance in this study. In addition, in the Kandel et al. (2004) study, the racial composition of the school predicted daily smoking for both African Americans and whites. Unfortunately, we did not measure this variable. We did include a measure of neighborhood quality, which included characteristics, such as racial tension. Also, we did not have measures of cultural or ethnic/racial identity, although this factor has been shown to affect racial and ethnic differences in cigarette smoking (Nichter, 2003). Other cultural factors may also account for increased smoking among African Americans, such as the commercial hip-hop culture which has adopted cigarette, cigar, and marijuana smoking, and the tobacco industry's increased sponsorship of African American community events and aggressive marketing to African American youth (Gardiner, 2001). We could not assess these influences within our data set, and, thus, more research is needed to examine cultural influences (Nichter, 2003).

Despite these limitations, this study had several strengths. It used prospective data and followed African American and white youth at least annually for 14 years. We utilized a new technique for examining both risk and protection. Our measures were collected from multiple sources and covered multiple domains across varying developmental periods. The findings, as well as those of previous studies, indicate that there are multiple factors that are related to the development of smoking behaviors including individual, family, and peer factors (Baker et al., 2004). Nevertheless, in this study we have identified several factors that were related to both the initiation and maintenance of cigarette smoking for African American and white youths and very few that were unique to either race. African American and white young men with low academic achievement and motivation, who are delinquent, who belong to delinquent peer groups, and / or who are high in hyperactivity, inattention, and impulsivity appear to be key targets for smoking prevention efforts in childhood and adolescence. For the most part, it appears that the same types of school-based smoking prevention programs (see Sussman, Dent, Stacy, Burton, and Flay, 1995) can be used with whites and African Americans in middle school and high school.

Acknowledgements

This research was supported, in part, by grants from the Robert Wood Johnson Foundation (043747), the National Institute on Drug Abuse (DA 17552; DA 411018), the Office of Juvenile Justice and Delinquency Prevention (96-MU-FX-0012), and the National Institute of Mental Health (MH 050778). Points of view in this document are those of the authors and do not necessarily represent the official position or policies of the U.S. Department of Justice. We acknowledge Rebecca Stallings for assistance in preparing the data files and Adam Thacker for his help with manuscript preparation. An earlier version of this paper was presented at the Society of Prevention Research annual meeting, May 28, 2004, Quebec City, Canada.

References

Achenbach, T.M., and Edelbrock, C.S. (1979). The child behavior profile: II. Boys ages 12-16 and girls ages 6-11 and 12-16. *Journal of Consulting and Clinical Psychology, 47*, 223-233.

American Psychiatric Association (1987). *Diagnostic and statistical manual of mental disorders*. Washington, DC: American Psychiatric Association.

Baker, T.B., Brandon, T.H., and Chassin, L. (2004). Motivational influences on cigarette smoking. *Annual Review of Psychology, 55*, 463-491.

Bauman K.E. and Ennett, S.T. (1994). Peer influence on adolescent drug use. *American Psychologist, 49*, 820-822.

Botvin, G.J., Baker, E., Botvin, E.M., Dusenbury, L., Cardwell, J., and Diaz, T. (1993). Factors promoting cigarette smoking among black youth: A casual modeling approach. *Addictive Behaviors, 18*, 397-405.

Breslau, N., Kilbey, M., and Andreski, P. (1991). Nicotine dependence, major depression, and anxiety in young adults. *Archives of General Psychiatry, 48*, 1069-1074.

Breslau, N., Kilbey, M., and Andreski, P. (1993). Nicotine dependence and major depression: New evidence from a prospective investigation. *Archives of General Psychiatry, 50*, 31-35.

Burke, J.D., Loeber, R., and Lahey, B.B. (2001). Which aspects of ADHD are associated with substance use in early adolescence? *Journal of Child Psychology and Psychiatry, 42*, 493-502.

Chaloupka, F.J. (2003). Contextual factors and youth tobacco use: Policy linkages. *Addiction, 98*, 147-149.

Chassin, L., Presson, C.C., Rose, J.S., and Sherman, S.J. (1996). The natural history of cigarette smoking from adolescence to adulthood: Demographic predictors of continuity and change. *Health Psychology, 15*, 478-484.

Chassin, L., Presson C.C., and Sherman S.J. (1990). Social psychological contributions to the understanding and prevention of adolescent cigarette smoking. *Personality and Social Psychology Bulletin, 16*, 133-151.

Chassin, L., Presson C.C., Sherman S.J., and Kim, K. (2002). Long-term psychological sequelae of smoking cessation and relapse. *Health Psychology, 21,* 438-443.

Chassin, L., Presson, C.C., Sherman, S.J., Montello, D., and McGrew, J. (1986). Changes in peer and parent influence during adolescence: Longitudinal versus cross-sectional perspectives on smoking initiation. *Developmental Psychology, 22,* 327-334.

Cohen, J., Cohen, P., West, S.G., and Aiken, L.S. (2003). *Applied multiple regression/correlation analysis for the behavioral sciences* (3rd ed.). Mahwah, NJ: Erlbaum.

Costello, E.J., and Angold, A. (1988). Scales to assess child and adolescent depression-Checklists, screens and nets. *Journal of the American Academy of Child and Adolescent Psychiatry, 27*, 726-737.

Derzon, J.H., and Lipsey, M.W. (1999). Predicting tobacco use to age 18: A synthesis of longitudinal research. *Addiction, 94*, 995-1006.

Diem, E.C., McKay, L.C., and Jamieson, J.L. (1994). Female adolescent alcohol, cigarette, and marijuana use: Similarities and differences in patterns of use. *The International Journal of the Addictions, 29*, 987-997.

D'Unger, A.V., Land, K.C., McCall, P.L., and Nagin, D.S. (1998). How many latent classes of delinquent/criminal careers? Results from mixed Poison regression analyses. *American Journal of Sociology, 103*, 1593-1630.

Edelbrock, C.S., and Achenbach, T.M. (1984). The teacher version of the Child Behavior Profile: I. Boys ages 6-11. *Journal of Consulting and Clinical Psychology, 52*, 207-217.

Flay, B., Hu, F.B., Siddiqui, O., Day, L.E., Hedeker, D., Petraitsi, J., Richardson, J., and Sussan, S. (1994). Differential influence of parental smoking and friends' smoking on adolescent initiation and escalation of smoking. *Journal of Health and Social Behavior, 35*, 248-265.

Flint, A.J., Yamanda, E.G., and Novotny, T.E. (1998). Black-white differences in cigarette smoking uptake: Progression from adolescent experimentation to regular use. *Preventive Medicine, 27*, 358-364.

Gardiner, P. (2001). African American teen cigarette smoking: A review. In D. Burns (Ed.), *Changing adolescent smoking prevalence: Where is it and why.* Tobacco Control Monograph 14 (pp. 213-226) (NIH Pub. No. 02-5086). Bethesda, MD: National Cancer Institute.

Glassman, A.H., Helzer, J.E., Covey, L.S., Cottler, L.B., Stetner, F., Tipp, J.E., and Johnson, J. (1990). Smoking, smoking cessation, and major depression. *Journal of the American Medical Association, 264*, 1546-1549.

Gorman, D., and White, H.R. (1995). You can choose your friends, but do they choose your crime? Differential association theories for crime prevention policy. In H. Barlow (Ed.), Criminology and public policy: Putting theory to work, pp. 131-155. Boulder, CO: Westview Press.

Gottfredson, D.C., and Koper, C.S. (1996). Race and sex differences in the prediction of drug use. *Journal of Consulting and Clinical Psychology, 64*, 305-313.

Griesler, P.C., and Kandel, D.B. (1998). Ethnic differences in correlates of adolescent smoking. *Journal of Adolescent Health, 23*, 167-180.

Gritz, E.R., Prokhorov, A.V., Hudmon, K.S., Chamberlain, R.M., Taylor, W.C., DiClemente, C.C., Johnston, D.A., Hu, S., Jones, L.A., Jones, M.M., Rosenblum, C.K., Ayars, C.L., and Amos, C. (1998). Cigarette smoking in a multiethnic population of youth: Methods and baseline findings. *Preventive Medicine, 27*, 365-384.

Hestick, H., Perrino, S.C., Rhodes, W.A., and Sydnor, K.D. (2001). Trial and lifetime smoking risks among African American college students. *Journal of American College Health, 49*, 213-219.

Hollingshead, A.B. (1975). *Four factor index of social status*. Unpublished manuscript. Department of Sociology at Yale University, MA.

Johnston, L.D., O'Malley, P.M., and Bachman, J.G. (2003). *Monitoring the Future: National survey results on drug use from the Monitoring the Future Study, 1975-2001. Vol. I, Secondary school students*. Bethesda. National Institute on Drug Abuse.

Jones, B.L., Nagin, D.S., and Roeder, K. (2001). A SAS procedure based on mixture models for estimating developmental trajectories. *Sociological Methods and Research, 29*, 374-393.

Juon, H.S., Ensminger, M.E., and Sydnor, K.D. (2002). A longitudinal study of developmental trajectories to young adult cigarette smoking. *Drug and Alcohol Dependency, 66*, 303-314.

Kandel, D.B., Chen, K., Warner, L.A., Kessler, R.C., and Grant, B. (1997). Prevalence and demographic correlates of symptoms of last year dependence on alcohol, nicotine, marijuana, and cocaine in the US population. *Drug and Alcohol Dependence, 44*, 11-29.

Kandel, D.B., and Davies, M. (1986). Adult sequelae of adolescent depressive symptoms. *Archives of General Psychiatry, 43*, 255-262.

Kandel, D.B., Kiros, G.-E., Schaffran, C., and Hu, M.-C. (2004). Racial/ethnic differences in cigarettes smoking initiation and progression to daily smoking: A multilevel analysis. *American Journal of Public Health, 94*, 128-135.

Landrine, H., Richardson, J.L., Klonoff, E.A., and Flay, B. (1994). Cultural diversity in the predictors of adolescent cigarette smoking: The relative influence of peers. *Journal of Behavioral Medicine, 17*, 331-346.

Lloyd-Richardson, E.E., Papandonatos, G., Kazura, A., Stanton, C., and Niaura, R. (2002). Differentiating stages of smoking intensity among adolescents: Stage-specific psychological and social influences. *Journal of Consulting and Clinical Psychology, 70*, 998-1009.

Loeber, R., Farrington, D.P., Stouthamer-Loeber, M., and Van Kammen, W.B. (1998). *Antisocial behavior and mental health problems: Explanatory factors in childhood and adolescence*. Mahwah, NJ: Lawrence Erlbaum Associates.

Mayhew, K.P., Flay, B.R. and Mott, J.A. (2000). Stages in the development of adolescent smoking. *Drug and Alcohol Dependence, 59*, s-61-s81.

Nagin, D.S. (1999). Analyzing developmental trajectories: A semiparametric, group-based approach. *Psychological Methods, 4*, 139-157.

Nagin, D.S. (2005). *Group-based modeling of development.* Cambridge, MA: Harvard University Press.Nagin, D.S., and Land, K.C. (1993). Age, criminal career, andpopulation heterogeneity: Specification and estimation of a nonparametic mixed Poisson model. *Criminology, 31*, 327-362.

Nagin, D.S., and Tremblay, R.E. (1999). Trajectories of boy's physical aggression, opposition, and hyperactivity on the path to physically violent and non-violent juvenile delinquency. *Child Development, 7*, 1181-1196.

Nagin, D.S., and Tremblay, R.E. (2001). Analyzing developmental trajectories of distinct but related behaviors: A group-based method. *Psychological Methods, 6*, 18-34.

National Center for Chronic Disease Prevention and Health Promotion. (2004). Adult cigarette smoking in the united states: Current estimates. Fact Sheet, May 2004 obtained on-line http://www.cdc.gov/tobacco/factsheets/AdultCigaretteSmoking_FactSheet.htm)

Newcomb, M.D., McCarthy, W.J., and Bentler, P.M. (1989). Cigarette smoking, academic lifestyle, and social impact efficacy: An eight-year study from early adolescence to young adulthood. *Journal of Applied Social Psychology, 19*, 251-281.

Nichter, M. (2003). Smoking: What does culture have to do with it? *Addiction, 98*, 139-145.

Patrick, D.L., Cheadle, A., Thompson, D.C., Diehr, P., Koepsell, T., and Kinne, S. (1994). The validity of self-reported smoking: A review and meta-analysis. *American Journal of Public Health, 84*, 1086-1093.

Patton, G.C., Hibbert, M., Rosier, M.J., Carlin, J.B., Caust, J., and Bowes, G. (1996). Is smoking associated with depression and anxiety in teenagers? *American Journal of Public Health, 86*, 225-230.

Raftery, A.E. (1995). Bayesian model selection in social research. *Sociological Methodology, 25*, 111-164.

Robinson, L.A., Klesges, R.C., Zbikowski, S.M., and Glaser, R. (1997). Predictors of risk for different stages of adolescent smoking in a biracial sample. *Journal of Consulting and Clinical Psychology, 65*, 653-662.

Roeder, K., Lynch, K.G., and Nagin, D.S. (1999). Modeling uncertainty in latent class membership: A case study in criminology. *Journal of the American Statistical Association, 94*, 766-776.

Rose, J., Chassin, L., Presson, C. C., and Sherman, S. J. (1996). Demographic factors in adult smoking status: Mediating and moderating influences. *Psychology of Addictive Behaviors, 10*, 28-37.

Schulenburg, J.E., and Maggs, J.L. (2002) A developmental perspective on alcohol use and heavy drinking during adolescence and the transition to young adulthood. *Journal of Studies on Alcohol, Supplement No. 14*, 54-70.

Schulenberg, J., Wadsworth, K.N., O'Malley, P.M., Bachman, J.G., and Johnston, L.D. (1996). Adolescent risk factors for binge drinking during the transition to young adulthood: Variable-and pattern-centered approaches to change. *Developmental Psychology, 32*, 659-674.

Storr, C.L., Ialongo, N.S., Kellam, S.G., Anthony, J.C. (2002). A randomized controlled trial of two primary intervention strategies to prevent early onset of tobacco smoking. *Drug and Alcohol Dependence, 66*, 51-60.

Stouthamer-Loeber, M., Loeber, R., Farrington, D.P., Zhang, Q., van Kammen, W., and Maguin, E. (1993). The double edge of protective and risk factors for delinquency: Interrelations and developmental patterns. *Development and Psychopathology, 5*, 683-701.

Stouthamer-Loeber, M., Loeber, R., Wei, E., Farrington, D.P., and Wilkstrom, P-O. (2002). Risk and promotive effects in the explanation of persistent serious delinquency in boys. *Journal of Consulting and Clinical Psychology, 70*, 111-123.

Stouthamer-Loeber, M., Wei, E., Loeber, R., and Masten, A.S. (2004). Desistance from persistent serious delinquency in the transition to adulthood. *Development and Psychopathology, 16*, 897-918.

Stouthamer-Loeber, M. and Van Kammen, W. (1995). Stouthamer-Loeber, M., and Van Kammen, W. B. (1995). Data collection and management: A practical guide. Newbury Park, CA.: Sage.

Sussman, S., Dent, C.W., Stacy, A.W. Burton, D., and Flay, B.R. (1995). Developing school-based tobacco use prevention and cessation programs. Thousand Oaks, CA: Sage Publications, Inc., 1995.

Unger, J.B., Rohrbach, L.A., Cruz, T.B., Baezconde-Garbanati, L., Howard, K.A. Palmer, P.H., and Johnson, C.A. (2001). Ethnic variation in peer influence on adolescent smoking. *Nicotine and Tobacco Research, 3*, 167-176.

US Department of Health and Human Services (1998). *Tobacco use among US racial/ethnic minority groups: A report of the surgeon general.* Atlanta, Georgia: USDHHS, CSC.

Wallace, J.M. and Muroff, J.R. (2002). Preventing substance abuse among African American children and youth: Race differences in risk factor exposure and vulnerability. *The Journal of Primary Prevention, 22*, 235-261.

White, H.R., Nagin, D., Replogle, E., and Stouthamer-Loeber, M. (2004). Racial differences in trajectories of cigarette use. *Drug and Alcohol Dependence, 76*, 219-227.

White, H.R., Pandina, R.J., and Chen, P-H. (2002). Developmental trajectories of cigarette smoking from adolescence to young adulthood. *Drug and Alcohol Dependence, 65*, 167-178.

Wilcox, P. (2003). An ecological approach to understanding youth smoking trajectories: Problems and prospects. *Addiction, 98*, 57-78.

Williams, J.G., and Covington, C.J. (1997). Predictors of cigarette smoking among adolescents. *Psychological Reports, 80*, 481-482.

Winefield, H.R., Winefield, A.H., and Tiggemann, M. (1992). Psychological attributes of young adult smokers. *Psychological Reports, 70*, 675-681.

www.monitoringthefuture.org. The Monitoring the Future Study, the University of Michigan.

In: Progress in Smoking and Health Research
Editor: T. C. Jeffries, pp. 71-87
ISBN: 978-1-60021-686-2

Chapter III

Smoking and Surgical Procedures Related to Dental Implantations

***Devorah Schwartz-Arad**[*1] **and Liran Levin**[2,3]*
[1] Department of Oral and Maxillofacial Surgery and [2] Department of Oral Rehabilitation, The Maurice and Gabriela Goldschleger School of Dental Medicine, Tel Aviv University, Tel Aviv, Israel. [3] Unit of Periodontology, Department of Oral and Dental Sciences, Rambam Medical Center, Haifa, Israel.

Abstract

Cigarette smoking is still considered a common habit in the Western world, even though it has come under increasing attack by numerous groups both within the United States and worldwide. Among smokers, increased plaque accumulation, higher incidence of gingivitis and periodontitis, higher rate of tooth loss, and increased resorption of the alveolar ridge, have been found in the oral cavity. The use of endosseous dental implants in various edentulous situations have increased over the past 10 years. Cigarette smoking may adversely affect wound healing, and thus jeopardize the success of bone grafting and dental implantation.

Bone grafts and sinus lift operations are both common and well documented procedures prior to dental implant placement. Autologous bone grafts for dental implants were originally described by Bränemark *et al.* in 1975, and is now a well-accepted procedure in oral and maxillofacial rehabilitation. A sinus lift operation has a predictable outcome with an implant survival rate of over 90% for 3 to 5 years. It is considered a safe treatment modality with only minor complications. Toxic by-products of cigarette smoking, such as nicotine, carbon monoxide and hydrogen cyanide, have been implicated as risk factors for impaired healing and thus may affect the success and complications of those surgical procedures.

[*] Correspondence and reprints to: Dr. Devorah Schwartz-Arad; Department of Oral and Maxillofacial Surgery; The Maurice and Gabriela Goldschleger; School of Dental Medicine; Tel Aviv University; Tel Aviv, Israel; Fax: +972-3-6409250; Email: dubish@post.tau.ac.il

Smoking also impairs wound healing in various surgical disciplines. It is the single most important risk factor for the development of post-operative complications in orthopedic surgery. In dermatology, smoking decreases the synthesis rate of collagen in skin, *in vivo,* and alters the balance of extracellular matrix turnover in skin. Tissue ischemia and wound-healing impairment, secondary to the influence of tobacco, are problematic for plastic surgeons.

An association between dental implants, grafting procedures (bone grafts, maxillary sinuses augmentation etc.), and history of smoking has been reported. A higher complication or failure rate was found in smokers with and without bone grafts.

The relationship between cigarette smoking and oral procedures with regard to dental implantations, i.e., sinus lift operations, onlay bone grafts and dental implantations, including the incidence of complications related to these procedures and long-term survival and success rates of dental implants among smokers and non-smokers will be described in this chapter.

This study was based on data from dental operations performed between the years 1995-2003, following accepted and well documented protocols. Criteria for patient inclusion in the study were: adequate information regarding age, gender, health status, pre- and post-operative radiographs, and follow-up for at least 6 months post-surgery.

All smoking habits were known at the time of operation. Current smokers were divided into two subgroups: number of cigarettes per day (less vs. more than 10) and duration of smoking (less vs. more than 10 years). Past smokers were defined as patients who stopped at least 6 months before the surgical procedure.

Introduction

Cigarette smoking has come under increasing attack by numerous groups, both within the United States and worldwide. This has been partially fueled by the recognition of the increasing number of diseases in which smoking has been directly or indirectly associated. Currently, there are approximately 50 million smokers in the United States [1]. The prevalence of smoking is higher among men (25.2%) than women (20.0%) and inversely related to age, from 28.5% aged 18-24 years to 9.3% aged $\geq$65 years [1]. The adverse effects of smoking on the cardiovascular system are common knowledge [2,3], and are implicated in the etiology of many cancers [2,4]. Smoking is now the leading avoidable cause of morbidity and mortality in the United States with more than 500,000 deaths per year in the United States alone [2].

Cigarette smoke has two phases: volatile and particulate. The volatile phase is the longer phase and accounts for 95% of the cigarette smoke. Nearly 500 different gases are released during this phase, including nitrogen, carbon monoxide, carbon dioxide, ammonia, hydrogen cyanide, and benzene. In the particulate phase, there are approximately 3,500 different chemicals released, including nicotine, nornicotine, natabine, and anabasine [5]. Without water, the remaining particulate matter or "tar" contains most of the carcinogens of cigarette smoke [6]. Nicotine, considered the addictive component of cigarette smoke, has been implicated in the pathogenesis of numerous diseases [6], increases platelet aggregation, decreases microvascular prostacyclin levels, and inhibits the function of fibroblasts, red blood cells, and macrophages [6,7]. Carbon monoxide has a stronger affinity for hemoglobin than oxygen, resulting in the displacement of oxygen from the hemoglobin and a lower oxygen tension in tissues [8]. Current and lifetime tobacco smoking are also associated with deterioration in bone quality [9].

Smoking and the Oral Cavity

Among smokers, an increase in plaque accumulation, a higher incidence of gingivitis and periodontitis, a higher rate of tooth loss and an increased resorption of the alveolar ridge have been found in the oral cavity [10]. The exact mechanisms in which tobacco exerts its influence on periodontal tissues are not completely explained. It is likely that smoking primarily has a systemic influence by altering the host response and/or by directly damaging the periodontal cells. Studies have shown that tobacco smoking is associated with decreased levels of salivary IgA antibodies [11] and serum IgG antibodies to *Prevotella intermedia* and *Fusobacterium nucleatum* [12], depressed numbers of helper lymphocytes [13], and impaired chemotaxis and phagocytosis of both oral [14] and peripheral [15] neutrophils. Additionally, nicotine has been shown to affect *in vitro* monocyte function [16] and gingival fibroblast proliferation [17], inhibit fibroblast synthesis of fibronectin and type I collagen [18], increase collagenase activity [17], and suppress proliferation of cultured osteoblasts while stimulating osteoblast alkaline phosphatase activity [19]. Impaired oxygen transport and metabolism caused by carbon monoxide, as well as enzyme poisoning by hydrogen cyanide, further reduce the oxidative metabolism needed for cellular repair [20].

Smoking and Endosseous Implants

The use of endosseous implants has increased over the past decade in some edentulous situations. Bain and Moy [21] assessed the various factors that predispose implants to failure in a group of 540 patients who received 2194 Bränemark implants. The most significant factor was smoking. De Bruyn and Collaert [22] found that smokers demonstrate a significantly higher failure rate before functional loading of implants than non-smokers. Lindquist *et al.* [23,24] compared marginal bone loss around osseointegrated dental implants among smokers and non-smokers. Among smokers who also had poor oral hygiene, marginal bone loss was nearly three times as great as that in non-smokers. Smokers can suffer detrimental effects around successfully integrated maxillary implants, with significantly greater bleeding index, greater mean peri-implant pocket depth, more frequent peri-implant inflammation and radiographically greater mesial and distal bone loss [25].

Implant failure is a result of a multifactorial process. Significant factors that influence prognosis include length and diameter of the implant [26], implant location [27], bone quality [28], and type of edentulous area treated [29].

It is difficult to assess adverse effects of smoking on the prognosis of implants on the basis of implant failure alone. Specific factors, such as type (coating, design, etc.) of implant and immediate versus late implantation can also be assessed and compared between smokers and non-smokers. These factors, related to clinical complications, enable the evaluation of the survival rate of the implants.

Smoking and Wound Healing

Cigarette smoking has long been suspected as adversely affecting wound healing. Arteriolar vasoconstriction and decreased blood flow are seen in response to smoking [21,22]. Toxic by-products, such as nicotine, carbon monoxide and hydrogen cyanide, have been implicated as risk factors for impaired healing [30].

Smoking impairs wound healing in various surgical operations. In orthopedic surgery such as hip or knee arthroplasty, smoking is the single most important risk factor for the development of post-operative complications, particularly those relating to wound healing, cardiopulmonary complications, and post-operative intensive care [31]. Smoking is also associated with an increased risk of complications in patients with open tibial fractures [32]. In dermatology, smoking proved to decrease the synthesis rates of types I and III collagens in skin, *in vivo,* and to alter the balance of extracellular matrix turnover in skin [33]. Tissue ischemia and wound-healing impairment secondary to the influence of tobacco is problematic for plastic surgeons, especially during elective facial esthetic procedures, cosmetic and reconstructive breast operations, abdominoplasty, free-tissue transfer, and replantation procedures [33]. Smoking also compromises healing after various mucogingival surgeries [26,27,35,36].

Smoking and Implant-Related Surgical Procedures

The most common augmentation procedures for the later use of dental implants include guided bone regeneration (GBR), sinus lift operation (SLO) and bone grafting. GBR is a common and well described procedure for augmentation with considerable long-term results [37,38]. SLO also has a predictable outcome with an implant survival rate of over 90% for 3-5 years [39-43]. It is considered a safe treatment modality, with only minor complications [44]. The use of autologous bone grafts with dental implants was originally described by Branemark *et al.* in 1975 [45], and is now a well-accepted procedure in oral and maxillofacial rehabilitation [46-49].

Notably, smoking is considered contraindicated for protocols such as bone regeneration and bone grafting [50]. The predictability and extent of periodontal regeneration are associated with cigarette smoking [51]. Smoking adversely affects treatment outcome, as measured by gains in clinical attachment levels of intra-bony defects treated by regenerative therapy [52]. An association between dental implants placed in augmented maxillary sinuses and history of smoking has been reported [53]. Smokers, after rehabilitation of severely resorbed maxillae with and without bone grafts, have a higher implant failure rate [21,54,55]. Cigarette smoking is detrimental to the success of osseointegrated implants in grafted maxillary sinuses regardless of the amount of cigarettes consumed [56].

The purpose of this chapter is to describe the relationship between cigarette smoking and surgical procedures related to dental implantations, i.e., sinus lift operations, bone grafts and dental implantations, including the incidence of complications related to these procedures and long-term survival and success rates of dental implants among smokers and non-smokers.

The facts presented will assist dental health professionals in treatment-planning decisions and provide them with important information to share with patients who use tobacco products.

Research

The studies presented were based on data from dental operations performed between the years 1995-2003, following accepted and well documented protocols. Criteria for patient inclusion into the studies were: adequate information regarding age, gender, health status, pre- and post-operative radiographs, and follow-up for at least 6 months post-surgery.

All smoking habits were known at the time of operation. Current smokers were divided into two subgroups regarding the number of cigarettes per day (mild smokers - less than 10; heavy smokers - more than 10) and duration of smoking (mild smokers - less than 10 years; heavy smokers - more than 10 years). Past smokers were defined as patients who stopped at least 6 months before the surgical procedure.

Smoking and Endosseous Dental Implants

The first study was designed to compare the incidence of the complications, such as premature spontaneous implant exposure (in a two-stage implantation procedure) [56-62], and survival and success rates related to dental implants among smokers and non-smokers. The influence of smoking was evaluated by analyzing data of 261 patients (18 to 67 years, mean 48 years) with 959 submerged implants placed during the years 1995 to 1998. There were 172 non-smokers with 579 implants and 89 smokers with 380 implants. One surgeon inserted all implants under sterile conditions, following a protocol described by Schwartz-Arad *et al.* [63-66]. An important parameter influencing premature implant exposure was the height of the cover screw above the crestal bone level (according to the implant design: internal or external connection), since all implants were placed at the crestal bone level. There were 386 implants with a high cover screw and 573 with a flat cover screw.

Time of implant placement (immediate vs. non-immediate) was another parameter that was examined as a potential parameter influencing implant success. Of the 959 implants, 288 were immediate.

Patients were divided into two groups: patients with no complications between the two surgical stages (implant placement and exposure), and those with complications: premature spontaneous implant exposure without surgical intervention (minor), premature spontaneous implant exposure with surgical intervention (major), or complete implant failure during surgical phase requiring implant removal [63-66].

The survival rate of each group was calculated. Two-way ANOVA test was used to analyze implant design and smoking. A statistically significant difference between the complication rate in the smoking and the non-smoking groups was found ($p<0.05$). Generally, there was a significantly higher incidence of complications ($p<0.05$) in both smoking groups (less than 10 per day or more than 10 per day) when the number of cigarettes per day was considered (table 1). When the number of years of smoking was considered, a significantly higher incidence ($p<0.04$) of complications was found as the number of smoking years increased (table 2). In the smokers group, there were more complications regardless of the time of implantation (immediate vs. non-immediate).

Table 1. Complication rate among non-smokers and smokers with regards to amount of cigarettes smoked per day

Group	Number of implants	No complications	Complications
Non-smokers	579	402 (69%)	177 (31%)
Smokers			
Less than 10/d	127	74 (58%)	53 (42%)
More than 10/d	253	131 (52%)	122 (48%)

Implant complications for all smokers vs. non-smokers $p<0.05$.

Table 2. Complication rate among non-smokers and smokers with regard to duration of smoking

Group	Number of implants	No complications	Complications
Non-smokers	579	402 (69%)	177 (31%)
Smokers			
Less than 10/y	103	66 (64%)	37 (36%)
More than 10/y	277	139 (50%)	138 (50%)

Increased relationship between complications and years of smoking $p<0.04$.

In a subsequent study, the influence of smoking on marginal bone loss around implants was examined using the same inclusion criteria as the previous work. In this study, 161 patients (aged 23 to 89 years, mean 57 years) received 646 implants, with a follow-up time ranging from 9.4 to 86.6 months (mean 45.5 months). There were 102 non-smokers (375 implants) and 59 smokers (271 implants). Of the implants, 391 (61%) were immediate ones.

Marginal bone level was measured on radiographs (orthopanthographs) using the implant threads as internal standard, a technique formerly suggested by Haas *et al.* [67]. Evaluation of marginal bone level was made by comparing the bone level at time of implant exposure with that of the most recent follow-up, and subtracting the two. The number of threads unsupported by bone in both the mesial and distal sides of each implant was counted, and the average number used for bone loss calculations. The accuracy level of this method is half a pitch of the implant thread. The number of threads was converted to millimeters using the given millimeter-per-thread for that particular implant. Information regarding the pitch of different implant systems was supplied by the manufacturers. An implant was considered successful if bone loss apical to the implant neck was less than 0.3 mm per year (starting from the first year).

The influence of smoking and other variables on bone loss was analyzed using the t-test and one-way ANOVA analysis. The cumulative survival rate was calculated with the Kaplan-Meier analysis. Success rate was calculated using the Chi-Square test.

In the maxilla, heavy smokers (more than 10 cigarettes per day) had the highest amount of bone loss (0.1897 ± 0.1825), followed by mild smokers (less than 10 cigarettes per day)

(0.123 ± 0.156) and non-smokers (0.046 ± 0.07) ($p<0.001$, table 3). In the mandible, there was no distinction between heavy and mild smokers, and both had greater marginal bone loss than non-smokers ($p<0.001$). Overall success rate for all implants was 93.2%. Non-smokers had a higher success rate (97.1%) than smokers (87.8%) ($p<0.001$) (table 4).

Table 3. Difference between smokers (S), mild smokers (MS) and non-smokers (Non-S)

		N	Mean	SD
Mandible*	Non-S	102	0.0487	0.09115
	MS	30	0.1502	0.15867
	HS	29	0.1390	0.1599
	total	161	0.0845	0.12831
Maxilla**	Non-S	102	0.0460	0.07035
	MS	30	0.1233	0.15559
	HS	29	0.1897	0.18247
	total	161	0.0867	0.12918

Tukey's method for multiple comparisons shows:
Mandible: Non-S ≠ MS, HS
Maxilla: Non-S ≠ MS ≠ HS
*$p< 0.001$
**$p< 0.001$.

Table 4. 5-year cumulative survival rate after loading (Kaplan-Meier analysis)

Year	Failures	Survival (in %)
1	0	100
2	2	99.7
3	1	99.5
4	0	99.5
5-7	0	99.5

Smoking and Implant-Related Surgical Procedures

This study was based on data obtained from 143 operations: 64 OBG (56 patients) and 79 SLO (72 patients). Information included complete medical and dental history, clinical and radiographic evaluation, and specific emphasis on smoking habits. OBG operations were performed in 12 (18.8%) smokers and 52 (81.3%) non-smokers, 4 to 5 months prior to dental implant placement following a modification of an operating protocol described by Misch [46]. SLO operations were performed in 30 (38%) smokers and 49 (62%) non-smokers, in which 55 operations (69.6%) involved simultaneous dental implantation. One surgeon performed all operations between the years 1995-2003 under sterile conditions, following a protocol described by Schwartz-Arad *et al.* [68]. Criteria for accepting patients into the study group were: adequate information regarding age, gender, health status, pre- and post-operative radiographs, and follow-up for at least 6 months post-surgery.

Smoking and non-smoking patients were divided into two groups: patients with and without complications. For the SLO, perforation of the Schneiderian membrane was the main intra-operative complication, followed by post-operative complications, mostly swelling, acute or chronic sinus infection, and bleeding.

For the OBG operations, minor complications were hematoma, swelling, inflammation, temporary paresthesia; major complications were graft exposure or graft mobility.

Statistical analysis included Pearson's chi square test of association and analysis of variance (ANOVA) using BMDP statistical software [68].

No relation was found between SLO complications and smoking and past smoking, including intra- and post-operative complications. Perforation of the Schneiderian membrane was the main intra-operative complication (37 patients, 46%), followed by post-operative complications consisting mostly of swelling (6 patients, 7%), acute or chronic sinus infection (4 patients, 5%), and bleeding (4 patients, 5%).

There were 23.1% complications following OBG in non-smokers compared to 50% complications in smokers. Major complications were found in one-third of the operations in smokers compared to 7.7% in the non-smokers ($p=0.04$). There was also a relation between complications and past smoking, although not statistically significant ($p=0.06$).

Discussion

Tobacco use is an important contributor to preventable morbidity and mortality in the United States [70]. A significant proportion of cardiovascular diseases, various oral and pulmonary neoplasms, non-malignant respiratory diseases, and peripheral vascular disorders are attributed to cigarette use. In the dental literature smoking has been shown to compromise healing after mucogingival surgery [26,27,37,38], and is associated with oral cancer, periodontal disease, leukoplakia, stomatitis nicotina and impaired gingival bleeding [71-73].

Smoking and Dental Implants

When dental implant failure and implant-related complications are considered, it is evident that non-smokers benefit significantly [74-78]. Smoking has been shown to be a contributing factor to implant failure between time of implant placement and second stage surgery [74]. Additionally, the failure rate among smokers was twice that of non-smokers [74].

Although the survival rate of immediate implantation is higher than non-immediate ones [63,65,66,79,80], smokers with an immediate implantation had a significantly higher rate of complications compared to non-smokers [63].

Smoking and Marginal Bone Loss (MBL)

Smokers have a greater MBL [81,82], which strongly concurs with the present findings. Our observations show that maxillary bone was more sensitive to tobacco exposure; heavy smokers had more MBL than mild smokers. It has been shown that the maxilla is more prone to the deleterious effect of smoking [21]. Lambert et al. [81] noted that in smokers, maxillary implants failed 1.6 times more than mandibular implants. De Bruyn and Collaert [22] and Esposito et al. [82] found that smokers had a higher implant failure rate in the maxilla. Presumably maxillary bone is compromised and, therefore more prone to the detrimental effects of smoking.

Our finding of greater MBL around implants in the posterior regions contradicts Lindquist et al. [2], who found bone loss around anterior sites almost twice as large as around the posterior sites.

Bone loss may be associated with smoking even in patients with good oral hygiene. In a group of 235 patients (72 smokers), radiographic analysis of bone height expressed as a percentage of root length, revealed lower mean bone levels for smokers (77.9-82.8%). This suggests that smoking is a risk factor for periodontal health [83]. In another radiographic study conducted on 210 Swedish dental hygienists with good oral hygiene and no periodontal disease, the distance from the cemento-enamal junction to the interdental septum was greatest in smokers, followed by former smokers and non-smokers [84]. A clinical and radiographic study of the condition of 257 dentally aware adults, aged 20-69 years, revealed that the condition of former smokers who quit was intermediate between current smokers and non-smokers. This suggests that former smokers have better periodontal health than current smokers, although worse than that of non-smokers [85]. The periodontal health condition of former smokers remained stable after 10 years [86]. Furthermore, the progression of bone loss is significantly reduced in individuals who stop smoking [87]. In post-menopausal women, smoking is a strong independent negative factor for alveolar bone loss [88]. In early onset periodontitis, smokers (mean smoking experience of 9.2 pack years) had significantly more maxillary bone loss than non-smokers [89].

Smoking and Oral Flora

It is unclear whether there is a consistent effect of smoking on the bacterial population selection, although recent studies suggest such an effect. The relationship between several bacterial strains associated with periodontal disease and smoking has been examined. In a study of 145 patients (83 smokers), Preber *et al.* [90] found that testing for *Actinobacillus actinomycetemcomitans*, *Porphyromonas gingivalis*, and *Prevotella intermedia* in pockets of 6 mm or more failed to show any difference between the groups. The use of DNA-hybridization for *P. gingivalis*, *P. intermedia*, *Prevotella nigrescens*, *Bacteroides forsythus*, *A. actinomycetemcomitans*, *Fusobacterium nucleatum*, *Treponema denticola*, *Peptostreptococcus micros*, *Campylobacter rectus*, *Eikenella corrodens*, *Selenomonas noxia*, and *Streptococcus intermedius* in a group of 33 smokers and 31 non-smokers with moderate-to-severe periodontal disease, both exhibited the same frequencies of the 12 species investigated [91]. In a microbiologic study of 272 subjects divided into never, past, and current smokers, a difference in the prevalence (percent of sites colonized) of species [92] rather than in counts or proportions, with the prevalence of *B. forsythus* and *P. nigrescens* significantly greater in the maxilla than the mandible where greater pocket depth and attachment loss were evident [93]. This may explain the greater severity of periodontal destruction in smokers. A similar distribution of pockets has been reported in a retrospective study of 183 patients in which pockets ≥5 mm were more prevalent in smokers, mainly in the maxillary anterior and premolars [94].

In a study of the subgingival microbial flora of 468 patients with periodontal disease, divided into untreated smokers, treated smokers, untreated non-smokers, and treated non-smokers, it was concluded that smoking is a determining factor for the composition of microbial flora and may be selective for *B. forsythus*, *P. micros*, *F. nucleatum* and *C. rectus* [95]. When bacteria were quantitated, it was found that smoking extends a favorable habitat for bacteria, such as *P. gingivalis*, *P. intermedia* and *A. actinomycetemcomitans* to shallow sites with a pocket depth ≤5 mm [95]. Several potential mechanisms in which smoke could influence the host control of bacteria were proposed. These include the effects of carbon monoxide, enhancing bacterial growth, which in turn provides growth factors for anaerobes, and damaging cells involved in protecting the periodontal environment, *e.g.*, neutrophils, which could be affected by the formation of advanced glycation end products by smoke.

Smoking and Implant-Related Procedures

Surgical outcomes can also be adversely affected as a result of cigarette smoking with intra- and post-operative pulmonary, cardiovascular, and cerebrovascular complications, as well as increased wound healing complications. These are found across the entire spectrum of surgical specialties [30-33].

Additionally to the fact that smoking causes a higher incidence of complications (spontaneous premature implant exposure) following implant placement [96], we found that smokers demonstrated significantly higher post-operative complications following OBG operations.

Smoking influence was less significant in SLO complications. Kan *et al.* [56] evaluated the effect of smoking on implant success in grafted maxillary sinuses. There was a higher cumulative implant success rate in non-smokers than in smokers. However, graft complications were not reported, as in our study.

There was no statistically significant difference between complications and past smoking. This finding indicates that the risk of complications can be reduced up to the normal non-smoker complication rate when smoking ceases. Numerous smoking cessation protocols have been proposed to improve the surgical outcome in smokers [97,98]. However, the effect of short-term smoking cessation on the risk of complicated tissue and wound healing or other complications of general surgery is still controversial [99,100].

It is beyond the scope of this chapter to discuss the possible mechanisms in which smoking increases failure rate and complications in both implant-related surgical procedures and dental implantation. It does not provide any insight into the mechanism associated with failures and complications in smokers. However, it is probable that these relate to any or all factors, such as systemic vasoconstriction, reduced blood flow, increased platelet aggregation, and polymorphonuclear leukocyte dysfunction, which have been identified in smokers [101-104]. Nicotine may have an effect on cellular protein synthesis and its modulation of γ_1 integrin expression and impair gingival fibroblast ability to adhere to and communicate with one another and with the extracellular matrix, thus impairing wound healing and/or exacerbating periodontal disease [104]. The volatile fractions of cigarette smoke, such as acrolein and acetaldehyde, could have a cytotoxic effect on human gingival fibroblasts, which results in capacity loss for adhesion and proliferation [106]. The consequences of this could be impaired maintenance, integrity, and remodeling of the oral connective tissue. These mechanisms are most crucial in implant-related procedures, such as OBG, in which primary tissue closure is essential for surgical success.

Smokers undergoing both implant-related surgical procedures and dental implantation should be encouraged by their dentists, oral and maxillofacial surgeons, or treating physicians to quit smoking, emphasizing that smoking can reduce the success rate.

Conclusion

Smokers had a higher incidence of failure rate and complications following dental implantation and implant-related surgical procedures. The risk of failure and complications are reduced once smoking ceases. Potential implant patients should be advised that smoking could have a detrimental effect on dental implantation and implant-related surgical procedures. Tobacco-associated surgical morbidity in the oral and maxillofacial surgical patient can be eliminated by educating and providing guidelines to smokers and by refusing to operate on individuals who fail to abstain.

References

[1] Husten, C; Jackson, K; Lee, C. Cigarette smoking among adults - United States. Morbidity and Mortality Weekly Report, 2004, 53, 427-431.

[2] Skurnik, Y; Shoenfeld, Y. Health effects of cigarette smoking. *Clinics in Dermatology,* 1998, 16, 545-556.

[3] Newby, DE; Wright, RA; Labinjoh, C; et al. Endothelial dysfunction, impaired endogenous fibrinolysis, and cigarette smoking: A mechanism for arterial thrombosis and myocardial infarction. *Circulation,* 1999, 99, 1411-1415.

[4] Routh, HB; Bhowmik KR; Parish, JL; Parish, LC. Historical aspects of tobacco use and smoking. *Clinics in Dermatology,* 1998, 16, 539-544.

[5] Hoffmann, D; Hoffmann, I. The changing cigarette, 1950-1995. *Journal of Toxicology and Environmental Health,* 1997, 50, 307-364.

[6] Zevin, S; Gourlay, SG; Benowitz, NL. Clinical pharmacology of nicotine. *Clinics in Dermatology,* 1998, 16, 557-564.

[7] Jorgensen, LN; Kallehave, F; Christensen, E; Siana, JE; Gottrup, F. Less collagen production in smokers. *Surgery,* 1998, 123, 450-455.

[8] Leow, YH; Maibach, HI. Cigarette smoking, cutaneous vasculature, and tissue oxygen. *Clinics in Dermatology,* 1998, 16, 579-584.

[9] Bernaards, CM; Twisk, JW; Snel, J; van Mechelen, W; Lips, P; Kemper, HC. Smoking and quantitative ultrasound parameters in the calcaneus in 36-year-old men and women. *Osteoporosis International,* 2004,15, 735-741.

[10] Scabbia, A; Cho, KS; Sigurdsson, TJ; Kim, CK; Trombelli, L. Cigarette smoking negatively affects healing response following flap debridement surgery. *Journal of Periodontology,* 2001, 72, 43-49.

[11] Bennet, KR; Read, PC. Salivary immunoglobulin A levels in normal subjects, tobacco smokers, and patients with minor aphthous ulceration. *Oral Surgery, Oral Medicine, Oral Pathology,* 1982, 53, 461-465.

[12] Haber, J. Cigarette smoking: A major risk factor for periodontitis. *Compendium of Continuing Education in Dentistry,* 1994, 15, 1002-1014.

[13] Ginns, LC; Goldenheim, PD; Miller, LG. T-lymphocyte subsets in smoking and lung cancer. Analyses of monoclonal antibodies and flow cytometry. *American Review of Respiratory Disease,* 1982, 126, 265-269.

[14] Kenney, EB; Kraal, JH; Saxe, SR; Jones, J. The effect of cigarette smoke on human oral polymorphonuclear leukocytes. *Journal of Periodontal Research,* 1977, 12, 227-234.

[15] Selby, C; Drost, E; Brown, D; Howie, S; MacNee, W. Inhibition of neutrophil adherence and movement by acute cigarette smoke exposure. *Experimental Lung Research,* 1992, 18, 813-827.

[16] Pabst, MJ; Pabst, KM; Collier, JA; et al. Inhibition of neutrophil and monocyte defensive functions by nicotine. *Journal of Periodontology,* 1995, 66, 1047-1055.

[17] Peacock, ME; Sutherland, DE; Schuster, GS; et al. The effect of nicotine on reproduction and attachment of human gingival fibroblasts in vitro. *Journal of Periodontology,* 1993, 64, 658-665.

[18] Tipton, DA; Dabbous, MK. Effects of nicotine on proliferation and extracellular matrix production of human gingival fibroblasts in vitro. *Journal of Periodontology,* 1995, 66, 1056-1064.

[19] Fang, MA; Frost, PJ; Iida-Klein, A; Hahn, TJ. Effects of nicotine on cellular function in UMR 106-01 osteoblast-like cells. *Bone,* 1991, 12, 283-286.

[20] Hanes, PJ; Schuster, GS; Lubas, S. Binding, uptake, and release of nicotine by human gingival fibroblasts. *Journal of Periodontology,* 1991, 62, 147-152.

[21] Bain, CA; Moy, PK. The association between the failure of dental implants and cigarette smoking. *International Journal of Oral and Maxillofacial Implants*, 1993, 8, 609-615.

[22] De Bruyn, H; Collaert, B. The effect of smoking on early implant failure. *Clinical Oral Implants Research,* 1994, 5, 260-264.

[23] Lindquist, LW; Carlsson, GE; Jemt, T. Association between marginal bone loss around osseointegrated mandibular implants and smoking habits: A 10 year follow-up study. *Journal of Dental Research,* 1997, 10, 1667-1674.

[24] Lindquist, LW; Carlsson, GE; Jemt, T. A prospective 15 year follow-up study of mandibular fixed prostheses supported by osseointegrated implants. Clinical results and marginal bone loss. *Clinical Oral Implants Research,* 1996, 7, 329-336.

[25] Haas, R; Haimbock, W; Mailath, G; Watzek, G. The relationship of smoking on peri-implant tissue: A retrospective study. *Journal of Prosthetic Dentistry,* 1996, 76, 592-596.

[26] Haas, R; Mensdorff-Pouilly, N; Watzek, G. Kaplan-Meier vergleichsanalysen von 3000 gesetzten implantaten in GOI gesellschaft fur orale implantologie (ed). *Jahrbuch Fur Orale Implantologie*. Berlin: Quintessenz 1994; 213-225.

[27] Hutton, JE; Heath, MR; Chai, JY; et al. Factors related to success and failure rates at 3-year follow-up in a multicenter study of overdentures supported by Bränemark implants. *International Journal of Oral and Maxillofacial Implants,* 1995, 10, 33-42.

[28] Dietrich, U; Lippold, R; Dirnmeyer, TH; Behneke, N; Wagner, W. Statistische ergebnisse zur implantatprognose am beispiel von 2017 IMZ - Implantaten unterschiedlicher indikationder letzten 13 jahre. *Zeit Zahnarztl Implant,* 1993, 9, 9-18.

[29] Mensdorff-Pouilly, N; Haas, R; Mailath, G; Watzek, G. The immediate implant: A retrospective study comparing the different types of immediate implantation. *International Journal of Oral and Maxillofacial Implants,* 1994, 9, 571-578.

[30] Silverstein, P. Smoking and wound healing. *American Journal of Medicine,* 1992, 93 (Suppl 1A), 22-24.

[31] Müller, AM; Pedersen, T; Villebro, N; Munksgaard, A. Effect of smoking on early complications after elective orthopaedic surgery. *Journal of Bone and Joint Surgery, British,* 2003, 85, 178-181.

[32] Adams, CI; Keating, JF; Court-Brown, CM. Cigarette smoking and open tibial fractures. *Injury,* 2001, 32, 61-65.

[33] Knuutinen, A; Kokkonen, N; Risteli, J; Vahakangas, K; Kallioinen, M; Salo, T; et al. Smoking affects collagen synthesis and extracellular matrix turnover in human skin. *British Journal of Dermatology,* 2002, 146, 588-594.

[34] Krueger, JK; Rohrich, RJ. Clearing the smoke: The scientific rationale for tobacco abstention with plastic surgery. *Plastic and Reconstructive Surgery,* 2001, 108, 1063-1073.

[35] Bergstrom, G; Floderus-Myrhed, B. Co-twin control study of the relationship between smoking and some periodontal disease factors. *Community Dentistry and Oral Epidemiology,* 1983, 11, 113-116.

[36] Krall, EA; Dawson-Hughes, B; Garvey, AJ; Garcia, RI. Smoking, smoking cessation and tooth loss. *Journal of Dental Research,* 1997, 76, 1653-1659.

[37] Cortellini, P; Tonetti, MS. Long-term tooth survival following regenerative treatment of intrabony defects. *Journal of Periodontology,* 2004, 75, 672-678.

[38] Zitzmann, NU; Scharer, P; Marinello, CP. Factors influencing the success of GBR. Smoking, timing of implant placement, implant location, bone quality and provisional restoration. *Journal of Clinical Periodontology,* 1999, 26, 673-682.

[39] Jensen, OT; Shulman, LB; Block, MS; Iacono, VJ. Report of the sinus consensus conference of 1996. *International Journal of Oral and Maxillofacial Implants,* 1998, 13 (Suppl), 5-45.

[40] Kirsch, A; Ackermann, KL; Hürzeler, MB; Hutmacher, D. Sinus grafting with porous hydroxyapatite. In: Jensen OT, editor. The Sinus Bone Graft, 1st ed. Chicago, IL: Quintessence; 1999; 79-94.

[41] Tong, DC; Drangsholt, M; Beirne, OR. A review of survival rates for implants placed in grafted maxillary sinuses using meta-analysis. *International Journal of Oral and Maxillofacial Implants,* 1998, 13, 175-182.

[42] Khoury, F. Augmentation of the sinus floor with mandibular bone block and simultaneous implantation: a 6-year clinical investigation. *International Journal of Oral and Maxillofacial Implants,* 1999, 14, 557-564.

[43] Hürzeler, MB; Kirsch, A; Ackermann, KL; Quinones, CR. Reconstruction of the severely resorbed maxilla with dental implants in the augmented maxillary sinus: a 5-year clinical investigation. *International Journal of Oral and Maxillofacial Implants,* 1996, 11, 466-475.

[44] Ziccardi, VB; Betts, NJ. Complications of maxillary sinus augmentation. In: Jensen OT, editor, The Sinus Bone Graft, 1st ed. Chicago, IL: Quintessence; 1999; 201-208.

[45] Bränemark, PI; Lindstrom, J; Hallen, O; Breine, U; Jeppson, PH; Ohman, A. Reconstruction of the defective mandible. *Scandinavian Journal of Plastic and Reconstructive Surgery,* 1975, 9, 116-128.

[46] Misch, CM. Ridge augmentation using mandibular ramus bone grafts for the placement of dental implants: presentation of a technique. *Practical Periodontics and Aesthetic Dentistry,* 1996, 8, 127-135.

[47] Misch, CM. Comparison of intraoral donor sites for onlay grafting prior to implant placement. *International Journal of Oral and Maxillofacial Implants,* 1997, 12, 767-776.

[48] Rissolo, AR; Bennett, J. Bone grafting and its essential role in implant dentistry. *Dental Clinics of North America,* 1998, 42, 91-116.

[49] Lynch, SE; Genco, RJ; Marx, R. Tissue Engineering: Applications in Maxillofacial Surgery and Periodontics, 1st ed. Chicago, IL: Quintessence Publishing; 1999; 83-98.

[50] Renouard, F; Rangert, B. Risk Factors in Implant Dentistry, 1st ed. Carol Stream, IL: Quintessence Publishing; 1999.

[51] Reynolds, MA, Bowers, GM. Periodontal regeneration following surgical treatment. *Current Opinion in Periodontology,* 1996, 3, 126-39.

[52] Rosen, PS; Marks, MH; Reynolds, MA. Influence of smoking on long-term clinical results of intrabony defects treated with regenerative therapy. *Journal of Periodontology,* 1996, 67, 1159-1163.

[53] Olson, JW; Dent, CD; Morris, HF; Ochi, S. Long-term assessment (5 to 71 months) of endosseous dental implants placed in the augmented maxillary sinus, *Annals of Periodontology,* 2000, 5, 152-156.

[54] Widmark, G; Andersson, B; Carlsson, GE; Lindvall, AM; Ivanoff, CJ. Rehabilitation of patients with severely resorbed maxillae by means of implants with or without bone grafts: a 3- to 5-year follow-up clinical report. *International Journal of Oral and Maxillofacial Implants,* 2001, 16, 73-79.

[55] Misch, CE; Scoretecci, G.M; Benner, KU. Implants and Restorative Dentistry. London: M. Duntz; 2001; 144-145.

[56] Kan, JY; Rungcharassaeng, K; Lozada, JL; Goodacre, CJ. Effects of smoking on implant success in grafted maxillary sinuses. *Journal of Prosthetic Dentistry,* 1999, 82, 307-311.

[57] Tal, H. Spontaneous early exposure of submerged implants: I. Classification and clinical observations. *Journal of Periodontology,* 1999, 70, 213-219.

[58] Schwartz-Arad, D; Grossman, Y; Chaushu, G. The clinical effectiveness of implants placed immediately into fresh extraction sites of molar teeth. *Journal of Periodontology,* 2000, 71, 839-844.

[59] Schwartz-Arad, D; Gulayev, N; Chaushu, G. Immediate versus non-immediate implantation for full arch fixed reconstruction following extraction of all residual teeth: A retrospective study. *Journal of Periodontology,* 2000, 71, 923-928.

[60] Schwartz-Arad, D; Yaniv, Y; Levin, L; Kaffe, I. A radiographic evaluation of cervical bone loss associated with immediate and non-immediate implants placed for fixed restorations in edentulous jaws, *Journal of Periodontology,* 2004, 75, 652-657.

[61] Levin, L; Herzberg, R; Dolev, E; Schwartz-Arad, D. Smoking and complications of onlay bone grafts and sinus lift operations. *International Journal of Oral and Maxillofacial Implants,* 2004, 19, 369-373.

[62] Schwartz-Arad, D; Samet, N; Mamlider, A. Smoking increases spontaneous exposure of dental implants between surgical stages. *Journal of Evidence-Based Dental Practice,* 2002, 2, 303-304.

[63] Schwartz-Arad, D; Samet, N; Samet, N. Single tooth replacement of missing molars: A retrospective study of 78 implants. *Journal of Periodontology,* 1999, 70, 449-454.

[64] Chaushu, G; Schwartz-Arad, D. Full-arch restoration of the jaw with fixed ceramometal prosthesis: Late implant placement. *Journal of Periodontology,* 1999, 70, 90-94.

[65] Schwartz-Arad, D; Chaushu, G. Full-arch restoration of the jaw with fixed ceramometal prosthesis. *International Journal of Oral and Maxillofacial Implants,* 1998, 13, 819-825.

[66] Schwartz-Arad, D; Chaushu, G. Immediate implant placement: a procedure without incisions. *Journal of Periodontology,* 1997, 68, 1110-1116.

[67] Haas, R; Mensdorff-Pouilly, N; Mailath, G; Watzek, G. Survival of 1,920 IMZ implants followed for up to 100 months. *International Journal of Oral and Maxillofacial Implants,* 1996, 11, 581-588.

[68] Schwartz-Arad, D; Herzberg, R; Dolev, E. The prevalence of surgical complications of the sinus graft procedure and its impact on implant survival. *Journal of Periodontology, 2004, 75,511-516.*

[69] Dixon, WJ. BMDP Statistical Software. San Francisco, CA: University of California Press; 1993.

[70] Centers for Disease Control and Prevention. Tobacco use: United States, 1900-1999. *Morbidity and Mortality Weekly Report,* 1999, 48, 986.

[71] Christen, AG. The impact of tobacco use and cessation on oral and dental diseases and conditions. *American Journal of Medicine,* 1992, 93, 25-31.

[72] Bergstrom, J; Eliasson, S. Noxious effect of cigarette smoking on periodontal health. *Journal of Periodontal Research,* 1987, 22, 513-517.

[73] Haber, J; Wattles, J; Crowley, M; et al. Evidence for cigarette smoking as a major risk factor for periodontitis. *Journal of Periodontology,* 1993, 64, 16-23.

[74] Gorman, LM; Lambert, PM; Morris, HF; Ochi, S; Winkler, S. The effect of smoking on implant survival at second stage surgery. *Implant Dentistry,* 1994, 3, 165-168.

[75] Morris, HF; Lambert, PM; Ochi, S. The influence of tobacco use on endosseous implant failures. In: Oral and Maxillofacial Surgery. Clinics of North America. London: WB Saunders Co; 1998; 255-274.

[76] McDermott, NE; Chuang, SK; Woo, VV; Dodson, TB. Complications of dental implants: identification, frequency, and associated risk factors. *International Journal of Maxillofacial Implants,* 2003, 18, 848-855.

[77] Wallace, RH. The relationship between cigarette smoking and dental implant failure. *European Journal of Prosthodontics and Restorative Dentistry,* 2000, 8, 103-106.

[78] Sennerby, L; Roos, J. Surgical determinants of clinical success of osseointegrated oral implants: a review of the literature. *International Journal of Prosthodontics,* 1998, 11, 408-420.

[79] Schwartz-Arad, D; Chaushu, G. The ways and wherefores of immediate placement of implants into fresh extraction sites: A literature review. *Journal of Periodontology,* 1997, 68, 915-923.

[80] Schwartz-Arad, D; Chaushu, G. Placement of implants into fresh extraction sites: 4 to 7 years retrospective evaluation of 95 immediate implants. *Journal of Periodontology,* 1997, 68, 1110-1116.

[81] Lambert, PM; Morris, HF; Ochi, S. The influence of smoking on 3-year clinical success of osseointegrated dental implants. *Annals of Peroidontology,* 2000, 5, 79-89.

[82] Esposito, M; Hirsch, JM; Lekholm, U; Thomsen, P. Biological factors contributing to failures of osseointegrated oral implants. (II) Etiopathogenesis. *European Journal of Oral Sciences,* 1998, 106, 721-764.

[83] Bergström, J; Eliasson, S. Cigarette smoking and alveolar bone height in subjects with a high standard of oral hygiene. *Journal of Clinical Periodontology,* 1987, 14, 466-469.

[84] Bergström, J; Eliasson, S; Preber, H. Cigarette smoking and periodontal bone loss. *Journal of Periodontology,* 1991, 62, 242-246.

[85] Bergström, J; Eliasson, S; Dock, J. Exposure to tobacco smoking and periodontal health. *Journal of Clinical Periodontology,* 2000, 27, 61-68.

[86] Chen, X; Wolff, L; Aeppli, D; Guo, Z; Luan, W; Baelum, V; Fejeskov, O. Cigarette smoking, salivary/gingival crevicular fluid cotinine and periodontal status. A 10-year longitudinal study. *Journal of Clinical Periodontology,* 2001, 28, 331-339.

[87] Bolin, A; Eklund, G; Frithiof, L; Lavstedt, S. The effect of changed smoking habits on marginal alveolar bone loss. *A longitudinal study. Swedish Dental Journal,* 1993, 17, 211-216.

[88] Hildebolt, CF; Pilgram, TK; Yokoyama-Crothers, N; Vannier, MW; Dotson, M; Muckerman, J; et al. Alveolar bone height and postcranial bone mineral density: negative effects of cigarette smoking and parity. *Journal of Periodontology,* 2000, 71, 683-689.

[89] Mullally, BH; Breen, B; Linden, GJ. Smoking and patterns of bone loss in early-onset periodontitis. *Journal of Periodontology,* 1999, 70, 394-401.

[90] Preber, H; Bergström, J; Linder, LE. Occurrence of periopathogens in smoker and non-smoker patients. *Journal of Clinical Periodontology,* 1992, 19, 667-671.

[91] Boström, L; Bergström, J; Dahlén, G; Linder, LE. Smoking and subgingival microflora in periodontal disease. *Journal of Clinical Periodontology,* 2001, 28, 212-219.

[92] Haffajee, AD; Socransky, SS. Relationship of cigarette smoking to the subgingival microbiota. *Journal of Clinical Periodontology,* 2001, 28, 377-388.

[93] Haffajee, AD; Socransky, SS. Relationship of cigarette smoking to attachment level profiles. *Journal of Clinical Periodontology,* 2001, 28, 283-295.

[94] van der Weijden, GA; de Slegte, C; Timmerman, MF; van der Velden, U. Periodontitis in smokers and non-smokers: intra-oral distribution of pockets. *Journal of Clinical Periodontology,* 2001, 28, 955-960.

[95] van Winkelhoff, AJ; Bosch-Tijhof, CJ; Winkel, EG; van der Reijden, WA. Smoking affects the subgingival microflora in periodontitis. *Journal of Periodontology,* 2001, 72, 666-671.

[96] Schwartz-Arad, D; Samet, N; Samet, N; Mamlider, A. Smoking and complications of endosseous dental implants. *Journal of Periodontology,* 2002, 73, 153-157.

[97] Bain, CA. Smoking and implant failure - benefits of a smoking cessation protocol. *International Journal of Oral and Maxillofacial Implants,* 1996, 11, 756-759.

[98] Miller, PD, Jr. Root coverage using the free soft tissue autograft following citric acid application. *International Journal of Periodontics and Restorative Dentistsry,* 1985, 5, 15-37.

[99] Sorensen, LT; Jorgensen, T. Short-term pre-operative smoking cessation intervention does not affect postoperative complications in colorectal surgery: a randomized clinical trial. *Colorectal Diseases,* 2003, 5, 347-352.

[100] Padubidri, AN; Yetman, R; Browne, E; Lucas, A; Papay, F; Larive, B; Zins, J. Complications of postmastectomy breast reconstructions in smokers, ex-smokers, and nonsmokers. *Plastic and Reconstructive Surgery,* 2001, 107, 342-349.

[101] Cryer, P; Haymond, MW; Santiago, JV; Shah, SD. Norepinephrine and epinephrine release and androgenic mediation of smoking associated homodynamic and metabolic events. *New England Journal of Medicine,* 1976, 295, 573-577.

[102] Sarine, CL; Austin, JC; Nickel, WO. Effects of smoking and digital blood flow volume. *Journal of the American Medical Association,* 1974, 229, 1327-1328.

[103] MacFarlane, GD; Herzberg, MC; Wolff, LF; Hardie, NA. Refractory periodontitis associated with abnormal polymorphonuclear leukocyte phagocytosis and cigarette smoking. *Journal of Periodontology,* 1992, 63, 908-913.

[104] Noble, RC; Penny, BB. Comparison of leukocyte count and function in smoking and non-smoking young men. *Infection and Immunology,* 1975, 12, 550-555.

[105] Snyder, HB; Caughman, G; Lewis, J; Billman, MA; Schuster, G. Nicotine modulation of in vitro human gingival fibroblast $\gamma 1$ integrin expression. *Journal of Periodontology,* 2002, 73, 505-510.

[106] Poggi, P; Rota, MT; Boratto, R. The volatile fraction of cigarette smoke induces alterations in the human gingival fibroblast cytoskeleton. *Journal of Periodontal Research,* 2002, 37, 230-235.

In: Progress in Smoking and Health Research
Editor: T. C. Jeffries, pp. 89-115
ISBN: 978-1-60021-686-2

Chapter IV

Smoking Cessation Strategies in New York City: 2002-2006

***Sarah B. Perl*[1], *Jennifer A. Ellis*[2], *Laura E. Vichinsky*[3], *Kelly Larson*[4], *Joslyn Levy*[5], *Lynn Silver*[6], *Mary T. Bassett*[7] *and Thomas R. Frieden*[8]**

[1] Bureau of Tobacco Control; [2] Bureau of Tobacco Control;
[3] Bureau of Tobacco Control; [4] Bureau of Chronic Disease;
[5] Bureau of Chronic Disease; [6] Bureau of Chronic Disease;
[7] Deputy Commissioner, Division of Health Promotion and Disease Prevention; [8] Commissioner; New York City Department of Health and Mental Hygiene

Abstract

In 2002, the New York City Department of Health and Mental Hygiene (DOHMH) launched an aggressive, comprehensive tobacco control program comprised of five components: taxation, legal action, cessation services, public education and evaluation. Smoking cessation has been delivered through two main approaches: the promotion of cessation behaviors, and the provision of specific population-based and targeted cessation services.

This chapter provides information on both the promotion of cessation behaviors and the provision of cessation services. It describes how cessation behaviors (e.g., making a quit attempt, adopting a smoke-free home policy) have been supported by the other four components of DOHMH's five-point tobacco control program (taxation, legal action, public education and evaluation) as well as provides details about the cessation services offered (giveaways of nicotine replacement therapy, face-to-face education of health care providers and their staff, and coordination of cessation services with the city's public hospital system).

By aggressively implementing a comprehensive tobacco control that includes the provision of cessation services and the promotion of cessation behaviors through taxation, legal action, public education and evaluation, New York City has been able to produce significant declines in smoking prevalence in less than 5 years.

Introduction

In 2002, the New York City (NYC) Department of Health and Mental Hygiene (DOHMH) launched an aggressive, comprehensive tobacco control program comprised of five components: taxation, legal action, cessation services, public education and evaluation. Smoking cessation has been delivered through two main approaches: the promotion of cessation behaviors, and the provision of specific population-based and targeted cessation services.

Smoking is the leading cause of preventable death in NYC, responsible for 1 in 3 preventable deaths, and 1 in 6 deaths overall (CDC, SAMMEC, 2006). One third of NYC's more than 1 million adult smokers will die prematurely from a smoking-related illness (Centers for Disease Control and Prevention, 2002); smokers who die from a smoking-related illness lose on average 14 years of life (CDC, 2002).

The role of cessation in efforts to reduce tobacco prevalence has been widely acknowledged. In combination with reductions in initiation rates, increases in cessation among current smokers are essential to successfully reduce adult smoking (Mendez, Warner and Courant, 1998). Moreover, for national adult smoking prevalence to even approach the Healthy People 2010 goal of 16%, it has been modeled that at least a 50% reduction in youth initiation and a doubling of adult cessation would need to occur between 2000 and 2010 (Mendez and Warner, 2000). An estimated 70% of smokers want to quit (CDC, 1997), and 66% of NYC smokers made a quit attempt in 2004 (NYC DOHMH, Community Health Survey, 2004).

This chapter provides information on both the promotion of cessation behaviors and the provision of cessation services. It describes how cessation behaviors (e.g., making a quit attempt, adopting a smoke-free home policy) have been supported by the other four components of DOHMH's five-point tobacco control program (taxation, legal action, public education and evaluation) as well as provides details about the cessation services offered (giveaways of nicotine replacement therapy, face-to-face education of health care providers and their staff, and coordination of cessation services with the city's public hospital system).

Promotion of Cessation Behaviors

Cessation is promoted by all the components of NYC's comprehensive tobacco control program. Cessation services by design promote cessation. But cessation behaviors are also promoted by the other four components of DOHMH's tobacco control program. The cessation behaviors that are promoted include actions taken by smokers that prompt them to make a quit attempt or increase their chance of successfully quitting (e.g., setting a quit date, getting medications, enlisting the social support of family and friends in their quit attempt (CDC, 2006a)). They also include actions taken by non-smokers that support a smoker in making a quit attempt and successfully quitting (e.g., adopting a smoke-free home policy, encouraging a smoker to quit, and informing a smoker about available cessation services.) The way taxation, legal action, education and evaluation promote cessation is described in greater detail below.

Taxation

In 2002, DOHMH began implementing its current comprehensive tobacco control program by focusing on making it harder to smoke. Raising the price of cigarettes -- typically through taxation -- is the single most effective strategy to prevent and reduce tobacco use (Jha and Chaloupka, 2000; CDC, 1998). Increasing the price of cigarettes promotes cessation behaviors (e.g., making a quit attempt) because it introduces a higher utility cost to maintaining a consistent level of cigarette consumption. In 2002, NYC increased the excise tax on cigarettes from $0.08 to $1.50 per pack one month following an NYS increase of $1.50, bringing the price per pack to almost $7, of which nearly 50% was tax. At that time, it was the highest combined tax in the nation. (As of 2006, NYC has the 6th highest combined U.S. tax.)

Taxation reduces smoking prevalence and promotes cessation behaviors because of the price elasticity of cigarettes, which is approximately -0.25 for adults (CDC, 1998). Teens are more price-sensitive than adults because they have less disposable income; estimated youth price elasticity is at least -0.5 (Powell, Tauras, and Ross, 2005; Ross and Chaloupka, 2003; Liang, Chaloupka, Nichter and Clayton, 2003). Thus, for adults, a 50 percent increase in the price of cigarettes leads to a 12.5% decrease in consumption. For teens, a 50 percent increase in the price of cigarettes leads to at least a 25% decrease in consumption.

Legal Action

Ample evidence on the hazards associated with exposure to secondhand smoke made passage of the Smoke-Free Air Act (SFAA) of 2002 – which prohibited indoor public smoking -- DOHMH's next priority to reduce tobacco use. The SFAA made virtually all workplaces in NYC smoke-free, including restaurants and bars. Despite significant concern that this law would reduce revenue in these food-service establishments a one-year assessment showed that tax receipts rose, employment increased and compliance with the law was more than 99%. Moreover, as a result of the new legislation, 150,000 fewer New Yorkers are exposed to secondhand smoke on the job (NYC Department of Finance et al., 2003).

The SFAA promotes cessation behaviors – including voluntary adoption of smoke-free home policies because of increased awareness of the hazards of secondhand smoke – by reducing the venues where smokers can use cigarettes, and by sensitizing those exposed to secondhand smoke to advocate for smoke-free environments.

Education

Public education -- about the dangers of both smoking and exposure to secondhand smoke and the benefits of quitting -- has contributed significantly to the promotion of cessation behaviors. Public education has been delivered by DOHMH through a variety of printed materials for health care providers and the public, as well as through coordinated media campaigns. In 2003, DOHMH launched "Everybody Loves a Quitter" – a media campaign that featured couples, families and friends congratulating their quitter because "Everyone loves a quitter when it's someone who has quit smoking." The campaign included both print and on-air components. Education – in print and on the air – promotes cessation by providing direct messages to smokers to quit, by enlisting friends and family of smokers to provide them with support, and by providing information on quit smoking services that are available in NYC to help smokers.

In 2006, DOHMH launched its largest media campaign to date; the campaign sought to increase smokers' awareness of reasons to quit, to provide supportive messages to quitters, and to direct those trying to quit to cessation services. Both the content and the size of the campaign were unprecedented for DOHMH. The campaign used seven different groups of ads. With the exception of the DOHMH-produced inspirational "Everybody Loves a Quitter" ads, all the ads were produced by other tobacco control programs and were hard-hitting. Ads that depict the health consequences of smoking in a graphic or emotion-provoking way are recalled as the most helpful by quitters (Biener et al., 2006).

The 2006 ads included three groups of testimonial ads from sick or dying smokers including Pam Laffin, a woman suffering from smoking-related emphysema, who died at 31; Mike Samms, a man battling smoking-related lung cancer, who died at 39; and Ronaldo Martinez, a man who underwent a tracheotomy at 39 as a result of smoking-induced laryngeal cancer (CDC, MCRC, 2006a; CDC, MCRC, 2006b, CDC, MCRC, 2006c). Another group of ads, titled "Every Cigarette Is Doing You Damage,"(CDC, MCRC, 2006d) featured graphic images of the effects of smoking on the lungs, arteries and brains of smokers. Another group of ads depicted the effects of secondhand smoke exposure. A final group of ads targeted to Chinese-speaking smokers delivered messages on both secondhand smoke exposure and the health consequence of smoking.

DOHMH aired the seven groups of ads between January and October 2006, at a volume of between 100 to 600 gross ratings points (GRPs) per week. (GRPs are an industry-specific standardized measure of the size of a campaign.) DOHMH did not air any ads between July and mid-September. Figure 1 shows the relationship between the number of GRPs aired and calls to 3-1-1, NYC's toll-free non-emergency government information line, by smokers seeking assistance in quitting for January through October 2006. (In order to assess response to the media campaign without conflating response to the NYC's 2006 nicotine patch giveaway discussed below, calls for enrollment in the giveaway are not shown on this graph.) As figure 1 demonstrates, calls for quit smoking assistance – one measure of responsiveness to advertisements – increased during weeks when DOHMH aired a large volume of GRPs.

In order to control for the role of seasonality in call volumes, the call volumes for January through June 2006 were compared with the same time period in 2005, during which DOHMH only aired ads to promote the 2005 nicotine patch giveaway discussed below. In 2006, the year of the large-scale media campaign, calls to 3-1-1 nearly quadrupled to 30,000, compared to January through June 2005, during which time about 7,500 calls were logged.

Media campaigns have traditionally been viewed as public education. However, media campaigns also promote cessation behaviors (Hyland et al, 2006). One recent population-based study found that quitters cited anti-tobacco television ads in helping them quit more often than other cessation aids including NRT, quitlines and professional help (Biener et al.,

2006). Another study identified a dose-response relationship between exposure to anti-tobacco media campaigns and quit attempts (Mudde, De Vries, 1999). While media campaigns can be effective in educating the public about the dangers of smoking and the benefits of quitting, their dual utility in also promoting cessation behaviors make them one of the strongest tools of comprehensive tobacco control.

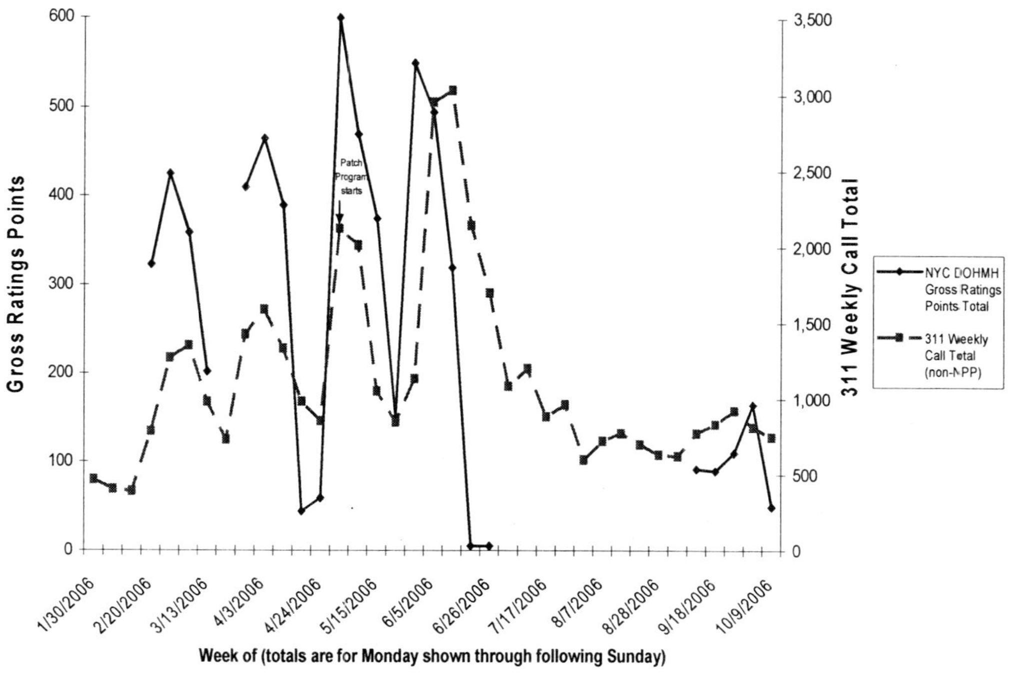

Figure 1. NYC Tobacco Control Weekly Media Ratings Points and Quit Smoking Service 311 calls through week of 10/9/2006 (Nicotine Patch Program Calls not shown).

Evaluation

Information about smoking prevalence and smoking behaviors in NYC – e.g., declines in adult smoking rates, increases in adoption of smoke-free home policies, declines in exposure to secondhand smoke at home and at work -- are publicized through press conferences and press releases to the media. Coverage of changes in these smoking-related behaviors promotes cessation behaviors – e.g., quitting, making a quit attempt, and adopting a smoke-free home policy – by providing reminders that smoking is a health hazard, by providing evidence that most NYC smokers have already quit, and by providing support that quit attempts can be successful (as most smokers make several quit attempts before they succeed)(Fiore et al., 2000).

In 2003, DOHMH reported a sharp decline in adult smoking prevalence in NYC after a decade during which the adult smoking prevalence had been stagnant. Between 2002 and 2003, smoking among NYC adults dropped from 21.6% to 19.2% -- an 11% decline (Frieden et al., 2005) which continued in 2004 to 18.4%. Between 2004 and 2005, adult prevalence leveled off; the 2005 adult prevalence of 18.9% was virtually identical to the 2004 rate of 18.4%.

DOHMH was able to document these changes in prevalence through a large-scale Community Health Survey (CHS) that tracks health-related behaviors, including smoking and smoking-related behaviors such as cessation attempts. Similar to the annual Behavioral Risk Factor Surveillance System, NYC's CHS is an ongoing telephone survey of 10,000 adults that provides both neighborhood and citywide estimates on a broad range of risk factors. The CHS has been conducted annually by DOHMH since 2002.

Data generated by the CHS and by other tobacco-related surveys provides opportunities to keep tobacco in the news. While public education through paid media is effective in delivering health-related messages to targeted audiences and the general public, generating earned media – by providing media outlets with data they turn into news stories – is an equally important approach. Having an earned media strategy that uses data to ensure that tobacco is a regular news story promotes cessation behaviors on a population scale by delivering messages through venues with a broad audience.

Promotion of Cessation Behaviors Conclusion and Future Direction

Taxation, legal action, education and evaluation promote cessation behaviors. DOHMH continues to pursue these four components of its comprehensive five-point tobacco control program. DOHMH is currently seeking to increase the NYC cigarette excise taxes by an additional 50 cents. Planning is underway to develop and air several DOHMH-produced ads for 2006 and 2007. Retaining the hard-hitting theme of its successful 2006 ads, DOHMH is reaching out to NYC smokers whose lives and health have been comprised by smoking to tell their personal stories. To complement the CHS measures of smoking-related behaviors in NYC, DOHMH has designed and implemented a longitudinal survey to provide further insight into the impact of specific elements of its comprehensive tobacco control program on a cohort of NYC smokers and recent quitters. DOHMH also promotes cessation though the provision of cessation services, such as giveaways of nicotine replacement therapy, face-to-face education of health care providers and their staff, and coordination of cessation services with the city's public hospital system. Details of these are described below.

Provision of Cessation Services

Between 2003 and 2006, DOHMH focused primarily on making it easier to quit through the provision of three cessation services to NYC smokers: giveaways of nicotine replacement therapy, face-to-face education of health care providers and their staff, and coordination of cessation services with the city's public hospital system. In accordance with recommendations from the 2000 U.S. Public Health Service Guidelines, each of these cessation strategies promoted increased access to and use of nicotine replacement therapy (NRT). Smokers who attempt to quit with the help of NRT are up to twice as likely to succeed as smokers who do not use medication (Fiore et al., 2000; Silagy, Lancaster, Stead, Mant and Fowler, 2004).

DOHMH's efforts to promote pharmacology-based cessation services were supported in part by a donation from Pfizer Inc. In 2004, Pfizer donated 325,000 boxes of NRT patches to DOHMH. The patches were repackaged into 100,000 six- or eight-week courses of therapy and distributed during 2004 and 2005.

Nicotine Replacement Therapy (NRT) Giveaways

In 2002, most states operated quitlines which made cessation assistance – including self-help materials, telephone counseling and some forms of nicotine replacement therapy (NRT) – more accessible to smokers trying to quit (CDC, 2004). But nationally, quitlines reach less than 6% of smokers, with most states reporting serving just 2-3% of smokers (CDC, 2003). The addition of NRT to the services provided by a quitline has been shown to increase call volume in multiple states and countries (An et al., 2006; Alberg et al., 2004). For example, New Zealand reported an overwhelming response to a program launched in 2000 through their quitline which made up to 8 weeks of subsidized NRT available to smokers making a quit attempt. The New Zealand campaign generated significant media attention, was viewed positively by smokers using the new quitline service, and increased the number of people accessing the New Zealand Quitline (Grigg and Glasgow, 2003).

In 2003, DOHMH began offering NRT to smokers for a limited time to determine if a direct-to-the-public giveaway was a viable avenue to increase success rates among smokers attempting to quit. Excluding 2004 – when DOHMH piloted distributing NRT primarily through its community- and clinic-based cessation partners – DOHMH has implemented a time-limited direct-to-the public NRT giveaway to NYC smokers annually. This section describes the details of each year DOHMH has conducted an NRT giveaway. Table 1 summarizes the major programmatic implementation differences between years.

In all three years, program eligibility remained consistent: enrollees needed to be NYC residents, be at least 18 years of age, smoke at least 10 cigarettes per day, be willing to make a quit attempt in the next 7 days, be willing to receive a follow-up call from DOHMH, not be currently using other forms of NRT, and have no medical contraindications for using NRT, such as a recent heart attack. Counseling calls following shipment of NRT patches to enrollees were attempted each year, based on evidence that combination therapy (medication combined with counseling) can be more effective that single modality interventions (Fiore et al., 2000). The counseling was delivered by telemarketers trained by DOHMH who used computer-based scripts. Telemarketers also collected information during the call on patch usage, adverse reactions, making or continuing a quit attempt and other cessation-related topics.

Table 1. NYC Nicotine Replacement Therapy (NRT) Program Implementation, 2003-2006

Year	2003	2005	2006
Partner	NYS Smokers' Quitline	NYC 3-1-1	NYC 3-1-1
NRT courses available	35,000	45,000	35,000
Length of program (days)	43	36	34
NRT provided	2 wks 21mg; 2 wks 14 mg; 2 wks 7 mg	6 wks 15mg	4 wks 21mg; option for 2 additional wks 14 mg
Other materials	• Letter from Health Commissioner (English and Spanish) • Patch use instruction sheet (English and Spanish) • NYS Smokers' Quitline stop-smoking guide • List of local smoking-cessation programs	• Letter from Health Commissioner (English and Spanish) • Patch use instruction sheet (English and Spanish) • NYC DOHMH Health Bulletin with tips on quitting smoking including a list of local smoking cessation programs	• Letter from Health Commissioner (English and Spanish) • Patch use instruction sheet (English and Spanish) • NYC DOHMH Health Bulletin with tips on quitting smoking including a list of local smoking cessation programs • Postcard to return to request an additional 2 weeks of patches
Follow-up provided	Calls at 3 weeks and 14 weeks to all enrollees (phone only)	Calls at 3 weeks to 10-20 cigarettes per day smokers (phone and email)	Calls at 3 weeks to 10-20 cigarettes per day smokers (phone and email)
Outreach: Press Releases, Press Conferences and Press Events	• 1 press release • 1 press conference	• 6 press releases • 2 press conferences	• 5 press releases • 1 press conference • 1 press event at 3-1-1

Table 1. (Continued).

Outreach: Earned Media Coverage	• Launch: multiple newspapers, and television and radio stations covered • Ongoing: some reported on progress throughout program	• Launch: multiple newspapers, and television and radio stations covered, but coverage was more descriptive and less in-depth • Ongoing: limited coverage of program process, but helped by multiple press releases	• Launch: multiple newspapers, and television and radio stations covered, but coverage was even less in-depth than 2005 • Ongoing: some coverage of program process, helped by multiple press releases and by Commissioner appearance at press event
Outreach: Paid Media	Neighborhood-specific outreach (areas with high smoking prevalence): fliers in community newspapers	Short television advertisements ("bumpers") informing NYC residents about the program and encouraging them to call 3-1-1 to see if they were eligible	Bumpers appended to major hard-hitting anti-tobacco media campaign that ran concurrently; various new venues, announcements and ads (during Major League Baseball, electronic message board at ferry terminal, TV news station "tickers.")

The main outcomes monitored for each program year are shown in table 2. Program enrollment for each year, including the number of people who began the screening process and the number who completed the screening relative to the total number eligible, is tracked closely. Callers dropped out of the screening primarily because they declined to answer eligibility criteria and optional demographic questions to facilitate assessing who was being reached by the program. Callers who were found eligible were sent NRT and supporting materials through the mail. Eligible callers from all three years with provided with 4 to 6 weeks of NRT. The percent of eligible NYC smokers (calculated using NYC Community Health Survey weighted population estimates) enrolled each year varied from 5% to 8% (with the difference being were primarily due to the amount of NRT available for distribution).

Table 2. NYC Nicotine Replacement Therapy (NRT) Program Outcomes, 2003-2006

Year	**2003**	**2005**	**2006**
Program Enrollment			
Called for patches	NA	87,000	55,000
Completed screening process	41,000	61,000	43,000
Eligible (% of screened)	35,000 (85%)	45,000 (74%)	35,000 (81%)
Eligible for counseling call (% of eligible)	35,000 (100%)	32,000 (71%)	24,000 (69%)
Received counseling call (% of eligible)	one call: 15,212 (45%) two calls: 5,128 (15%)	19,800 (62%)	12,300 (51%)
% of eligible NYC smokers enrolled	5.0%	8.4%	6.6%
Estimated # quits attributable to program*	6,300	8,100	6,300
Estimated # smoking-related deaths averted**	2,100	2,700	2,100
Program Cost			
Cost of patches	$2.5 million	No cost (donated)	$1.6 million
Cost of outreach	No costs	$1.2 million	$1.4 million
Cost of counseling	$100,000	$315,000	$340,000
Cost of materials development and mailing	$200,000	$440,000	$320,000
Total Cost	$2.8 million	$2.0 million	$3.7 million
Cost per quit (approximate)	$440	$240	$580
Cost per death averted (approximate)	$1,333	$724	$1743

*Estimated program-attributable quits based on 18% attributable quit from 2003 program evaluation (Miller et al., 2005)

** Estimated deaths averted based on assumption that one-third of quitters would have died from a smoking-related illness (Fiore et al., 2000).

The overall cost of the program, estimated cost per program-attributable quit and estimated cost per smoking-related death averted are also shown in table 2. The cost of each program ranged from $2.0 million to $3.7 million. Differences in costs are primarily due to the donation of the medication (as in 2005) and the amount of paid media outreach necessary to create sufficient call volume (as in 2005 and 2006). Costs per quit and death averted are based on findings from the 2003 evaluation, showing that the program-attributable quits are about 18% of those enrolled (Miller et al., 2005), and evidence showing that about one third of smokers die from a smoking-related illness (Fiore et al., 2000).

Although tables 1 and 2 summarize some of the variations in program implementation throughout the three years of the program, the section below provides details on changes to the program and differences in program outcomes.

2003 NRT Giveaway

The key component of the 2003 giveaway that is different from other years of the program is the intensive evaluation conducted by DOHMH in coordination with New York State Smokers' Quitline and the Roswell Park Cancer Institute. Two follow-up studies were conducted with subgroups of 2003 NRT patch recipients: one at 6 months following enrollment and one at 12 months following enrollment (Miller et al., 2005; Cummings et al., 2006). Quit rates and other data were calculated based on self-reported responses to questions about smoking status and cessation behavior.

The 6-month evaluation assessed smoking status among 1,305 randomly selected participants (response rate=60%). Results of the 6-month evaluation suggest that applying the conservative assumption that all non-responders continued to smoke yielded a quit rate of 20%, more than three times the quit rate of a comparison group (6%) comprised of people who were eligible for NRT but did not receive it because of incorrect addresses. However, if it is assumed that non-responders quit at the same rate as responders, then the quit rate of 33% is almost six times the 6% quit rate of the comparison group (Miller et al., 2005).

In addition to overall quit rates, the 6-month evaluation included analyses of demographic and program characteristics associated with higher quit rates. These analyses informed subsequent patch giveaway programs. In particular, a logistic regression analysis of quit rates at 6-month follow-up showed a significant interaction ($p = .02$) between receipt of counseling call and level of smoking at baseline. Smokers of 10-19 cigarettes per day who received counseling quit at a higher rate (50.3%) than those smokers of 10-19 cigarettes per day who had not received counseling (27%). Similarly, smokers of 20 cigarettes per day who received counseling quit at a higher rate (38.4%) compared to those smokers of 20 cigarettes per day who had not received counseling (31.7%). In contrast, smokers of more than 20 cigarettes per day who received counseling quit at essentially the same rate (29%) as those who did not receive counseling (27.2%).

2005 NRT Giveaway

In 2005, three differences in program implementation merit further explanation. First, the 2005 program was conducted in collaboration with the NYC Department of Information Technology and Telecommunications (DoITT), which runs 3-1-1, the toll-free NYC non-emergency government information line. This collaboration allowed DOHMH to keep all programmatic activities local and created greater flexibility in both program design and implementation.

The second major difference in the implementation of the 2005 program was the decision to provide counseling calls only to patch recipients who smoked between 10 and 20 cigarettes per day. This decision was made in direct response to the 2003 findings noted above showing that the counseling call was only effective for those who smoked 10 to 20 cigarettes per day at enrollment.

Third, in 2005, counseling was also offered both over the phone and through a secure website hosted by DOHMH. Patch recipients who provided their email addresses at enrollment were sent an email about one month after receiving NRT. The email provided a link to DOHMH's secure website, where a computer-based application delivered counseling and collected information based on participants' answers to cessation-related questions. Of the 32,000 callers eligible for counseling, about 13,500 (42%) provided email addresses. Of the 13,500 participants who provided an email address, 1,860 (14%) responded to the email and obtained counseling through the website.

Providing multiple venues for participants to access counseling may increase the number of participants who accept counseling. Because NRT coupled with counseling can be more effective than NRT alone (Fiore et al., 2000), offering counseling through multiple methods may increase overall program quit rates.

2006 NRT Giveaway

In 2006, DOHMH conducted its third citywide NRT distribution. As in 2005, the 2006 giveaway was conducted in collaboration with 3-1-1. The two major additional differences in the implementation of the 2006 program were the methods used for outreach, the inclusion of a postcard in the mailed NRT to access additional NRT and the requirement that eligibility include agreement from callers that they could be contacted by DOHMH at any time in the future (instead of just for 12 months).

As mentioned above, in January 2006, DOHMH launched a large, hard-hitting anti-tobacco media campaign, airing graphic ads on both cable and broadcast television at a very high volume. This media campaign generated significant press coverage. One anti-smoking ad featured plaque being squeezed out of the artery of a smoker (CDC, MCRC, 2006d). Another ad featured a man in the shower cleaning his tracheotomy hole, the results of a diagnosis of smoking–related larygeal cancer at age 39 (CDC, MCRC, 2006c). Because this campaign extended through June 2006, it overlapped with the 2006 NRT giveaway. The campaign served as a vehicle to alert smokers to the availability of medication through the 2006 giveaway.

The second major difference in the implementation of the 2006 NRT giveaway was the decision to send each enrollee a 4-week supply of patches along with a postcard to return to request an additional 2 weeks of patches. This programmatic change was made primarily in response to literature showing that distribution of fewer than 6 weeks of patches may results in less waste of NRT and comparable quit rates among participants (Cummings et al., 2006). Similar findings emerged from the 12-month evaluation of the 2003 program, showing that less than 20% of participants used all 6 weeks of patches provided (Cummings et al., 2006). Of the 35,000 participants who received 4 weeks of NRT patches, 3,600 (10%) requested the additional two weeks of patches. The low volume of requests for additional patches may have been due to recipients not understanding the purpose of the included postcard or not feeling that additional NRT would be helpful. A 6-month evaluation of the 2006 program is underway to address these questions.

The third difference was that during intake in 2003 and 2005, the eligibility requirements included agreement from callers to be contacted by DOHMH during the next year for follow up to assess smoking status. In 2006, the time period for re-contacting callers was unbounded so that DOHMH could contact smokers at any time in the future to assess smoking status, and use the list for outreach to offer future cessation interventions.

NRT Giveaway Conclusions and Future Directions

Since 2003, DOHMH has distributed 115,000 courses of NRT (about 4.4 million individual patches) to NYC smokers through annual giveaways. Based on the 20-33% quit rate established in evaluating the 2003 efforts, these giveaways have helped between 23,000 and 38,000 smokers quit. Assuming one-third of these smokers will not die from a smoking-related illness (Fiore et al., 2000), the giveaways have prevented between 7,500 and 12,500 NYC smoking-related deaths. The cost per quit ranged from $240 and $580, depending primarily on the costs of outreach and medication for each year. The cost per premature death prevented ranged from $725 to $1,740.

Planning is currently underway to evaluate 2006 effort. The evaluation design is similar to that employed in 2003; those receiving patches will be compared with those who did not receive patches due to an undeliverable address. This design will allow for determination of the quit rate in a large-scale giveaway implemented after several years of comprehensive tobacco control programming had been in place. Additionally, although participants who requested the additional 2 weeks of patches available in the 2006 program are likely systematically different from those who did not, analyses will be conducted to assess any difference in quit rates between the two groups. Because this program was not designed as a randomized controlled trial, this analysis will not allow for conclusive understanding of the change in quit rates resulting from the additional 2 weeks of patches. However, if quit rates are comparable, DOHMH could distribute 4-week courses of patches to an additional 10% more smokers (4,000) seeking assistance for the same cost.

Planning is also underway for DOHMH's 2007 direct-to-the-public giveaway. Innovations for the 2007 effort will include provision of NRT medications (gum) for smokers who use fewer than 10 cigarettes, new outreach venues to reach groups that under-enroll in the giveaways (e.g., men and young people aged 18-24), facilitating household enrollment so that multiple smokers in the same home can enroll simultaneously, reaching out to 2006 enrollees to provide another course of medication to facilitate a new quit attempt and running the giveaway program for a limited number of days (instead of a limited number of courses of medication).

Public Health Detailing

The second cessation service implemented by DOHMH was face-to-face education of health care providers and their staff. Visits with health care providers and their staff present a unique opportunity to provide cessation education, medication and counseling to smokers.

More than 70% of smokers see a physician every year, averaging 5.3 visits annually (US Department of Health and Human Services, 1994). Because of this sustained access to smokers, health care providers and their staff can play an important role in influencing patient smoking behavior. As little as three minutes of clinician time spent providing smokers with brief cessation intervention can be effective in increasing tobacco quit rates (Fiore et al., 2000).

National guidelines for the treatment of tobacco use recommend that all health care providers identify, track and offer treatment to patients who smoke (Fiore et al., 2000). Counseling, nicotine replacement therapy (NRT) and other medications can double quit rates (Fiore et al., 2000). However, only 67% of doctors speak to their patients about their smoking behavior, and in 1995 only 29% of health care providers provided counseling to smokers (up from 20% in 1991). The proportion of smokers provided NRT was .6% in 1991, 3% in 1993, and 1.3% in 1995 (Thorndike, Rigotti, Stafford and Singer, 1998). Given that clinical interventions to reduce smoking have been underutilized, the introduction of programs to encourage the delivery of evidence-based cessation interventions by health care providers is a promising strategy for reducing the prevalence of smoking.

The goal of DOHMH's Public Health Detailing program is to encourage and assist health care providers to deliver evidence-based interventions for health promotion and disease prevention (Larson et al., 2006). The program relies on face-to-face meetings in physicians' offices, an approach pioneered by the pharmaceutical industry. Outreach visits, combined with social marketing techniques such as using commercial-quality educational materials, have been shown to positively impact physician behavior (O'Brien et al., 1997).

In 2003, DOHMH adapted the outreach model used in pharmaceutical detailing to promote ("sell") key public health interventions to health care providers and their staff. The Public Health Detailing program continued DOHMH's long history of promoting clinical best practices and built on its "brand" strength as a technical expert with no vested interests. DOHMH publications, such as *City Health Information* (NYC DOHMH, 2006), a monthly bulletin sent to all physicians in NYC, have been distributed to licensed NYC health care providers since the 1980s, and DOHMH's expertise in the design and implementation of public health interventions is nationally recognized.

The launch of DOHMH's Public Health Detailing program was supported by its collaboration with Pfizer Inc. The partnership with Pfizer enabled DOHMH to draw on the pharmaceutical company's detailing expertise to adapt this private sector marketing strategy for the field of public health (Larson et al., 2006) and in particular to develop a staff training program on communications and selling skills specific to health care providers and their staff. As previously mentioned, Pfizer donated a significant amount of NRT to DOHMH; the detailing program provided a venue to distribute the Pfizer-donated NRT.

Public Health Detailing began by promoting the use of three highly effective essential clinical preventive services known to be underutilized: influenza vaccination, colon cancer screening and smoking cessation. DOHMH representatives conducted topic-specific campaigns for 10-12 weeks each, making unscheduled visits to health care practices. Employing a "total office call" approach at each practice, representatives met with health care providers (physicians, nurse practitioners and physician assistants) and their staff (nurses, medical assistants, managers and clerks). The program targeted three underserved areas of

NYC -- East and Central Harlem, North and Central Brooklyn and the South Bronx. These three communities, in which DOHMH had established District Public Health Offices, were selected because they have the highest rates of risk behaviors, morbidity and mortality and the lowest rates of treatment for a range of conditions compared to other NYC communities. Each of the Public Health Detailing representatives was assigned to one of these communities. Co-locating the detailing program with the district office enabled the detailing representatives to benefit from the staff's knowledge of the neighborhoods' particular characteristics and health issues, and provided the district offices with a new venue to communicate with health care providers.

District Public Health Office Smoking Cessation Campaign

Launched in May 2004, the smoking cessation campaign focused on delivering three key recommendations: 1) assess smoking status and readiness to quit at every visit; 2) provide brief cessation counseling and 3) prescribe medications to assist patients in becoming tobacco-free. Recommendations were delivered in person and supported by materials designed especially for the detailing campaign. At each practice, representatives distributed Public Health Detailing "action kits." The action kit has the high-quality look and feel of a commercially developed product. Each kit contains 1) clinical tools to support delivery of evidence-based care, such as flow sheets, reminder stickers and questionnaires; 2) peer-reviewed journal articles and evidence-based care guidelines; and 3) patient education materials to display in waiting or exam rooms, such as brochures, palm cards and posters. Detailing action kits were distributed along with prescription pads for NRT and small incentive items, such as pens, post-it pads and bags.

Detailing representatives participated in an intensive one-week training session prior to the start of the campaign to ensure their ability to convey the recommended health interventions clearly and credibly. Training for the cessation campaign included: content on tobacco-related illness and smoking cessation, review of the action kit materials, communications skills to promote campaign recommendations, techniques and responses to potential objections encountered during the interactions, strategies for obtaining a commitment to implement campaign recommendations or utilize campaign materials, and procedures for documenting detailing activities (Larson et al., 2006).

The 12-week campaign targeted nearly 200 sites in the three DPHO neighborhoods. All practice types, including hospital ambulatory care centers, community health centers and private practices, were included. The goal was to reach all health care providers and their staff and to meet with each of those individuals twice -- conducting one initial visit and one follow-up visit. The detailing representatives completed visits at 151 of the 200 targeted sites (75%). About 580 individuals, including 260 physicians, 20 nurse practitioners, 20 physician assistants, and 280 other staff, received at least one detailing visit, and more than 330 of the 580 received a follow-up visit (57%). The length of the average detailing visit with health care providers was 9.6 minutes. About 300 providers accepted the offer of NRT for their patients, resulting in the distribution of 3,500 six-week courses of NRT (Larson et al., 2006).

Citywide Smoking Cessation Campaign

Based on the positive provider feedback to the district office campaign, DOHMH launched a citywide detailing campaign in April 2005. The campaign coincided with the 2005 NRT giveaway. The eight-week campaign targeted health care practices throughout the five boroughs of NYC; practices in the three previously detailed high-risk DPHO neighborhoods were excluded. Fifty-five representatives were hired on a temporary basis to reach an estimated 2,300 practices. As in the previous smoking cessation campaign, detailing representatives met with health care providers and their staff to promote the three key recommendations, distribute actions kits, which were redesigned for the 2005 campaign to match the DOHMH "Everybody Loves a Quitter" media campaign (see picture 1 for action kit cover), and supply NRT to providers to distribute to their patients.

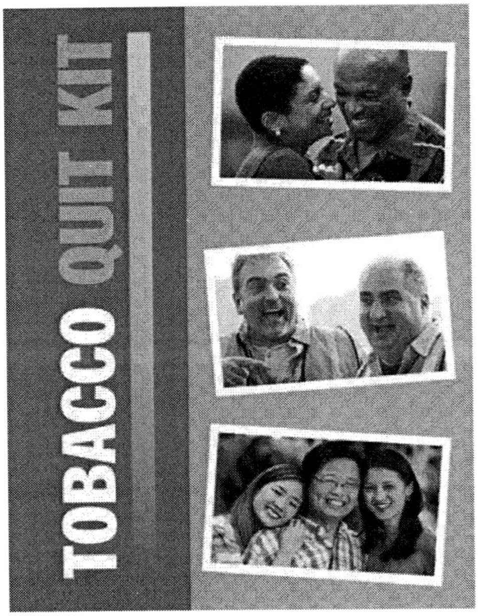

Picture 1. Cover of Citywide Public Health Detailing Smoking Cessation Action Kit.

The 2005 Citywide Smoking Cessation campaign reached 2,250 practices. About 8,600 individuals received at least one detailing visit with more than 6,000 (70%) receiving a second visit. About 3,000 primary care physicians were reached, representing about 40% of NYC primary care physicians (United Hospital Fund of New York, 2004). On average, the length of detailing visits with health care providers was 10 minutes. A total of 6,750 six-week courses of NRT were distributed to providers.

Evaluation was based primarily on self-reports from health care providers. A set of standardized questions was asked at the initial visit (baseline) and at the follow-up visit to evaluate any changes in self-reported knowledge or practice (Larson et al., 2006). Areas assessed included cessation counseling practices and techniques promoted by the detailing campaign: assessing smoking status at every visit, providing brief cessation counseling, and making referrals to cessation resources. Outcomes from the 2005 citywide campaign include:

- An increase in the proportion of physicians who reported assessing smoking status at every visit (from 62% at baseline to 81% at follow-up visit (see figure 2).
- An increase in the proportion of physicians who reported using referrals to 3-1-1, NYC's toll-free non-emergency information line which provides quit smoking assistance, from 8% of physicians at baseline to 47% at follow-up visit (see figure 2).

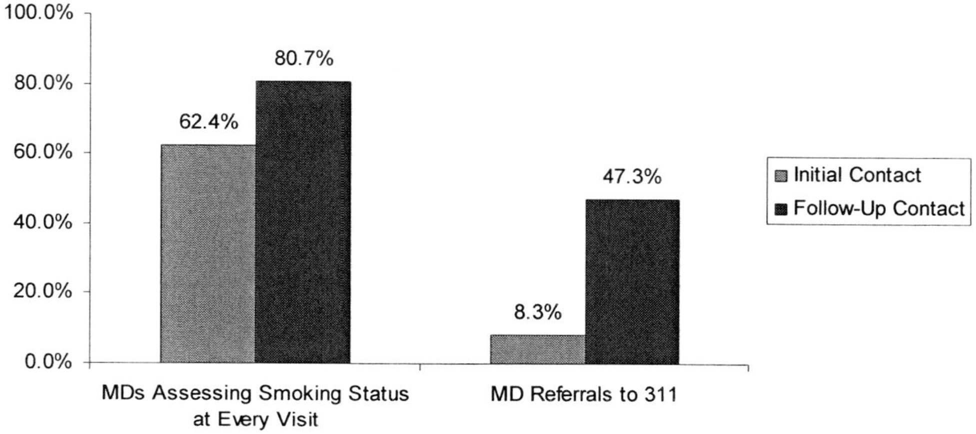

Figure 2. 2005 Public Health Detailing Citywide Campaign Selected Outcomes.

Representatives assessed provider and staff interest in and receptivity to the campaign and they submitted written comments documenting their practice visits. Practice providers and their staff appeared to be both familiar with the NRT giveaway and informed about DOHMH's smoking cessation efforts. Receptivity to the detailing campaign recommendations was generally high.

Public Health Detailing Conclusions and Future Directions

Planning is currently underway for a smoking cessation detailing campaign to be launched in January 2007 targeting select facilities within NYC's public hospital system, the Health and Hospitals Corporation (HHC). The pilot will focus on six HHC facilities (3 hospitals and 3 ambulatory care clinics) in the borough of Brooklyn.

This campaign will expand Public Health Detailing's target audience to include not only primary care practices, but also OB/GYN, dental, mental health, adolescent and drug treatment practices. The key recommendations will be adapted to address characteristics specific to the HHC system. HHC has an electronic medical record that prompts assessment of smoking status at every visit, so compliance with this recommendation will likely be high. In addition, HHC has 14 smoking cessation programs; referral to a cessation program has become an increasingly frequent intervention. However, there is anecdotal evidence that patients do not follow through on referrals, underscoring the need for the integration of cessation counseling into primary care. Detailing representatives will emphasize the second and third campaign recommendations -- promoting brief cessation counseling and prescribing medications -- and add a fourth recommendation encouraging selective referral to the smoking cessation programs. If the six-site pilot proves successful, an HHC-wide detailing campaign will be considered.

DOHMH's Primary Care Information Project (PCIP) also holds great promise to promote clinical cessation services. Launched in 2005, PCIP promotes the use of electronic health records (EHRs) that incorporate decision support at the point of care. Point-of-care reminders based on detailed clinical algorithms translate patient data into simple prompts and "order sets" (which include recommended procedures, education materials and patient referrals) to guide providers through smoking assessment and cessation interventions tailored to each patient. EHRs will also generate reports to ensure the delivery of services (e.g., patients due for follow up) and to facilitate service delivery improvement (e.g., percent of providers prescribing quit smoking medications).

Use of Cessation Registries in a Large Public Hospital System

The third cessation service implemented by DOHMH was coordination of cessation services with the city's public hospital system. The NYC HHC is the largest municipal health care system in the nation. HHC, which was created in 1970 as a public benefit corporation, is comprised of 11 acute care hospitals, 6 diagnostic and treatment centers, 4 long-term care facilities, a certified home health care agency, and more than 80 community health clinics. For DOHMH, collaborating with HHC to enhance the delivery of cessation services represented a unique opportunity to reduce smoking rates among some of NYC's most vulnerable residents. HHC serves 1.3 million New Yorkers annually, including more than 450,000 uninsured New Yorkers. HHC provides care to all, regardless of ability to pay.

In 2001, HHC created 14 smoking cessation programs to serve its patients. HHC promoted a model through which health care providers screened patients for tobacco use and readiness to quit and then referred them to the smoking cessation programs for intensive treatment. HHC provided training for health care providers and tobacco cessation program staff and implemented an HHC-wide marketing strategy to recruit patients. In 2002, HHC and DOHMH agreed to collaborate on the development of a registry to increase the number of HHC patients who were screened for cessation, who were provided cessation medications, and the number who quit smoking.

Tools of the Cessation Registry

The cessation registry was comprised of three main tools: a patient treatment card, a registry book and a quarterly report. Additional tools included the distribution of joint letters providing progress updates, and the use of quality improvement meetings to review relevant data.

Patient Treatment Card

The patient treatment card is an individual smoker medical record that enables health care providers to collect and analyze data on all smokers including demographics, insurance coverage, nicotine dependence, readiness to quit, screening criteria for medications, and prescribed treatment including, medication(s), dosage, and counseling. The implementation of the patient treatment card institutionalized the collection of a standard set of indicators that could be analyzed to better understand which subpopulations (gender, age, race, amount smoked, type of treatment provided) were being helped and which ones remained challenging. The patient treatment card serves as a reminder to providers to deliver all aspects of cessation treatment including assessing tobacco use, prescribing medication and counseling, and conducting follow-up (Fiore et al., 2000). Completion of a patient treatment card for each smoking cessation program patient promotes assessment, treatment and prescribing, especially prescribing NRT, as usual and customary practice, as described in the 2000 U.S. Public Health Service Guidelines (Fiore et al., 2000).

Patient treatment card data allows for system-wide and hospital-specific aggregation of the number of patients assessed, the number treated, and the number prescribed NRT. These three measures became the benchmarks for monitoring, evaluating and improving the performance of HHC smoking cessation programs and for ensuring that patients received the best possible cessation treatment available.

Registry Book

The registry book is modeled after the type used to track treatment of TB patients (Pio and Chaulet, 1998). The ledger format prompts staff to enter key data from the patient treatment card and then summarize select demographic data (e.g., age and gender) as well as end-of-treatment outcomes and follow-up outcomes, typically at 4-6 months. Similar to the patient treatment card, the registry seeks to standardize both clinical practice and data collection across multiple HHC smoking cessation program sites. A fully utilized cessation registry would serve as a management tool for the program, enabling staff to ensure systematic monitoring, outreach, and follow-up of every patient started on cessation treatment and to self-monitor how well they are reaching their own cessation services goals. The registry book helps organize the work of the cessation programs into one manageable document that could be maintained over time and aggregated to assess trends, determine areas of challenge, and identify best practices that could be shared across smoking cessation program sites.

Quarterly Report

The quarterly reports consists of a series of charts and graphs that compare and rank outcomes from the individual smoking cessation program sites and provide an aggregate assessment of outcomes across all sites. Several key indictors have been tracked since the inception of the DOHMH and HHC collaboration including:

- Number of patients started on treatment and number of patients who received cessation medications (aggregated across all sites)
- Number of smokers documented to have quit (aggregated across all sites)
- Number of patients started on treatment (ranked by site)
- Number and proportion of smokers documented to have quit (ranked by site)

The quarterly reports were circulated among smoking cessation program staff as well as among hospital administrators including individual facility medical directors and other high-ranking personnel at regular HHC quality improvement meetings.

Data Collection, Reporting and Outcomes

Formal data collection and reporting began in January 2003 and has been maintained for 14 quarters over three and a half years (2003-2006). Figure 3 shows, for all HHC sites, the total number of patients who have started on treatment and the total number who have received cessation medications for each quarter since formal data collection began.

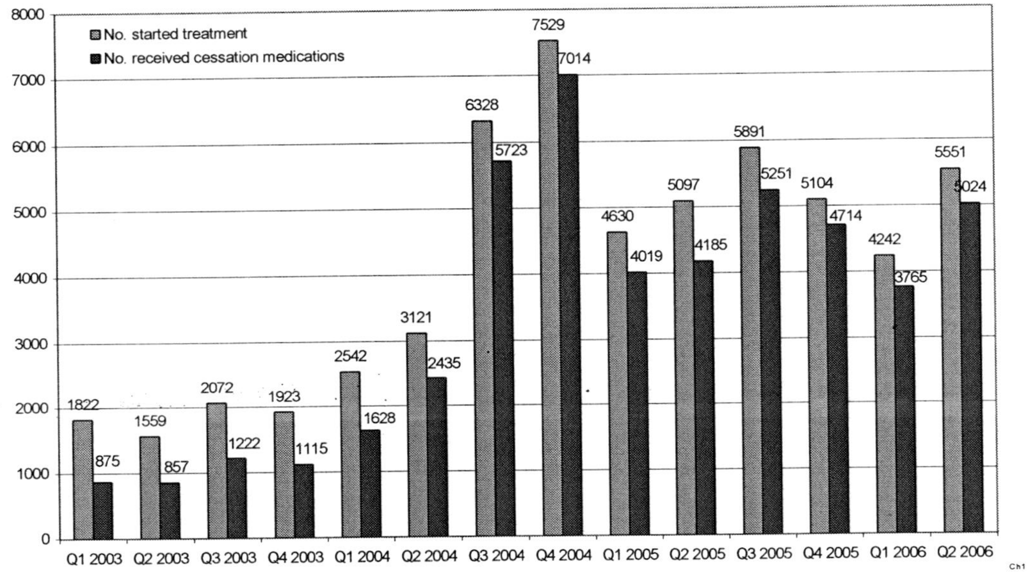

Figure 3. Tobacco Cessation in HHC Quit Smoking Programs, Patients Started on Treatment and Patients who Received Cessation Medications by Quarter, Q1 2003-Q2 2006.

Table 3 and figure 3 demonstrate the consistent success of the HHC registry in increasing both the number of patients started on treatment as well as the number who have been treated with cessation medications, increasing their chances of quitting successfully. The reporting also enabled each site to compare its performance to the performance of other sites. Figure 4 shows for each HHC smoking cessation program the number of patients documented to have quit smoking for the last two quarters for which data are available (12 programs are shown because two sites group their data with other sites).

Data from the quarterly reports show that during the 14 months of the collaboration, the quarterly number of patients started on treatment increased more than two and a half times between 2003 and 2006 (from 1,850 to 4,900); the quarterly number of patients who received cessation medications increased more than four times between 2003 and 2006 (from 1,020 to 4,500); and the annual percent of patients started on treatment who received cessation medication increased from 55% in 2003 to 90% in 2006.

Table 3. HHC Registry Outcomes, 2003-2006

	2003	2004	2005	2006 (1st half)
Number of patients started on treatment	7400	19,500	20,700	9800
Average number of patients started on treatment each quarter	1850	4880	5180	4900
Number of patients who received cessation medication	4070	16,800	18,200	8800
Average number of patients who received cessation medications each quarter	1020	4200	4540	4400
Percent (%) of patients started on treatment who received cessation medications	55%	86%	88%	90%

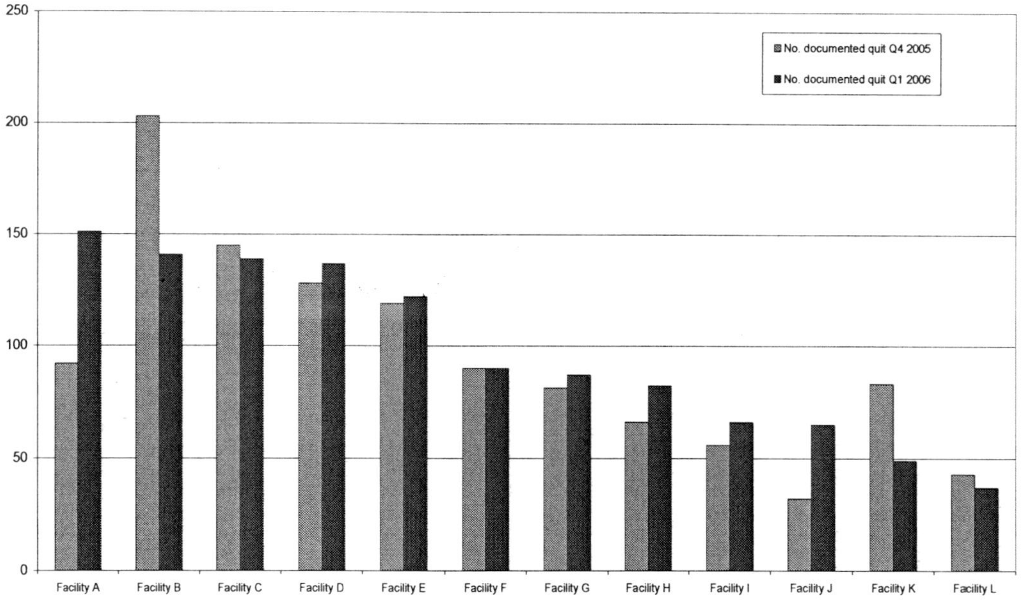

Figure 4. Patients Documented to Have Quit Smoking by HHC Smoking Cessation Program Q4 2005 and Q1 2006.

Cessation Registry Conclusions and Future Directions

In 2004, when DOHMH received the donation of NRT from Pfizer, it began supporting HHC's cessation services by providing HHC with NRT to distribute. In 2004, DOHMH provided HHC with 15,000 courses of NRT. In 2005, DOHMH provided HHC with 5,000 courses of NRT. And in 2006, DOHMH provided HHC with 10,000 courses of purchased NRT. The combination of provision of NRT and ongoing attention paid to the smoking cessation programs' key indicators (patients started on treatment, patients provided medications and patients quit) helped produce the substantial increases in the outcomes of interest, ensuring that more HHC patients were screened for tobacco use and provided with evidence-based cessation treatment to help them quit smoking.

The DOHMH-HHC collaboration continues to promote cessation services. As of this writing, HHC and DOHMH are planning a retrospective analysis of the collaboration to determine which smokers have been helped by the smoking cessation programs and how the collaboration can use its data to refine the delivery of cessation services.

Conclusion

Cessation is a critical component of comprehensive tobacco control. Cessation saves lives (Anthonisen NR, et al., 2005). Cessation services are cost effective compared to other public health interventions (CDC, 1999; Cromwell, Bartosch, Fiore, Hasselblad and Bake, 1997). Finally, in the wake of efforts that make it harder to smoke – such as higher prices through taxation and restrictions on where people can smoke through smoke-free workplace legislations – helping smokers quit by providing cessation services is the responsible thing to do. Government intervention in what are considered lifestyle choices is an area of considerable debate. Most of the outcry against interventions to curb smoking has been orchestrated by the tobacco industry, which spends more than of $15 billion annually in the United States alone to promote its products (Federal Trade Commission, 2005). The tobacco industry spends significant resources trying to defeat tobacco excise taxes and smoke-free air laws nationally (Campaign for Tobacco Free Kids, 1999; CTFK, 2006a). Governments also benefit financially from the collection of higher tobacco taxes (CTFK, 2006b) and would appear remiss were they not to invest in aiding smokers in their effort to quit.

DOHMH's efforts to provide cessation services and promote cessation behaviors through its five-point tobacco control program have likely helped many more smokers quit than are reflected in calls to enroll in the NRT giveaway programs, patients enrolled in HHC tobacco cessation programs or calls to 3-1-1 for quit smoking assistance. Because smoking is a chronic relapsing condition, which often requires multiple quit attempts to achieve permanent abstinence (Fiore et al., 2000), prompting smokers to make quit attempts may be as important as providing them with medications to increase success. DOHMH's cessation efforts, particularly the direct-to-the public NRT giveaways and the large anti-tobacco media campaigns, because they generated a significant amount of press attention, serve to encourage all smokers to make a quit attempt as well as provided a subset of smokers with medication to assist them in their quit attempt. Exposure to pharmaceutical-industry advertisements for smoking cessation products has been found to increase both quit attempts and quit success with and without use of the products being advertised (Avery, Kenkel, Lillard and Mathios, 2006). Cessation product advertising was found to prompt more "cold turkey" quit attempts than NRT-supported quit attempts (Avery, Kenkel, Lillard and Mathios, 2006). DOHMH's cessation efforts were responsible for product-assisted quit attempts, but were also most likely responsible for prompting additional unaided quit attempts – a benefit beyond what cessation program-specific data reflects.

In NYC, most people who have ever smoked have already quit. Since implementing its five-point comprehensive tobacco control program in 2002, NYC has experienced a prevalence decline of 13%. Prevalence was stagnant in NYC for about a decade between 1993 and 2002 at about 22%. In 2005, the most recent year for which data are available,

NYC adult smoking prevalence was 18.9%, lower than the national median smoking prevalence of 20.5% (CDC, 2006b). Youth smoking rates have also declined dramatically. In 2005, the rate of smoking among public high school students had dropped 36% since 2001, to a prevalence of 11% -- a steeper rate of decline than documented nationally (20% decline between 2001 and 2005), and a prevalence less than half the national average of 23% for 2005 (CDC, 2006c). By 2005, nearly 200,000 fewer New Yorkers were smoking than in 2002.

The primary components of comprehensive tobacco control are higher priced cigarettes, restrictions on where people can smoke, large anti-tobacco media campaigns and cessation interventions (CDC, 1999). The theoretical basis for comprehensive tobacco control is that the components work better in concert than any individual effort on its own (Jha et al., 2006; Bialous, 2006). In keeping with this understanding of comprehensive tobacco control, it is difficult to quantify the relative contribution of each element in reducing initiation and bringing down prevalence. Nearly half (45.3%) of NYC smokers surveyed in 2003 reported that they had reduced the number of cigarettes smoked, thought about quitting, tried to quit, or quit in response to the 2002 tax increase (Frieden et al., 2005). The U.S. states – California, Massachusetts -- that implemented large comprehensive tobacco control program have seen steeper declines in smoking prevalence than the rest of the country (Bitton, Fichtenberg and Glantz, 2001). By aggressively implementing a comprehensive tobacco control that includes the provision of cessation services and the promotion of cessation behaviors through taxation, legal action, public education and evaluation, NYC has been able to produce significant declines in smoking prevalence in less than 5 years.

References

Alberg, A.J., Stashefsky, M.R., Burke, A., Rasch K.A., Stewart, N., and Kline, J.A. (2004). The influence of offering free transdermal nicotine patches on quit rates in a local health department's smoking cessation program. *Addictive Behavior*, 29(9), 1763-1778.

An, L.C., Schillo, B.A., Kavanaugh, A.M., Lachter, R.B., Luxenberg, M.G., and Wendling, A.H. (2006). Increased reach and effectiveness of a statewide tobacco quitline after the addition of access to free nicotine replacement therapy. *Tobacco Control,* 15(4), 286-93.

Anthonisen, N.R. (2005). The effects of a smoking cessation intervention on 14.5-year mortality: a randomized clinical trial. *Annals of Internal Medicine*, 142, 233-239.

Avery, R., Kenkel, D., Lillard, D.R., and Mathios, A. (2006). Private Profits and Public Health: Does Advertising Smoking Cessation Products Encourage Smokers to Quit? *National Bureau of Economic Research*, Working Paper No. 11938.

Bialous, S. (2006). Tobacco use cessation within the context of tobacco control policy: opportunities for nursing research. *Nursing Research,*55(4 Suppl 1),S58-63.

Biener L., Reimer R.L., Wakefield M., Szczypka G., Rigotti N.A., Connolly G. (2006). Impact of smoking aids and mass media among recent quitters. *American Journal of Preventative Medicine,* 30(3),217-24.

Bitton A., Fichtenberg C., Glantz S. (2001). Reducing smoking prevalence to 10% in five years. *Journal of the American Medical Association,* 286, 2733–2734.

Campaign for Tobacco-Free Kids Factsheet. (1999). Tobacco Industry Interference With State Efforts to Prevent and Reduce Tobacco Use. Retrieved December 11, 2006 from http://tobaccofreekids.org/research/factsheets/pdf/0078.pdf.

Campaign for Tobacco-Free Kids Factsheet. (2006a). Voters Across America Rebuff Big Tobacco, Approve Ballot Measures To Reduce Smoking, Save Lives. Press Release. Retrieved December 19, 2006 from *http://tobaccofreekids.org/Script/ DisplayPress Release.php3?Display=954*.

Campaign for Tobacco-Free Kids Factsheet. (2006b). Raising State Tobacco Taxes Always Increases State Revenues and Always Reduces Tobacco Use. Retrieved December 11, 2006 from http://tobaccofreekids.org/research/factsheets/pdf/0098.pdf.

Centers for Disease Control and Prevention. (1997). Cigarette Smoking Among Adults – United States,1995. *Morbidity and Mortality Weekly Report*, 46(51), 1217-1220.

Centers for Disease Control and Prevention. (1998). Response to increases in cigarette prices by race/ethnicity, income, and age groups--United States,1976-1993. *Morbidity and Mortality Weekly Report,* 47(29), 605-9.

Centers for Disease Control and Prevention. (1999). Best Practices for Comprehensive Tobacco Control Programs – August 1999.Atlanta GA: US Department of Health and Human Services, Centers for Disease Control and Prevention, National Center for Chronic Disease Prevention and Health Promotion, Office on Smoking and Health.

Centers for Disease Control and Prevention and American Legacy Foundation. (2003). Tobacco Use Quitlines. Atlanta, GA: U.S. Department of Health and Human Services, Centers for Disease Control and Prevention, National Center for Chronic Disease Prevention and Health Promotion, Office on Smoking and Health.

Centers for Disease Control and Prevention. (2004). Telephone Quitlines: A Resource for Development, Implementation, and Evaluation. Atlanta, GA: U.S. Department of Health and Human Services, Centers for Disease Control and Prevention, National Center for Chronic Disease Prevention and Health Promotion, Office on Smoking and Health.

Centers for Disease Control and Prevention.(2005). Annual smoking-attributable mortality, years of potential life lost, and economic costs—United States. *Morbidity and Mortality Weekly Report*, 51, 300–303.

Centers for Disease Control and Prevention. Smoking-Attributable Mortality, Morbidity, and Economic Costs (SAMMEC). (2006). Adult SAMMEC and maternal and child health (MCH) SAMMEC software. Retrieved Nov 14, 2006 from http://apps.nccd.cdc.gov/ sammec/.

Center for Disease Control and Prevention. (2006a). How and why to quit smoking today. Retrieved Dec. 12, 2006 from http://www.cdc.gov/tobacco/news/QuitSmoking.htm#quit.

Centers for Disease Control and Prevention. (2006b). Tobacco use among adults -- United States. *Morbidity and Mortality Weekly Report,* 55(42), 1145-1148.

Centers for Disease Control and Prevention. (2006c). Cigarette Use Among High School Students -- United States. *Morbidity and Mortality Weekly Report,* 55(26), 724-726.

Centers for Disease Control and Prevention. Media Campaign Resource Center. (2006a). "Krystell-Memorial." Retrieved on December 18, 2006 from *http://apps.nccd.cdc.gov/ MCRC/SearchDetail.asp?SearchType=0 and PageSize=20 and Group=1 and SID= and*

NewType=0 and Media=0 and Theme=0 and FreeText=Pam+Laffin and OrderBy= and Req= and Page=1 and ProgName= and CatalogID=747

Centers for Disease Control and Prevention. Media Campaign Resource Center. (2006b). "Before and After." Retrieved on December 18, 2006 from *http://apps.nccd.cdc.gov/MCRC/SearchDetail.asp?SearchType=0 and PageSize=20 and Group=1 and SID= and NewType=0 and Media=0 and Theme=0 and FreeText=Mike+Sams and OrderBy= and Req= and Page=1 and ProgName= and CatalogID=1303.*

Centers for disease control and prevention. Media Campaign Resource Center. (2006c). "Shower." Retrieved on December 18, 2006 from *http://apps.nccd.cdc.gov/MCRC/SearchDetail.asp?SearchType=0 and PageSize=20 and Group=1 and SID= and NewType=0 and Media=0 and Theme=0 and FreeText=shower and OrderBy= and Req= and Page=1 and ProgName= and CatalogID=867*

Centers for Disease Control and Prevention. Media Campaign Resource Center. (2006d). "Artery." Retrieved on December 18, 2006 from *http://apps.nccd.cdc.gov/MCRC/SearchDetail.asp?SearchType=0 and PageSize=20 and Group=1 and SID= and NewType=0 and Media=0 and Theme=0 and FreeText=Every+Cigarette+ and OrderBy= and Req= and Page=1 and ProgName= and CatalogID=198*

Cromwell, J., Bartosch, W.J., Fiore, M.C., Hasselblad, V., and Baker, T. (1997).Cost-effectiveness of the clinical practice recommendations in the AHCPR guideline for smoking cessation. *Agency for Health Care Policy and Research,* 278, 1759-1766.

Cummings, K. M., Fix, B., Celestino, P., Carlin-Menter, S., O'Connor, R., and Hyland, A. (2006). Reach, efficacy, and cost-effectiveness of free nicotine medication giveaway programs. *Journal of Public Health Management and Practice*, 12(1), 37-43.

Cummings, K.M., Hyland, A., Fix, B., Bauer, U., Celestino, P., Carlin-Menter, S., et al. (2006). Free nicotine patch giveaway program 12-month follow-up of participants. *American Journal of Preventive Medicine*, 31(2), 181-184.

Federal Trade Commission. (2005). Federal Trade Commission Cigarette Report for 2003.

Fiore, M.C., Bailey, W.C., and Cohen, S.J. (2000). Treating Tobacco Use and Dependence. Clinical Practice Guideline. Rockville MD: US Department of Health and Human Services. Public Health Service.

Frieden, T.R., Mostashari, F., Kerker, B.D., Miller, N., Hajat, A., and Frankel, M. (2005). Adult tobacco use levels after intensive tobacco control measures: New York City, 2002-2003. *American Journal of Public Health*, 6, 1016-23

Grigg, M., and Glasgow, H. (2003). Susidised nicotine replacement therapy [Letter to the Editor]. *Tobacco Control,* 12, 238-9.

Hyland A., Wakefield M., Higbee C., Szczypka G., Cummings K.M. (2006). Anti-tobacco television advertising and indicators of smoking cessation in adults: a cohort study. *Health Education Research*, 21(3), 348-54.

Jha, P., and Chaloupka, F. (2000). The economics of global tobacco control. *British Medical Journal,* 321, 358-361.

Jha, P.,Chaloupka, F.J., Moore, J., Gajalakshmi, V., Gupta, P.C., Peck, R. et al. (2006). Tobacco Addiction. *Disease Control Priorities in Developing Countries*. 2nd ed., ed. New York: Oxford University Press. 869–886.

Larson, K., Levy, J., Rome, M.G., Matte, T.D., Silver, L.D., and Frieden, T.R. (2006). Public health detailing: a strategy to improve the delivery of clinical preventive services in New York City. *Public Health Report,* 121(3), 228-34.

Liang L, Chaloupka F, Nichter M, Clayton R. (2003). Prices, policies and youth smoking, May 2001. *Addiction*. 98 (Suppl 1), 105-22.

Mendez D, Warner KE, Courant PN. (1998). Has smoking cessation ceased? Expected trends in the prevalence of smoking in the United States. *American Journal of Epidemiology,* 148(3), 249-58.

Mendez D., and Warner K.E. (2000). Smoking prevalence in 2010: why the Healthy People goal is unattainable. *American Journal of Public Health,* 90(3), 401–3.

Miller N, Frieden TR, Liu SY, Matte TD, Mostashari F, Deitcher DR, Cummings KM, Chang C, Bauer U, Bassett MT. (2005). Effectiveness of a large-scale distribution programme of free nicotine patches: a prospective evaluation. *Lancet*, 365(9474), 1849-54.

Mudde A.N., De Vries H. (1999). The reach and effectiveness of a national mass media-led smoking cessation campaign in the Netherlands. *American Journal of Public Health,* 89(3), 346-50.

New York City Department of Health and Mental Hygiene. (2004). Community Health Survey 2004. Retrieved November 6, 2006 from *https://a816-health3ssl.nyc.gov/ survey/index2004.htm.*

New York City Department of Health and Mental Hygiene. (2006). City Health Information. Retrieved December 19, 2006 from *http://www.nyc.gov/html/doh/html/pub/ pub.shtml? y=chi*

New York City Department of Health and Mental Hygiene, NYC Community Health Profiles. (2006). Retrieved November 6, 2006 from *http://www.nyc.gov/html/ doh/html/data/data.shtml#3*

NYC Department of Finance, NYC Department of Health and Mental Hygiene, NYC Department of Small Business Services, NYC Economic Development Corporation. (2004). "The State of Smoke-Free New York City: A One-Year Review." Retrieved Dec. 18, 2006 from *http://www.nyc.gov/html/doh/pdf/smoke/sfaa-2004report.pdf.*

O'Brien MA, Oxman AD, Davis DA, Haynes RB, Freemantle N, Harvey EL. (1997). Educational outreach visits: effects on professional practice and health care outcomes. *Cochrane Database of Systematic Reviews*, 4: CD000409.

Pio A. and Chaulet P. (1998). *Tuberculosis Handbook*. Geneva: World Health Organization World Health Organization. WHO/TB/98.253

Powell, L.M., Tauras, J.A., and Ross, H. (2005). The importance of peer effects, cigarette prices and tobacco control policies for youth smoking behavior. *Journal of Health Economics,* 5, 950-68.

Ross, H., and Chaloupka, F.J. (2003). The effect of cigarette prices on youth smoking. *Health Economics*, 12(3), 217-30.

Silagy, C., Lancaster, T., Stead, L., Mant, D., and Fowler, G. (2004). Nicotine replacement therapy for smoking cessation (Cochrane Review). *Cochrane Database of Systematic Reviews,* 3: CD000146.

Centers for Disease Control and Prevention. Smoking-Attributable Mortality, Morbidity, and Economic Costs (SAMMEC): adult SAMMEC and maternal and child health (MCH)

SAMMEC software. Retrieved November 14, 2006 from *http://apps.nccd.cdc.gov/sammec/*.

Thorndike A.N., Rigotti N.A., Stafford R.S., Singer D.E. (1998). National Patterns in the Treatment of Smokers by Physicians. *Journal of the American Medical Association*, 279(8), 604-608.

United Hospital Fund of New York. (2000). The New York City Physician Workforce. Profile of the Supply and Distribution of Physicians Practicing in NYC in 2000: Profiles by Borough, Neighborhood, and Specialty 2004.

US Department of Health and Human Services. (1994). Current Estimates from the National Health Interview Survey, 1993. Hyattsville, MD: Public Health Service, Centers for Disease Control, National Center for Health Statistics. Department of Health and Human Services Publication No. (PHS) 95-1518.

In: Progress in Smoking and Health Research
Editor: T. C. Jeffries, pp. 117-139
ISBN: 978-1-60021-686-2

Chapter V

Effectiveness of a Smoking-Cessation Intervention and Comprehensive Environmental Changes: A New but Classical Experience from Japan

Takashi Kadowaki, Akira Okayama, Hideyuki Kanda, Makoto Watanabe, Kayoko Hishida, Tomonori Okamura and Hirotsugu Ueshima

Abstract

Male smoking prevalence is considerably high in many Asian countries including Japan, but there have been few reports on effectiveness of smoking cessation measures. In this article, we examined the following four fundamental questions that public health professionals often face;

1) To what extent do smokers quit smoking? In many situations, we encourage smokers to quit smoking regardless of their intention to quit. In one of these situations, we implemented a smoking-cessation intervention in a workplace setting (263 male smokers, smoking prevalence: 62.9%) in a cross-over design, and ascertained that the cessation rate was 12.9% and 3.1% in the intervention and control groups, respectively.

2) To what extent do smokers maintain their cessation of smoking after having quit for more than four weeks? Many smokers successfully quit smoking, but later relapse. After our cross-over intervention study was completed, we then observed all ex-smokers who quit smoking at least once for more than four weeks, and ascertained that no relapse occurred after three years had passed since cessation and that 45% of them continued smoking cessation.

3) Is a small-scale intervention effective in reducing smoking prevalence? In smoking cessation programs, we are usually able to reach only a small portion of smokers, and most of them voluntarily participate in the program. We ascertained that small-scale annual interventions for smoking cessation repeated for ten years yielded lower smoking prevalence than doing no intervention at all.

4) Are comprehensive environmental changes as effective as direct intervention? It is usually hard to compare these two measures, because environmental changes affect all smokers, making concurrent comparison impossible. Smokers in Japan have experienced environmental changes since 2002, such as a price increase and implementation of laws. In the occupational setting described above, indoor smoking was banned in 2003. We compared the smoking abstinence rate in the intervention period and during the period of comprehensive environmental changes. We ascertained that the smoking abstinence rate was 8.9% and 7.1% in the periods of intervention and environmental changes, respectively, and revealed that comprehensive environmental changes are fairly effective in promoting smoking cessation.

Introduction

Many Asian countries have a high smoking prevalence among men in particular. Of note, among the developed countries, Japan is the only one with a male smoking prevalence of more than 40%. However, the reduction in smoking prevalence has accelerated in recent years; for a 7% reduction of male smoking prevalence, it took more than ten years from 61% (in 1990) to 54% (in 2000), but four years from 54% (in 2000) to 47% (in 2004) [1].

It is important for health care providers to conduct effective smoking cessation programs, especially in regions with high smoking prevalence. However, there has been little evidence of the effectiveness of such interventions from regions with high smoking prevalence, including Japan. In this chapter, we present the effectiveness of a smoking cessation program in a relatively small occupational setting in Japan and also examine a comprehensive intervention including support for current smokers and environmental changes. In the following sections, we address these four study questions: (1) Can a smoking cessation program reduce male smoking prevalence?; (2) Does the effectiveness of such an intervention last over time?; (3) Is repeated conduct of such small-scale interventions effective in reducing smoking prevalence?; (4) Are comprehensive environmental changes as effective as an intervention among smokers?

Section 1: Effectiveness of a Smoking Cessation Intervention

Smoking is expected to kill 10 million people annually worldwide by 2030, and over 70% of these deaths will be in the developing world [2]. In populations with such high smoking prevalence, it is important to provide all smokers with smoking cessation programs, including those who seem healthy and those who may not currently be willing to quit smoking. .It is usually more feasible to conduct programs that do not include costly components such as nicotine replacement therapy.

In order to determine the effectiveness of an intervention among all smokers regardless of their willingness to quit smoking, we conducted a randomized controlled intervention trial in an occupational setting [3].

Methods

Study Population

We performed an intervention study in a factory that employed 542 workers (423 men and 119 women) in 1997. We first conducted a self-administered questionnaire survey. The questionnaire included questions regarding their smoking status, smoking history, degree of nicotine addiction (Fagerström Tolelance Questionnaire [4], or FTQ), willingness to quit smoking. Through this questionnaire, 267 smokers (263 men and 4 women) were identified. Due to the small number of women, we excluded female smokers from the study, although they received the same intervention. We randomly allocated all the male smokers into an intervention group (n=132) and a control group (n=131).

Smoking Cessation Intervention

All the smokers in the intervention group underwent five months of intervention starting in January, 1997.

First, we approached all the smokers in the intervention group regardless of their willingness to quit smoking. Each smoker was asked to visit the health consulting room in the factory to attend a face-to-face counseling session with a health care provider during working hours. The health care provider discussed harmful effects of tobacco and the benefits of cessation, and encouraged each smoker to quit. Smokers underwent a measurement of carbon monoxide (CO) concentration in expiratory air with a Smokerlyzer® [5] during the counseling session. If a smoker expressed a desire to quit, he was asked to choose a date on which he would quit smoking, and record that date on a signed Smoking Cessation Declaration. Then the health care provider additionally explained situations where he might want to re-start smoking, and how to deal with such situations. For those who did not sign the Declaration, we monitored their smoking status without active intervention.

The five month program included periodic visits to work sites by health care providers for encouragement, leaflet distribution, and group discussions. The five-month intervention materials (counseling materials, pamphlets, and follow-up leaflets) are described elsewhere [6].

After the five month intervention period, we conducted the same self-administered questionnaire survey in all of the workers to identify those who succeeded in smoking cessation. The smoking status of each non-respondent was individually confirmed. Successful smoking cessation was defined as self-reporting of quitting for more than four weeks and an expiratory CO concentration of less than 9 ppm. Those who succeeded in smoking cessation in both intervention and control groups were asked to visit the health consulting room to undergo an expiratory CO concentration.

Delayed Intervention

For the purpose of offering each smoker an opportunity to consider smoking cessation, we made an equivalent intervention in the control group after the initial intervention was completed. During this delayed intervention period, the original intervention group was left without any active intervention.

Evaluation of Smoking Status

As to the evaluation of nicotine dependence, we classified the FTQ score into low (score 0-3), medium (score 4-6), and high (score 7-) nicotine dependence. Non-respondents and incomplete respondents to FTQ questions were excluded from the FTQ analysis.

In order to compare those who succeeded in smoking cessation and who did not after the delayed intervention, we combined the two groups and divided them into "successful" and "non-successful" groups. Those who were lost to follow-up were included in non-successful group for this analysis.

Those who initially reported being non-smokers in the self-administered questionnaire but later contradicted themselves about their status (n=3) were categorized as current smokers, though we did not conduct any intervention approach for them.

We assumed that those who were lost to follow-up (retired, moved to some other branch, or left the company for some reason) did not change their initial smoking habit. If a subject was originally a habitual smoker and quit once during the intervention period before leaving the factory, we classified him as restarting habitual smoking after he left. However, in the calculation of smoking prevalence, we included only those who remained at the worksite in order to show the actual smoking rate of those in the same setting at each step.

Results

Baseline Characteristics

The smoking prevalence was 62.9% among male workers. The distribution of smoking status is presented in table 1. As for the randomization into the intervention and control groups, the two groups showed no significant differences with regard to the number of subjects, age, beginning age of habitual smoking, number of cigarettes consumed per day, FTQ score, and proportion of those who had any previous experience with smoking cessation (table 2).

Table 1. Smoking status and age distribution at baseline survey

		Smoker	Ex-smoker	Never-smoker	Total
n (%)		263 (62.2)	59 (13.9)	101 (23.9)	423 (100.0)
Age ± standard deviation		33.3 ± 9.6	38.2 ± 9.2	34.1 ± 9.8	34.2 ± 9.7
Age distribution (n)					
Age	18-24	43	1	16	60
	25-34	115	22	45	182
	35-44	64	19	21	104
	45-54	32	14	16	62
	55-60	9	3	3	15

Table 2. Comparison of baseline characteristics between the intervention and control group after the random allocation

	Intervention group n = 132	Control group n = 131	p-value
Age ± standard deviation	33.5 ± 10.1	33.2 ± 9.2	0,84
Age of onset of habitual smoking ± standard deviation	18.8 ± 3.8	18.6 ± 2.3	0,648
Number of cigarettes per day ± standard deviation	19.3 ± 7.2	19.6 ± 6.5	0,742
FTQ score ± standard deviation	4.3 ± 1.9	4.6 ± 2.0	0,225
Number of those with previous quit attempts (%)	59 (44.7)	59 (45.0)	0,974
Number of those who always inhale deeply (%)	65 (49.2)	72 (55.0)	0,497
Willingness to quit smoking at baseline (%)			
Negative (not at all/ in the future)	124 (93.9)	122 (93.1)	0,808
Positive (before long/ currently trying)	8 (6.1)	9 (6.9)	

Intervention

Each subject was first asked to attend an individual counseling session. Among the 132 intervention subjects, 125 (94.7%) agreed to receive the counseling, and 63 (47.7%) signed a Smoking Cessation Declaration. The counseling took three minutes longer for those who signed the Declaration (16.0 ± 4.1 minutes) than those who did not (13.0 ± 5.4 minutes) (p=0.0005).

Among those who signed the Declaration, 71.4% (n=45) and 28.6% (n=18) were able to stop smoking for one day and for one week, respectively. The cessation rate at the five-month survey was 12.9% and 3.1% in the intervention and control groups, respectively (p=0.003), confirmed by the questionnaire (response rate: 93.4%) and the expiratory CO measurement of less than 9 ppm (table 3).

At the five month survey, the proportion of those who reduced the number of cigarette consumption per day (including those who quit) was significantly larger in the intervention group than in the control group (p=0.016) (table 3). Those with lower FTQ score showed a higher cessation rate in both groups, and even in the medium FTQ score group the cessation rate tended to be higher in the intervention group (p=0.055) (table 3). As for the willingness to quit smoking, the proportion of those who did not express a willingness to quit significantly decreased in the intervention group, while the distribution did not show a significant change in the control group (table 3).

Delayed Intervention

As to the delayed intervention, for the original control group (n=131), there were 123 smokers left after excluding those who were lost to follow-up (n=4) and those who had already quit smoking (n=4). After undergoing the equivalent intervention, 16 subjects (13.0%) succeeded in smoking cessation at the end of the delayed intervention (figure 1).

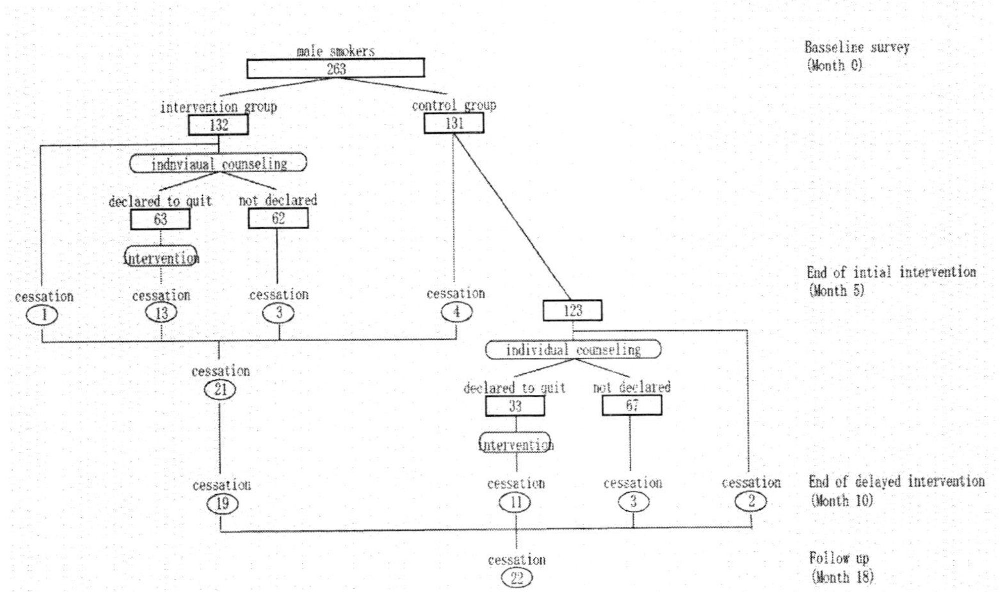

Figure 1. Flow chart of the smoking cessation program, the number of smoking subjects, and the number of those who quit smoking at each stage. All the male smokers (n = 263) were divided into an intervention group (n = 132) and a control group (n = 131). Among those in the intervention group, 125 subjects received an individual counseling session and 63 subjects signed the Smoking Cessation Declaration. There were 17 and 4 subjects who succeeded in smoking cessation in the intervention and control groups, respectively, at Month 5. At the end of the delayed intervention for the control group at Month 10, 19 subjects in the intervention group continued smoking cessation, and 16 subjects in the control group quit smoking. At month 18, 22 subjects continued smoking cessation. Figures in the rectangles show the number of smoking subjects, and those in the ovals show the number of subjects on smoking cessation at each stage.

Table 3. Comparison between the intervention and control groups before and after the five month intervention period regarding smoking cessation rate, changes in number of cigarettes per day, FTQ, and willingness to quit smoking

	Intervention group			Control group			
Cessation rate (%)	12.9 (17/132)			3.1 (4/131)			(p = 0.003)
Cessation rate by nicotine dependence measured by FTQ score (%)							
Low (0 - 3)	18.6 (8/43)			7.3 (3/41)			(p = 0.125)
Medium (4 - 6)	12.3 (8/65)			2.2 (1/46)			(p = 0.055)
High (7 -)	5.0 (1/20)			0.0 (0/19)			(p = 0.323)
Proportion of those who quit/reduced cigarette consumption per day (%)	30.3 (40/132)			17.5 (23/131)			(p = 0.016)
Willingness to quit smoking	Baseline	at 5 months	p-value	Baseline	at 5 months	p-value	
Negative (not at all/ in the future)	93,9	81,0	0,002	93,1	90,8	0,494	
Positive (before long/ currently trying)	6,1	6,1	1,000	6,9	6,1	0,793	
Succeeded in smoking cessation	-	12,9	-	-	3,1	-	

Comparison of Successful and Unsuccessful Subjects

A comparison of all subjects in both groups between those who succeeded and those who did not succeed in quitting revealed that smokers were more likely to abstain from smoking if the number of cigarette consumed per day was smaller and if the onset age of habitual smoking was higher (table 4). The proportion of those who signed the Declaration was significantly higher in the successful group. Among those who had no intention of cessation at baseline (n=60), and signed the Declaration at the counseling session (n=19), the cessation rate was 15.8% (n=3). As for age, there was no significant relationship between the age group and the smoking abstinence rate through our intervention. As for the willingness to quit, there was an increasing tendency between the willingness to quit and the cessation rate; 6.9% of those who had no intention to quit succeeded, and the cessation rate significantly increased as the willingness to quit increased (p=0.002).

Table 4. Comparison of the successful and non-successful groups in smoking cessation during our intervention

	Succeeded n = 37*	Non-succeeded n = 226**	p-value
Age ± standard deviation	33.7 ± 9.3	33.3 ± 9.7	0,807
Age of beginning habitual smoking ± standard deviation	20.7 ± 5.4	18.4 ± 2.5	<0.001
Number of cigarettes per day ± standard deviation	16.8 ± 7.6	19.9 ± 6.6	0,009
FTQ score ± standard deviation	3.9 ± 2.1	4.6 ± 1.9	0,048
Number of those with previous quit attempts (%)	20 (54.1)	98 (43.4)	0,225
Number of those who always inhale deeply (%)	17 (45.9)	120 (53.1)	0,416
Number of those who signed Declaration (%)	25 (67.6)	72 (31.9)	<0.001

* Including subjects in both groups who succeeded in smoking cessation during the initial five month intervention and those in the control group who succeeded in smoking cessation during the following delayed intervention.

** Including those who were lost to follow-up.

Table 5. Distribution of the subjects according to their willingness to quit smoking at baseline and the cessation rate of each category

Willingness to quit at baseline	Not at all	In the future	Before long	Currently trying
n*	131	115	13	4
(Distribution among all subjects (%))	(49.8)	(43.7)	(5.0)	(1.5)
Succeeded in cessation**	9	23	3	2
(Cessation rate in each category (%))	(6.9)	(20.0)	(23.1)	(50.0)

* Including those who were lost to follow-up.

** Including subjects in both groups who succeeded in smoking cessation during the initial five month intervention and those in the control group who succeeded in smoking cessation during the following delayed intervention.

In the comparison between those who continued and discontinued smoking cessation after quitting at least once during our intervention, there was no significant difference in age, onset age of habitual smoking, number of cigarettes per day, FTQ score, previous quit attempts, deep inhalation of smoke, and signing the Declaration.

Message from this Section

We assessed the effectiveness of a smoking cessation intervention in all smokers, regardless of their willingness to quit smoking, through a randomized controlled trial. Attempts to approach those with high nicotine dependence and those with little willingness to quit smoking are also effective as compared with leaving them without any intervention, although the cessation rate is naturally lower than among those with lower nicotine dependence and higher willingness to quit smoking. Even among smokers who failed to quit smoking, the number of cigarettes consumed and the willingness to quit smoking may be improved through an intervention. Although there are measures to improve the smoking cessation rate such as nicotine replacement therapies, health care providers, especially in developing countries with high smoking prevalence, face the challenge of decreasing smoking prevalence without any costly measures. We can expect a smoking cessation rate of 13% through intervention programs of five months including individual counseling, group discussion, and periodic leaflet distribution.

Section 2: Long-Term Duration of Smoking Cessation

The intervention programs without nicotine replacement therapy for all smokers regardless of their willingness to quit smoking are effective, as was shown in the previous section. We are also interested in whether quitters can continue smoking cessation for a long period of time.

Many smokers cite weight gain after smoking cessation as a primary reason for not trying to quit smoking [7]. There have been reports on weight gain following smoking cessation from observational studies, but no study has examined an intervention and consequent weight gain in smokers who achieved smoking cessation.

We followed up those smokers who successfully quit smoking at least once after the intervention presented in Section 1, and examined their long-term smoking cessation and consequent weight gain [8].

Methods

Study Population

At the end of the delayed intervention period, a total of 35 out of the 251 baseline smokers (n = 19 from the intervention group and n = 16 from the control group combined) had abstained from smoking for more than four weeks at Month 10, after excluding 12 subjects who left the worksite for some reason unrelated to health or smoking status during the initial ten months. Thus, the subjects of the present study were those 251 subjects remaining at Month 10 who were originally all smokers and who had received individual counseling from a physician in 1997, including the 35 subjects who successfully quit smoking.

Outcome Measurements

For this Section, the main outcomes were: the cessation rates among those who quit smoking during our intervention program (n = 35) at each follow-up survey; and changes in the body mass index (BMI) of the abstainers who continued cessation until the end of the study period.

To determine the cessation rates, smoking status was monitored regularly. Smoking status at Month 18 was checked using a self-reported written questionnaire for all subjects, and absence of urine cotinine, a nicotine metabolite which remains longer than lung CO (NicCheck [9]), was demonstrated for those who had reported continuing cessation since the ten-month survey. After Month 18, the abstainers' smoking status was regularly monitored through self-reported written questionnaires completed during annual health checkups at Months 30, 42, 54 and 66. During this observation period, subjects did not receive any active smoking cessation intervention at the worksite, although smoking cessation may have been recommended at the annual checkups.

Cessation rates were determined in all previous smokers who had achieved cessation at Month 10 (n = 35) and in subgroups stratified by nicotine dependence or willingness to quit smoking at baseline.

Height and weight were recorded at the annual checkups, and the subject's BMI was calculated as body weight (in kg) divided by the square of body height (in m). For the baseline BMI, we used the measurements recorded at the annual checkup in 1996 before the initial intervention. We compared the BMI changes of two groups: the continuous abstainers who continued smoking cessation until the end of our study period; and the continuous smokers who never tried smoking cessation during our study period.

We excluded those who were lost to follow-up at each survey, because we believed that none of the subjects left the company for reasons related to health or smoking status, and that classifying those who had left the company as recidivists would skew the real rate of abstinence.

Results

The total number of subjects and the number able to maintain smoking cessation at each survey are shown in table 6. The cessation rates after three years were approximately 8-10% in subjects who had received support for smoking cessation.

When we looked closely at the 35 subjects who had successfully stopped smoking for more than four weeks at Month 10, the cessation rates reduced substantially at the first year, but became stable after three years (table 6). There was actually no change in the number of continuous abstainers between Months 42 and 66, but one of the recidivists left the site by the Month 54, which accounted for the apparent improvement in the rate.

For the original smokers whose nicotine dependence was not low (FTQ $\geq$ 4) and who abstained from smoking at Month 10, 61.5% continued smoking cessation throughout our study period. For the original smokers who initially were not willing to quit smoking, 47.6% continued smoking cessation throughout our study period.

Table 6. Number and proportion of subjects who maintained smoking cessation at each follow-up survey among all original smokers and among 35 abstainers who once achieved smoking cessation

Survey months after initial intervention	Among original smokers	Among 35 abstainers
Month 10	35/251	35/35
	(13.9%)	(100.0%)
Month 18	22/230	13/31
	(9.6%)	(58.1%)
Month 30	18/202	13/28
	(8.9%)	(46.4%)
Month 42	17/202	11/25
	(8.4%)	(44.0%)
Month 54	19/197	11/24
	(9.6%)	(45.8%)
Month 66	19/180	11/24
	(10.6%)	(45.8%)

Table 7 shows changes in body weight and BMI, comparing continuous abstainers (n=11) with continuous smokers (n=128). At baseline, there was no statistical difference between the prospective continuous abstainers and habitual smokers in height (171.0cm vs. 171.3cm), weight (64.3kg vs. 63.8kg) or BMI (22.0 kg/m^2 vs. 21.7 kg/m^2). In the abstainers, BMI increased by up to 1.55 kg/m^2 on average, but then gradually decreased. Among the 11 abstainers, four lost weight, two gained less than 1 kg/m^2 on the BMI index, and one gained more than 3 kg/m^2 on the BMI index (figure 2).

Table 7. Changes in body weight and body mass index in continuous abstainers who quit smoking through the intervention and continuous smokers who never stopped habitual smoking

	Continuous abstainers (n=11)			Continuous smokers (n=128)			
Survey months	Body weight (kg)	Body weight change (kg)	BMI change (kg/m^2)	Body weight (kg)	Body weight change (kg)	BMI change (kg/m^2)	P-value*
after initial intervention	[Minimum, Maximum]	[Minimum, Maximum]	[Minimum, Maximum]	[Minimum, Maximum]	[Minimum, Maximum]	[Minimum, Maximum]	of BMI change
Baseline	64.3±6.7	0	0	64.2±9.3	0	0	
	[56.0, 80.0]			[44.2, 104.6]			
Month 18	67.0±8.2	3.5±2.7	1.10±0.77	64.9±9.4	0.7±2.4	0.13±0.84	0,001
	[59.0, 88.6]	[-1.6, 8.6]	[-0.36, 2.52]	[45.4, 105.3]	[-6.9, 6.8]	[-2.57, 2.35]	
Month 30	68.9±7.4	4.6±4.0	1.55±1.30	65.0±9.7	0.6±3.2	0.26±1.12	<0.001
	[61.0, 87.2]	[0.1, 12.3]	[0.10, 4.12]	[43.5, 103.7]	[-11.6, 9.7]	[-4.02, 3.38]	
Month 42	68.3±8.4	4.0±5.1	1.36±1.64	65.1±9.5	0.7±3.3	0.32±1.11	0,005
	[58.6, 89.9]	[-2.5, 12.6]	[-0.92, 3.78]	[46.8, 100.6]	[-8.5, 9.3]	[-2.87, 3.66]	
Month 54	68.1±8.7	3.9±5.6	1.26±1.77	65.4±9.7	1.1±3.5	0.33±1.19	0,017
	[58.6, 89.7]	[-3.3, 11.5]	[-1.17, 3.76]	[45.5, 100.3]	[-8.3, 10.7]	[-2.94, 3.54]	
Month 66	67.2±8.3	2.9±5.2	1.00±1.64	65.3±9.5	0.9±3.6	0.28±1.19	0,063
	[58.7, 87.0]	[-5.0, 10.2]	[-1.54, 3.26]	[44.6, 99.0]	[-7.6, 9.8]	[-2.60, 3.41]	

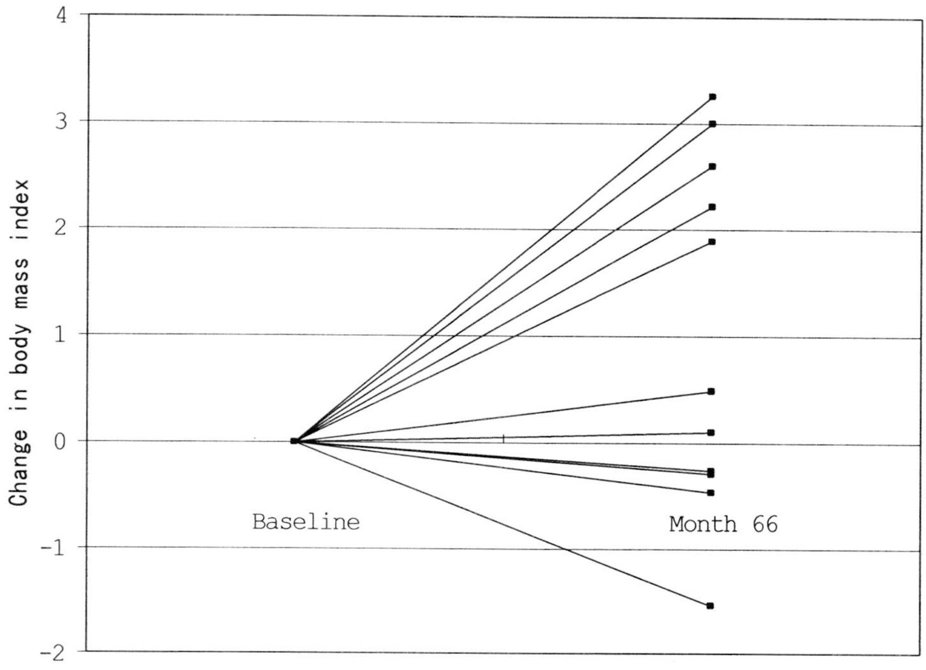

Figure 2. Change in body mass index of 11 continuous abstainers who abstained from smoking throughout the study period. Among those who achieved smoking cessation from the intervention, four lost weight, two gained less than 1 kg/m^2 on the BMI index, and one gained more than 3 kg/m^2 on the BMI index in five years.

Message from this Section

We clarified that once subjects had stopped smoking for more than four weeks, the continuation rate was 45%. The cessation rate did not change after three years regardless of their baseline willingness to quit smoking or their nicotine dependence. With regard to the BMI change, there was an increase of up to 1.55 kg/m^2 on average, but BMI gradually decreased and stabilized at a gain of about 1 kg/m^2 over five years. The results also showed that the cessation rates in those with high nicotine dependence and less willingness to quit smoking were not statistically different after one year, although those with lower nicotine dependence and those who were positive about smoking cessation were more likely to quit at the initial stage, as was shown in Section 1. Even if the smokers originally had high nicotine dependence and less willingness to quit smoking, their cessation rates were better than the natural trend of one percent decline per year at that time [10]. The results may serve as a template for smokers' prognoses when health care providers plan to promote smoking cessation among similar populations.

Section 3: Repeated Conduct of Smoking Cessation Programs

The effectiveness of a smoking cessation program and its long-term duration have been presented in the previous sections. However, in reality, such intervention programs may likely to be small in scale, and it is difficult to reach all smokers in any program. Nevertheless, we could still reduce smoking prevalence if we conduct such small-scale intervention programs repeatedly. In this section, we examined the effectiveness of annual smoking cessation programs using a similar intervention in other settings in Japan [11].

Methods

Study Setting

Smoking cessation programs using a similar intervention on a smaller scale were conducted annually in August to October, for ten consecutive years (1993 to 2002) in a chemical plant in Hyogo, Japan. The number of employees was approximately 1,500 and 95% of the workers were male. We recruited smokers who were willing to quit smoking through posters, company circulars and intranet emails. Participants received a smoking cessation intervention program of approximately two months. The main outcome is male smoking prevalence in this plant.

As a control, smoking prevalence of male workers in the same company's other plants in Shiga and Ibaraki from 1995 to 2002 was employed. The two other plants are within the same industry and have identical health care systems, but they do not conduct annual interventions on smoking cessation.

Intervention Protocol

The intervention protocol consisted of one group session, and correspondence via postal or in-house mail instead of periodic visits by health care providers.

Participants initially attended a group session of approximately one hour, where the health care providers and participants discussed harmful effects of tobacco, past experience of abstinence, and merits of smoking cessation. They also discussed how to quit smoking and overcome nicotine withdrawal symptoms. Then each participant decided the starting date of smoking cessation and signed a declaration form stating that they would quit smoking on the determined date.

Participants received letters of encouragement and self-help leaflets five to seven times on how to quit smoking. They received the first set of materials prior to the determined date as a reminder of starting smoking cessation, the second set three or four days later when abstainers tend to suffer from the strongest nicotine withdrawal symptoms, and the subsequent materials once every one or two weeks periodically for approximately two months. Each participant was asked to fill in and send back a questionnaire card clarifying the smoking status along with brief comments every time they received a letter of encouragement and self-help leaflets. Subsequent materials were selected in accordance with the smoking status confirmed in the questionnaire responses. In principle, nicotine replacement therapy was not part of the intervention but subjects may have obtained nicotine gum at the Health Care Center if they wanted it.

Determination of Smoking Cessation

At the end of the intervention program approximately two months after the initial meeting, participants were invited to the closing session where they discussed their experience of achieving smoking cessation and their resolution of continuing abstinence. They also underwent a measurement of an expired CO concentration. Smoking cessation was considered to be achieved when 1) a participant declared abstinence of more than four weeks in the closing session as well as in the periodic communication and 2) had an expired CO concentration of less than 9 ppm.

Outcomes Measurements

The main outcome of this study is the male smoking prevalence in the intervention and control worksites of our present study. Smoking prevalence was monitored through self-administered questionnaires provided at the annual health checkups. The control data of 1993 and 1994 were not available due to technical reasons within data management system. Thus we decided to regard the 1995 data as our baseline. Age distributions were adjusted for that of the intervention group at the end of the study.

Results

The number of male employees and age distributions in the intervention and control worksites in 1995 and 2002 are shown in table 8. As described previously, although the intervention started in 1993, we used the 1995 data as the baseline, because the data of 1993-94 in the control group were not available. At baseline, subjects in the intervention group were younger, but the distribution did not differ significantly. At the end of the study, both the mean and distribution of age ranks showed borderline significance.

The number of participants in the intervention program, participation rate among smokers, and cessation rate in each year are displayed in table 9. The trends of crude smoking prevalence in the intervention and control worksites are shown in figure 3. The male smoking prevalence of the intervention worksite decreased from 56.2% in 1993 and 52.6% in 1995 to 47.0% in 2002, while in the control worksite it decreased from 58.2% in 1995 to 57.8% in 2002. After adjusting each smoking prevalence for the age distribution of the intervention group at the end of the study, the smoking prevalence changed from 51.4% to 47.0% in the intervention group while it changed from 58.3% to 58.1% in the control group. Although we cannot compare the smoking prevalence in 1993 and 94, the intervention worksite showed significant decline as compared to the control in both crude and age-adjusted rates in the last two years of the study.

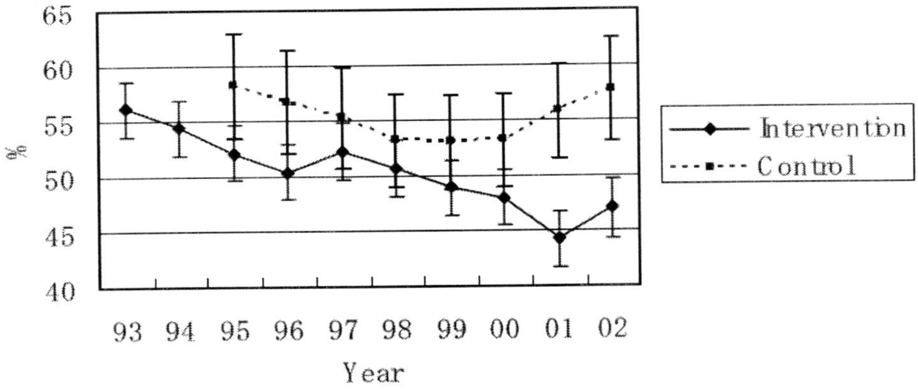

Figure 3. Trends of male smoking prevalence and 95% confidence interval in the intervention worksite in Hyogo in 1993-2002 and the control worksite in Shiga and Ibaraki in 1995-2002 are shown. The male smoking prevalence of the intervention worksite decreased from 56.2% in 1993 and 52.6% in 1995 to 47.0% in 2002, while in the control worksite it decreased from 58.2% in 1995 to 57.8% in 2002.

Message from this Section

The findings suggest that a small-scale intervention can reduce the smoking prevalence in the long run when repeated annually. Even though the proportion of smokers actually willing to participate in the program was not very large, we succeeded in having motivated smokers quit smoking every year, resulting in a reduction of smoking prevalence. Although the impact of each annual intervention may be small, by repeating small-scale intervention annually, the smoking prevalence can be reduced more efficiently than the lack of an intervention at all.

Section 4: Comprehensive Environmental Changes and Smoking Prevalence

Environmental changes such as designation of smoking areas, legislation and price increase, and health education for smokers are both important measures of reducing the prevalence of smoking. It is, however, practically impossible to concurrently compare the effectiveness of these two measures, because environmental changes necessarily affect all smokers.

Table 8. Age distribution of male workers at the smoking cessation intervention and control worksites in 1995 and 2002

	1995			2002		
	Intervention	Control	p-value*	Intervention	Control	p-value*
Number of male workers	1509	419	0,041	1378	434	0,066
Mean age (Standard deviation)	38.5 (11.4)	39.8 (11.9)		39.4 (10.7)	38.3 (11.4)	
Age range (minimum-maximum)	19-67	19-64		20-64	20-69	
Age distribution (%)						
18-29	28,3	24,8	0,234	22,2	26,6	0,096
30-39	26,0	24,6		30,1	24,8	
40-49	25,8	26,7		24,1	30,5	
50-	19,8	23,9		23,6	18,1	

* P-values were obtained through Student's t-test for age and Chi-squre test for the ditribution of age groups.

Smokers in Japan have experienced nationally implemented environmental changes since 2002. The Japanese government enacted a new law called Health Promotion Law in August, 2002 and began enforcing it in May, 2003. This law was enacted to promote public wellness through specifying fundamental actions concerning the comprehensive promotion of public health. One of the articles reads as follows:

Article 25: Protection from Passive Smoking

Administrators of facilities used by the general public, such as schools, gymnasiums, hospitals, theaters, pavilions, assembly halls, exhibition halls, department stores, offices, public facilities, and eating and drinking places, shall endeavor to take necessary measures to protect users of these facilities from being exposed to passive smoking. (Passive smoking refers to unwillingly inhaling others' tobacco smoke in indoor or equivalent environments.)

After the enforcement of this law, many facilities, including occupational settings, banned indoor smoking or initiated designated smoking areas. In July, 2003, the government raised the tobacco tax by approximately 20 Japanese yen (nearly equivalent to 19 U.S. cents) per pack.

Cumulative environmental changes are likely to affect smokers and help a considerable number of them quit smoking. Public health approaches to tobacco control can affect large numbers of individuals at minimal cost. Smoke-free workplaces and increasing the cost of cigarettes through increased taxation are two cost-effective approaches to tobacco control. Evidence from countries of varying economic levels shows that price increases on cigarettes are highly effective in reducing demand [12]. However, the effectiveness of such measures is lower than direct intervention targeting smokers [13].

Apart from these environmental changes, health education on smoking cessation is also effective to reduce the smoking prevalence, as was presented in Sections 1 and 2. While such interventions may be more effective than public health approaches, they can usually reach only a small proportion of smokers [13].

In this Section, we examined the study question; "Can comprehensive environmental changes be as effective as health education in a setting where smoking prevalence is considerably high?" As mentioned above, it is hard to compare these two measures, because one affects all smokers and the other can reach a relatively small proportion of smokers. We can, however, still compare them if we involve all smokers in health education in a limited setting, although we need to give up parallel comparison and allow different time frames. We compared the smoking cessation rates of two time periods: the time period of health education for all smokers regardless of their willingness to quit smoking that was presented in Section 1, and the time period of environmental changes including legislation, price increase and designation of smoking areas in an occupational setting in Japan [14].

Methods

Study Population

The study setting is the same factory as we presented in Sections 1 and 2. Subjects in this study were male workers in a factory in Shiga, Japan, who were habitual smokers at the beginning of each study period: the time period of health education (1997 – 1999) and the time period of environmental changes (2002 – 2004). Those who left the worksite for some reason unrelated to smoking status during the pertinent time period were excluded from the study. The time frame of this study is displayed in figure 4. The Time Period of Health Education (1997 – 1999) indicates the period of conducting a smoking cessation program presented in Section 1.

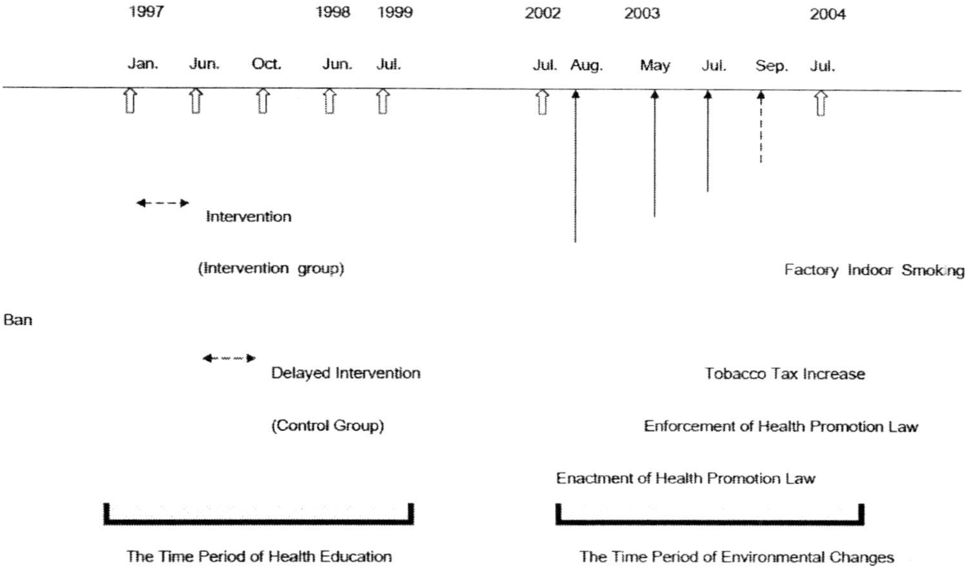

Figure 4. Time frame of events the factory experienced and smoking status survey in 1997-99 and 2002-04

N.B. ⇧ : Smoking status survey was done.

The Time Period of Environmental Changes (2002-2004)

For the time period of environmental changes, we set the time frame of 2002 to 2004 to include all the cumulative changes in the smoking environment at the worksite (figure 4). As mentioned above, the Japanese government enacted the Health Promotion Law in August, 2002, and enforced it in May, 2003. The tobacco tax was increased in July, 2003. In addition, the Health and Safety Committee of the factory decided to ban indoor smoking as of September 1, 2003, in accordance with Article 25 of the Health Promotion Law. Since then, smokers at the factory were allowed to smoke only at designated smoking areas outside the buildings. We identified smokers through a self-administered questionnaire at their annual health check-up in July, 2002, when no environmental change had yet begun. We reassessed the smoking cessation rate at the annual health check-up in July, 2004, when the cumulative environmental changes were over. We did not conduct any health education programs for smokers during the time period of environmental changes.

Confirmation of Smoking Status

In the beginning of each period, male smokers were self-identified in self-administered written questionnaires. Successful smoking cessation was ascertained by a urine test of nicotine metabolites [9]. The smoking cessation rate was calculated as the proportion of those who were ascertained to have quit smoking among those baseline smokers who remained employed in the factory through the entire pertinent period (and this may make the result apparently different from Section 1).

Results

At the beginning of the time period of health education in January, 1997, there were 263 male smokers. By the end of the period in July, 1999, 61 of the baseline smokers had left the worksite for some reason unrelated to smoking status, and the remaining 202 baseline smokers were included in the analysis of the time period of health education. Among the 202 smokers in the period of health education, 18 (8.9%) quit smoking by the end of the period in 1999.

At the beginning of the time period of environmental changes in July, 2002, there were 202 male smokers. Among the 202 smokers, 159 were from the previous period and 43 newly entered the worksite. By the end of the period in July, 2004, 32 of the baseline smokers had left the worksite for some reason unrelated to smoking status, and the remaining 170 baseline smokers were included in the analysis of the time period of environmental changes. Among those 170 male smokers, 141 experienced both periods. Among the 170 baseline smokers in the period of environmental changes, 12 (7.1%) quit smoking by the end of the period in 2004.

Table 9 shows the age distribution and the number and proportion of men who quit smoking in each age group. There was no difference in the cessation rate between these two time periods in a chi-square test (P=0.513). The age distribution in the beginning of the two periods were significantly different (P=0.007). The age-adjusted cessation rate of the period of environmental changes, having the health education subjects as the reference group, was 7.0%. There was no significant difference in the cessation rates after age adjustment between health education and environmental change groups (P=0.189).

Table 9. Age distributions and cessation rates in the occasions of health education and smoking environmental changes

	Health Education (Reference Group)				Environmental Changes (Comparison Group)			
	Baseline Smokers		Abstainers		Baseline Smokers		Abstainers	
	(1997)		(1999)		(2002)		(2004)	
Age group	n	(% in population)	n	(% in age group)	n	(% in population)	n	(% in age group)
18-24	32	(15.8)	1	(3.1)	11	(6.5)	0	(0.0)
25-34	102	(50.5)	8	(7.8)	92	(54.1)	8	(8.7)
35-44	49	(24.3)	8	(16.3)	37	(21.8)	4	(10.8)
45-60	19	(9.4)	1	(5.3)	30	(17.6)	0	(0.0)
Total	202	(100.0)	18	(8.9)	170	(100.0)	12	(7.1)

Message from this Section

We evaluated the effectiveness of cumulative environmental changes including designation of smoking places, and price increase on tobacco that Japan has experienced in recent years, comparing them to health education in a limited specific setting. We found that cumulative environmental changes are fairly effective, and may yield a similar proportion as health education on smoking cessation rates.

Conclusion

Smoking cessation intervention without nicotine replacement therapy regardless of the smokers' willingness to quit is effective in populations with high smoking prevalence such as those in developing countries. Even though the scale of intervention is small, repeating the intervention can yield reduced smoking prevalence. Once smokers achieve cessation of more than four weeks, the relapse is likely not to occur after three years, and 45% of former smokers continue smoking cessation for more than three years. Comprehensive environmental changes, as well as intervention on smoking cessation, may yield fair effectiveness on reducing smoking prevalence. The series of these outcomes may serve as a projection of the expected results when health care providers conduct smoking cessation activities in similar situations.

Reference

[1] Mackay J, Eriksen M, and Shafey O (2006). The Tobacco Atlas. (2nd edition). Atlanta: The American Cancer Society

[2] World Health Organization (1999). The Health Report 1999. Geneva: World Health Organization

[3] Kadowaki T, Watanabe M, Okayama A, et al. (2000). Effectiveness of smoking-cessation intervention in all of the smokers at a worksite in Japan. *Ind. Health,* 38,396-403.

[4] Heatherton TF, Kozlowski LT, Frecker RC, et al. (1991). The Fagerstrom test for nicotine dependence: a revision of the Fagerstrom Tolerance Questionnaire. *Br. J. Addict,* 86, 1119-27.

[5] Jarvis MJ, Belcher M, Versey C, et al. (1986). Low cost carbon monoxide monitors in smoking assessment. *Thorax,* 41, 886-8.

[6] Kadowaki T, Okayama A, et al. (2007) Health education for smoking cessation (*kinnenn-wo-shienn-suru-kenko-kyoiku, in Japanese*). Tokyo: Hoken-dojin-sha

[7] Filozof C, Fernandez Pinilla MC, et al. (2004). Smoking cessation and weight gain. *Obes. Rev.* 5, 95-103

[8] Kadowaki T, Watanabe M, Okayama A, et al. (2006). Continuation of smoking cessation and following weight change after intervention in a healthy population with high smoking prevalence. *J. Occup. Health,* 48, 402-406.

[9] Eswara AR, Nochur SV, and Mossman DJ. (1996). Detection of nicotine and its metabolism in urine. *Am. J. Health Behav,* 20, 335-45
[10] Kawane H. (1998). The tobacco epidemic in Japan (letter). *Thorax.* 53, 328
[11] Kadowaki T, Okamura T, Funakoshi T, et al. (2004). Effectiveness of annual intervention for smoking cessation on an occupational setting in Japan. *Environ. Health Prev. Med,* 9, 161-164.
[12] World Health Organization (2003). Tools for Advancing Tobacco Control in the XXIst century: Policy Recommendations for Smoking Cessation and Treatment of Tobacco Dependence, Tools for Public Health. Geneva: World Health Organization
[13] Parrott S, Godfrey C, Raw M, et al. (1998). Guidance for commissioners on the cost-effectiveness of smoking cessation interventions. *Thorax,* 53, S1-S38.
[14] Kadowaki T, Kanda H, Watanabe M, et al. (2006). Are comprehensive environmental changes as effective as health education for smoking cessation? *Tob. Control,* 15, 26-29

In: Progress in Smoking and Health Research
Editor: T. C. Jeffries, pp. 141-155
ISBN: 978-1-60021-686-2

Chapter VI

Smoking Cessation: Different Intervention Techniques between Sexes

*Ioannis Gkiozos, Georgios Papaetis and Kostas Syrigos**
Oncology Unit, 3rd Department of Medicine, Athens Medical School,
Sotiria General Hospital, Athens, Greece

Abstract

With 4.9 million people being killed each year due to smoking worldwide, tobacco is the only product that kills half its consumers. Across the E.U. countries, it is estimated that around 106.000 women die prematurely each year as a result of smoking. Women are affected by the main smoking-related diseases in the same way as men, but are also at risk of developing a number of gender-specific problems including cancer of cervix and problems related to reproductive health and osteoporosis.

An important question regarding quitting smoking is whether men and women should receive different cessation treatments. Although smoking cessation clinical trials reveal that the same pharmacotherapy treatments (Bupropion SR, Nicotine Replacement Therapies) benefit both men and women, there is strong evidence that the approach should be different towards female smokers. In fact, women may face different stressing parameters and barriers to quitting that may be useful to address in treatment decisions. These include greater likelihood of depression, greater weight control concerns, and hormonal cycle abnormalities. This suggests that women may benefit from tobacco dependence treatments that address these topics, although only few studies have examined programs targeted to one gender.

* Address for Correspondence: Konstantinos N. Syrigos, MD, PhD; Assistant Professor of Oncology in Medicine; Athens University School of Medicine; Head, Oncology Unit, Third Department of Medicine; Building Z, Sotiria General Hospital; Mesogion 152; 115 27 Athens, Greece; Tel: +30 210 7475 034 / Fax: +30 210 7781 035; Email: knsyrigos@usa.net / ksyrigos@med.uoa.gr

With regard to motivation in a smoking cessation program for females, one should underline benefits such as physical appearance and lower incidence of osteoporosis. In particular, women, who are candidates to become pregnant, may be more receptive to stop smoking because of the serious risks imposed on the fetus.

In conclusion, different smoking cessation treatment strategies with augmented psychosocial interventions and more intensive counseling about weight gain, osteoporosis, physical appearance, depression, and pregnancy may be needed for female smokers in order to achieve better abstinence rates.

Introduction

According to the *2001 Report of the Surgeon General on Women and Smoking,* smoking is the leading known cause of preventable death and disease among women [1]. In addition, a woman's annual risk for death more than doubles among continuing smokers compared with persons who have never smoked in all age groups from 45 to 74 years [1].

Although women are affected in the same way as men regarding the main smoking-related diseases, they do face specific gender-related health problems such as increased risks for conception delay, decreased fertility, moderate risk for ectopic pregnancy, spontaneous abortion, osteoporosis, cancer of cervix and vulvae. Moreover, female smokers are a target-group of the tobacco industry marketing which influences there susceptibility to and initiation of smoking especially among girls.

In the world of women-smokers, it is understood that there are many gender-related differences concerning health problems, as well as differences in the reasons of smoking and in the risk rates of developing smoking-related diseases. A reasonable question which is raised is if there are any different interventional techniques in smoking cessation programs between the two sexes in order to achieve better abstinence rates among women.

Research on gender differences in smoking cessation was initiated partially in response to the *1980 Report of the Surgeon General on Women and Smoking*, which stated, 'women have more difficulty in giving up smoking than men, both at the end of treatment and at long-term points of measurement," and partially in response to national survey (NHIS, AUTS) findings from the mid-1960s to mid-1980s which indicated that women had lower quit ratios than men. The quit ratio describes the proportion of ever smokers who are now former smokers (former smokers/ever smokers). Gender differences in the quit ratio have always existed: for men, rising from 31.4% (1965) to 48.7% (1987) to 51.6% (1991); and for women, rising from 24.6% (1965) to 40.1% (1987) to 44.7% (1991) [2,3]. On the other hand, gender differences in the pattern of quitting do not exist, as demonstrated by changes in average quit ratios. According to the 1990 *Surgeon General's Report on the Health Benefits of Smoking Cessation*, quit ratios were reported to increase 0.70% per year for men and 0.76% per year for women over the time period from 1965 to 1987.

Thus, the average annual rate of increase in quitting is similar for men and women. However, do these studies of the previous years reveal any differences between the two sexes and, if so, in which fields? Which are the differences between the two sexes regarding the abstinence rates and the type of pharmacotherapy? Do any specific physiological, psychological, and behavioral factors for women exist that influence the quit ratios? Are there any gender differences in smoking cessation associated with employment and joblessness? Can pregnancy-specific programs enable women to increase cessation rates? Are female-smokers more concerned about physical appearances and body-weight than male-smokers? Do tobacco-control programs with gender-sensitive approaches need to be developed for adolescent boys and girls? All these issues of the last decade have been questioned in regards to implementing effective, possible gender-sensitive, smoking cessation programs.

Different Pharmacologic Approaches to Smoking Cessation between Two Sexes

Generally, men and women have responded similarly to smoking cessation attempts and interventions [4] but, differences in abstinence or relapse rates have been reported for women [5,6] in unaided quit attempts [7], community interventions [8], and large clinical trials [9,10] . The US National Clinical Practice Guideline for the treatment of nicotine dependence recommends the use of pharmacotherapy with behavioral treatments, but does not make treatment recommendations based on gender with the exception with pregnant women [11]. Nicotine plays an integral role in the vicious circle between the continuous use of tobacco and a steady level of carcinogenic exposure for both sexes [12]. Nicotine Replacement Therapy (NRT) is effective in both men and women as demonstrated by a recent meta-analysis [13], and there is no clinical rational for not using these products in both genders.

However, there are reports of significant differences in women's responses to pharmacotherapies [9-11]. The most common pharmacotherapy using NRT shows that women often, but not always, respond more poorly than men. This suggests that non-nicotinic therapies may be more effective for women [14] than men or that NRT is more effective for men [15,16] than women.

What may partially account for the relatively better outcomes for women in these trials may be the suppression of several important factors related to smoking for women. For example, olfactory and taste stimuli are associated with smoking pleasure for women but not for men and bupropion may change the taste in cigarettes. A change in cigarette taste may result in negatively reinforced smoking behavior, especially for women, by reducing pleasure stimuli. While efficacy of bupropion for smoking cessation is independent of a history of depression, bupropion seems to reduce cessation-related depression, post-cessation appetite, weight gain, irritability and a negative affect [17,18].

Another trial [19] did not reveal any evidence for gender differences either in response to 7 weeks 300 mg bupropion treatment plus brief counseling or after 52 weeks of bupropion vs. placebo for relapse prevention. The authors suggested that bupropion is a promising pharmacotherapy for preventing relapse.

A recent placebo-controlled trial of bupropion with behavioral counselling [20] demonstrated that although women have more difficulty than men in quitting smoking, bupropion may attenuate this gender disparity particularly among females who are lighter smokers. According to the prolonged abstinence data, women tended to respond more poorly than men on placebo plus behavioral counselling but female lighter smokers had better abstinence rates to men on bupropion plus counselling.

In another study [21], women and elderly tobacco users were much less likely to receive prescriptions for cessation medications, while patients requesting treatment for tobacco-cessation and those with tobacco-caused diagnoses were more likely. Women using the Veterans Health Administration (VA) Smoking Cessation Services [22] were less likely to receive a prescription for nicotine patches, probably due to gender differences in knowledge, attitudes, or beliefs on the part of either the patient or the provider. Women may be less willing to use a medication to address a habit compared to men. It was seen that a year after the first attempt to quit, female smokers were less likely to have successfully quit smoking. On the other hand, male veterans were more likely to report problems associated with quitting, which is an important piece of information for providers to initiate pharmacotherapy [23].

A recent study [24] assessed the efficacy of two forms of pharmacotherapy (nicotine and phenylpropanolamine gums in addition to a 13-week cognitive behavioral smoking cessation program targeted for women. The results suggested that although the pharmacological interventions had no effect on cessation rates and post-cessation weight gain, the behavioral component of the intervention was effective in increasing the odds of quitting smoking in weight-concerned women.

A double-blinded, placebo-controlled trial [25] evaluated the efficacy of naltrexone (a primary mu-opioid receptor antagonist that is currently FDA-approved for the treatment of opioid and alcohol dependencies) as an adjunct to standard smoking cessation treatments. A preliminary study showed that naltrexone produced an overall modest improvement in smoking cessation rates. Potentially interesting sex differences were also observed (women showing a worse outcome compared to men) in the placebo group but not in the naltrexone group. Although this finding was statistically significant at 8 weeks, it was no longer significant at the 6-month follow-up, which may suggest a need for longer durations of treatment.

Regarding the type of Nicotine Replacement Therapy, individual NRT formulations have proven efficacy in smokers motivated to make a quit attempt, and there is little direct evidence that one nicotine product is more effective than another. Thus the decision about which product to use should be guided by individual preferences [26].

In conclusion, despite the evidence from various studies that differ in design, sample characteristics and intensity of the interventions, researchers to date have not found consistent gender-specific differences in the effectiveness of pharmacotherapy treatment in smoking cessation programs. Further investigation is still needed.

The Role of Physiological Factors between Two Sexes in a Smoking Cessation Program

Smoking has a multifactorial dependence: physical, psychological and social. The interaction between nicotine addiction, sociodemographic characteristics and behavioral factors is relevant to the success of smoking cessation [27]. The exploration of differences in nicotine sensitivity, tolerance and dependence as a function of gender began only the last decade.

Although there is no clear consensus, some interesting findings have emerged showing gender differences in nicotine-induced thermogenesis, satiety, heart rate, tolerance and perception of muscle tension. Therefore, the experience of smoking and the withdrawal distress may be somewhat different for women than to men.

A study [28] showed that nicotine enhanced thermogenesis during moderate physical activity for men but not for women and that among women, energy expenditure did not increase when nicotine consumption preceded exercise. In another study, female smokers were noted to work harder than male smokers to obtain food reinforces when they were deprived of cigarettes [29]. This is consistent with the idea that nicotine may enhance feelings of satiety, thus reducing food consumption and this may contribute to lower weight among smokers.

Women also experienced significantly more impairment than men in the detection of forearm muscle tension in smoking versus non-smoking conditions [30]. Thus, in some women, nicotine may be used to block the perception of muscle tension. This may encourage smoking in situations that often result in increased muscle tension (for example: anxiety, pain, headaches, depression). It was also noted that smoking may reduce fatigue or improve concentration to a greater extent for women than for men [31].

Regarding the withdrawal distress, studies have shown that there are significantly more symptoms in women than in men and that females were more likely than males to report that relapses were associated with anxiety or craving [32]. Moreover, gender differences were reported in the severity of withdrawal symptoms among nicotine users. Over an eight-week period, women experienced more severe withdrawal symptoms than men, particularly those who received the lowest doses of nicotine gum (2mg) [33]. On the other hand, the Transdermal Nicotine Study Group reported no differences in nicotine withdrawal symptoms between men and women [34].

Women also face unique biological processes which may affect the course and outcome of cessation. Commonly reported symptoms of smoking withdrawal include depression, irritability, anxiety, lethargy, tension, decreased concentration and weight changes [35]. These symptoms are similar to those reported by many women during menstrual distress. A study reported that women who quit smoking in the luteal phase (ovulation to day prior to menses) of their menstrual cycle experienced greater withdrawal than women who quit during the follicular phase (day 1 of the menses to day 15). When withdrawal scores of men were compared to women who quit in the luteal phase, women reported significantly more withdrawal symptoms [36]. These findings imply that the phase of a woman's menstrual cycle should be considered when selecting a quit day, especially if she experiences a high level of premenstrual distress.

Female smokers are more prone to early menopause than nonsmokers and may also experience more menopausal symptoms. Moreover, postmenopausal women who smoke have lower bone densities and an increased risk for hip fractures compared to women who do not smoke. As a result of these hormonal changes, menopausal women may experience fluctuations in affect, greater difficulties in weight control and changes in body image. Cumulatively, these factors may negatively influence the likelihood of cessation.

The Role of Behavioral and Psychological Factors between Two Sexes in a Smoking Cessation Program

Concerning the behavioral level, a number of psychological and socially-mediated factors may affect cessation among women. These factors include: fear of weight gain, need for social support, and reliance on cigarettes for control of negative affect or stress management, confidence in ability to quit (self-efficacy).

More women than men fear weight gain if they quit smoking [37,38]. However, few studies have found a relationship between weight gain concerns and smoking cessation among either women or men. Further actual weight gain during cessation does not predict relapse to smoking [39].

A large population-based prospective study (n=4,981) evaluated current and previous weight loss efforts and smoking behavior at baseline and at a two-year follow-up [40]. The researchers found that a change in weight and current or previous dieting were not related to relapse or cessation in men or women. Nevertheless, women who had a history of participation in weight loss programs were significantly more likely to quit smoking than men who also had a history of attending weight loss programs.

In clinical trials, attempts to suppress post-cessation weight gain have been generally unsuccessful [38,41] leading some investigators to conclude that, instead of developing intensive interventions to prevent weight gain, a more prudent strategy might be followed to help smokers to accept this relatively small weight gain[42].

On the other hand, another study revealed that if smoking cessation is followed by a moderate increase in the level of physical activity, then weight gain is minimized [43].

Further interventional trials are warranted to confirm that physical activity or incorporating a weight control program into a smoking cessation program are attractive options for women considering quitting. Additionally, weight control programs may be particularly important for the subgroup of women who use smoking to manage weight [44].

Smoking cessation and the social support derived from family and friends improve cessation rates, but it is inconclusive whether there are gender differences in the role of social support on long-term smoking cessation [39]. While women report that social support (behaviors or acts provided by others that include emotional, instrumental, informational and appraisal support) is of great importance to them, studies that incorporate social support components have not generally shown significant gender differences in cessation outcomes[45].

However, a population-based survey of smokers [46] revealed that the importance of social support in quitting was rated higher among women than men. This means that among women, successful quitters were significantly more likely to report greater social support than those who relapsed, whereas this difference was only marginally significant among men. Finally, women rated empathetic support (encouragement, listening) as more helpful than instrumental support (for example: suggesting alternatives to smoking).

A recent study investigated the effect of the partner smoking status on the success of a cessation program. Significant differences were found in the abstinence rates at 12 months by the partner smoking status: abstinence was achieved by 28.3% of patients with a smoking partner and by 46.5% of patients without a smoking partner. The subjects whose partner was smoking at the beginning of the program appeared to be more likely to relapse than the subjects without smoking partners and this was more pronounced in women than in men [47].

Women tend to use social support more than men to cope with stress and when making lifestyle behavioral changes. Findings from two population-based surveys [48,49] revealed that women making quit attempts are more likely than men to use cessation programs that provide some type of assistance, such as from mental health professionals and prefer formal smoking cessation groups or help from health professionals.

Moreover, there are specific socioeconomic conditions for subgroups of female smokers, like African-American women, which face stressing parameters for smoking cessation, such as a different cultural norm for smoking or a lack of social support and isolation. These women stated that smoking cessation would be feasible if it where a component of broader social support efforts to improve their lives [50]. Detailed research needs to clearly conceptualize social support and examine which types of support are beneficial for men and women.

Regarding the role of the negative affects (stress, anxiety, anger, fear, sadness, depression) on both sexes to smoking habit, few studies have evaluated gender differences. Women smoke more often in stressful and "high arousal" situations [45] and are more likely to relapse in the face of stressful life events, particularly health and financial stressors [51], whereas men relapse more often in positive situations such as social events or as part of relaxation. Studies which support these findings also report that women are more likely than men to expect that smoking will improve their mood [52] and they are more likely to relapse at home when they report a negative mood (in contrast to men who are more likely to report relapses outside of the home, when their mood is positive) [53] .

Special attention should be paid to the assessment and treatment of depressed female smokers, particularly with the use of pharmacological and behavioral therapies. Studies have shown that smokers with major depression, who were more nicotine-dependent, were less successful in quitting, experienced more withdrawal symptoms and were more likely to relapse compared to non-depressed smokers [54, 55, 56. These findings are significant for women given that the incidence of depression is higher in women than in men.

A recent study [57] evaluated the gender differences in smoking cessation associated with employment and joblessness through young adulthood in the US. There were findings that joblessness is more strongly associated with persistence in smoking among women than it is among men and that the lower likelihood of cessation among women who have exited the labor force is due to the associated reductions in social and economic resources. One explanation for that lower likelihood may be the combined strains of material deprivation and parenthood, to which women are unwilling to add to the stress associated with smoking cessation. Women may indeed benefit from a smoking cessation program designed to deal with negative affects and how to cope with them in a different way than men.

Women smokers also seem to be less self-confident than men to attempt to quit smoking. It was found [58] that men were significantly more likely to report plans to quit completely in the next 12 months, while women were significantly more likely to report intentions to cut down on the number of cigarettes smoked in the next 12 months. Although the above study did not find significant differences between the two sexes concerning their self-confidence in making a quit attempt, the researchers noted that women seemed to be less committed to quitting and responded more negatively than men to cessation failures. Therefore, it is critical to help females view relapse as a learning experience for future quit attempts and not as a sign of failure.

Pregnancy: A Unique Chance for a Successful Smoking Cessation Program

Women who smoke have increased risk for conception delay and for both primary and secondary infertility. Female smokers during pregnancy also risk pregnancy complications, premature birth, low-birth weight infants, stillbirth infant mortality and have a modest increase in risks for ectopic pregnancy (fallopian tube or peritoneal cavity pregnancy) and spontaneous abortion. Moreover, studies show a link between smoking and the risk of sudden infant death syndrome (SIDS) among the offspring of women who smoke during the pregnancy [1]. Despite increased knowledge of the adverse health effects of smoking during pregnancy, it is estimated that pregnant women continue to smoke throughout their pregnancies ranging from 12% (based on birth certificate data) up to 20% (based on survey data). If they manage to quit during pregnancy, most return to smoking after pregnancy- up to 67% by the 12th month after delivery. However, smoking during pregnancy appears to have decreased from 1989 to 2000. *According to the Treating Tobacco Use and Dependence clinical practise guideline* [11] an evidence-based recommendation for brief pregnancy-tailored counselling for routine use in prenatal care has been found to double or triple pregnant smokers' quit rates compared with simply advising them to quit.

Pregnant smokers who are unable to quit with the help of the five A's (Ask, Advise, Assess, Assist, Arrange) may benefit from other clinical practise guidelines and intensive counselling from a provider with special training in the treatment of tobacco dependence and the appropriate use of effective pharmacotherapies. Pharmacotherapies are recommended for consideration only among pregnant women who smoke heavily and are unable to quit using counselling alone and when the potential benefits and likelihood of quitting outweigh the potential risks [59]. Bupropion is specifically contraindicated in pregnancy as well as other antidepressants which are subject to special caution. The treatment of choice for pregnant women is nicotine replacement therapy (NRT). Any safety concerns about this treatment can be discounted by the fact that the alternative for most women is continued smoking and hence, continued fetal exposure to nicotine and other toxins. In order to avoid unnecessary exposure of the fetus to nicotine, it is probably advisable to avoid the longer-acting NRT formulations, such as 24 hour transdermal patches [60]. Additionally, further research is still needed to evaluate the safety of NRT_S during pregnancy.

Programs that encourage women to stop smoking before, during and after pregnancy deserve high priority for two reasons: during pregnancy women are highly motivated to stop smoking and they still have many remaining years of potential life.

Smoking Cessation between Young People

While smoking has declined among adults in Europe over recent years, there has been little decline among 11 to 15 year olds [61,62]. In addition, smoking among young people has become increasingly gendered, with regular (weekly) smoking in girls being higher than boys in 19 out of 31 European countries. It is now widely accepted that tobacco control strategies aimed at reducing smoking among young people need to adopt a more gender-sensitive approach [63-66], although their development is hampered by our limited understanding of the reasons behind gender differences in youth smoking.

A wide range of factors influence young people to start and continue smoking. These are related to young people's individual characteristics (e.g. attitudes, beliefs, self-esteem, risk-taking, age, educational attainment), their close personal environment (e.g. family and friends' smoking, school ethos) and their wider social and cultural environment (e.g. social norms, tobacco promotion, access to cigarettes) [67,68].

Several studies have found gender differences in relation to some of these factors. These include differences relating to body image (girls are more concerned about body image and believe that smoking can control weight), affect control (girls more likely to smoke so as to cope with negative feelings) and self-esteem (poor self-esteem being more influential in girls' smoking) [69]. Girls who initiate smoking are also more likely to have parents or friends who smoke and have weaker attachments to parents and family and stronger attachments to peers and friends.

A study of Scottish 11- and 13- years olds [70] found that smoking was most common among 'top girls' who were described as 'good-looking', 'loud' and 'cool' and used smoking as a marker of their membership of this group, and by 'bottom girls' who smoked to be like 'top girls' and attain their status. In contrast, high status boys were less vulnerable to smoking as it conflicted with their wish to be fit and they could secure a cool identity through other activities, notably sports.

A recent qualitative study [71] which used single-sex focus groups to explore the gendered nature of the meaning and function of smoking among Scottish 15- to 16- years old smokers found that young people were ambivalent about their smoking and that this was somewhat different for boys and girls. These differences related to their social worlds, pattern of social relationships, interests, activities and concerns, the meanings they attached to smoking, and the role smoking played in dealing with the everyday experience of being a boy or girl in their mid-teens. Of particular importance was how different, according to gender, smoking was identified as, in reference to the working image/status, where adolescents had to go through in order to achieve a socially and culturally acceptable image.

Research evidence on sex-linked differences is unclear or inconsistent for the most of these factors and there is a need for further evaluation in order to achieve better abstinence rates or to avoid smoking in adolescence. In conclusion, tobacco-control programs need to develop broader gender-sensitive approaches to health promotion which are congruent with adolescent boys' and girls' experiences of smoking and their wider social worlds. Moreover, health professionals could consider becoming involved in anti-tobacco educational programs at schools that promote acquisition of social influence skills for young people. This is best achieved by involving young people in the development and evaluation of such programs. It is also important that such interventions occur before smoking (and being a smoker) becomes fully integrated into young people's notions of self.

Marketing Cigarettes to Women

Tobacco advertising gearing towards women began in the 1920_s and the number of women aged 18 to 25 years who began smoking increased significantly in the mid-1920_s. In 1960, about 10% of all cigarette advertisements appeared in popular women's magazines and by 1985 cigarette this increased by 34%. In 1999, expenditures for domestic cigarette advertising and promotion reached $8.24 billion increasing 22.3% from the $6.73 billion spent in 1998 [72].

Tobacco marketing targets women and men smokers in different ways: messages to women tend to link smoking with maturity, confidence, sexual attractiveness, and beauty, particularly in developing countries [73]. Advertising is used in part to reduce women's fear of the health risks from smoking by presenting information on nicotine and tar content or by using positive images (e.g. models engaged in exercise or pictures of white capped mountains against a background of clear blue skies). The promotion of 'mild' and 'light' cigarettes has typically involved associations with weight control with the connotation that there is a benefit in smoking with less of the 'bad' effects. In fact, this is far from the truth and bans on the use of these terms as well as a global control on tobacco advertising are being sought.

Conclusion

Even though it is known that smoking cessation clinical guidelines and treatments benefit both men and women, further insight raises the reasonable question as to whether or not the approaches should be tailored to suit the sexes, in particular by altering the intervention techniques towards female smokers. There are many studies that have evaluated different pharmacotherapeutic treatments between the two sexes, but there is still conflicting evidence about gender-specific differences in the effectiveness of pharmacotherapy treatment in smoking cessation.

Female smokers experience different withdrawal symptoms than male smokers which may be because of the different role of physiological factors which interact during smoking. Women also seem to smoke for different reasons than men e.g. to cope with negative feelings, control weight, in response to depression and the need for 'time out' in caring responsibilities. Pregnancy is a unique chance for women for a successful smoking cessation attempt knowing the adverse health effects of smoking to fetal and neonatal growth and development. Of particular importance are young girls smokers who are not smoking for the same reasons as the older female smokers. Tobacco-control programs in schools with the involvement of young smokers are needed for these adolescents. Gendered differences between women and men in smoking triggers and associations (in the form of tobacco advertising) also affect the likelihood of successful quits.

It is essential that all the above differences between women/men and girls/boys are factors underling smoking initiation and continuation and are fully understood in order to achieve better abstinence rates in a smoking cessation program for female smokers.

References

[1] US Department of Health and Human Services. *The Health Consequences of Smoking for Women, A Report of the Surgeon General.* US Public Health Service, Office of the Assistant Secretary for Health, Office on Smoking and Health; 2001.

[2] Syrigos KN, Nutting C, Roussos C, Tumors of the chest. Biology, Diagnosis and Management. Verlag, New York, May 2006.

[3] CDC. Cigarette smoking among adults-United States, 1991.*MMWR.* 1993;42:230-233.

[4] Whitlock EP, Vogt TM, Hollis, JF, Lichtenstein E. Does gender affect response to a brief clinic-based smoking intervention? *American Journal of Preventive Medicine.* 1997;13:159-66.

[5] Pomerleau CS. Smoking and nicotine replacement treatment issues specific to women. *Am. J. Health Behav.* 1996;20:291-9.

[6] Escopedo LG, Peddicord JP.Smoking prevalence in US birth cohorts: the influence of gender and education. *American Journal of Public Health.* 1996;86:231-6

[7] Ward KD, Klesges RC, Zbikowski SM, Bliss RE, Garvey AJ. Gender differences in the outcome of an unaided smoking cessation attempt. *Addict. Behav.* 1997;22:521-33.

[8] Royce JM, Corbett K, Sorensen G, Ockene J. Gender, social pressure and smoking cessation: the Community Intervention Trial for Smoking Cessation (Commit) at baseline. *Soc. Sci. Med.* 1997:44:359-70.

[9] Bjornson WM, Rand C, Connett JE, et al. Gender differences in smoking cessation after three years in the Lung Health Study. *Am. J. Public Health.* 1995;85:223-30.

[10] Nides MA, Rakos RF, Gonzales D, Murray RP, Tashkin DP, Bjornson-Benson WM. Predictors of initial smoking cessation and relapse through the first 2 years of the Lung Health Study. *Journ. Consult. Clin. Psychol.* 1995;63:60-69.

[11] Fiore MC, Baile WC, Cohen SJ, et al. Treating tobacco use and dependence: clinical practice guideline. Rockville, MD: *US. Department of Health and Human Services, Public Health Service*, June 2000.

[12] Mauer C, Syrigos KN. Biology of tobacco and smoking. In Tumors of the Chest : Biology, Diagnosis and Management. Eds : Syrigos KN, Nutting C, Roussos Ch. Springer-Verlang, New York, 2006, pp 23-39.

[13] Cepeda-Benito A, Reynoso JT, Erath S. Meta-analysis of the efficacy of nicotine replacement therapy for smoking cessation: differences between men and women. *Journ. Consult. Clin. Psychol.* 2004;72:712-22.

[14] Perkins KA.Nicotine discrimination in men and women.*J Pharmacol Biochem Behav* 1999;64:295-9.

[15] Killen JD, Fortmann SP, Newman B,Varady A. Evaluation of a treatment approach combining nicotine gum with self-guided behavioural treatments for smoking relapse prevention. *Journal of Consulting and Clinical Psychology.* 1990;58:85-92.

[16] Hatsukami D, Skoog K, Allen S,Bills R. Gender and the effects of different doses of nicotine gum on tobacco withdrawal symptoms. *Experimental and Clinical Psychopharmacology*. 1995;3:163-173.

[17] Shiffman S, Johnston JA, Khayrallah M, et al. The effect of bubropionn on nicotine craving and withdrawal. *Psychopharmacologia*. 2000;148:33-40.

[18] Borrelli B, Spring B ,Niaura R, Hitsman B, Papandonatos G. Influences of gender and weight gain on short-term relapse to smoking in a cessation trial. *Journal of Consulting and Clinical Psychology*, 2001;69 *3,511/515.

[19] Gonzales D, Bjornson W, Durcan MJ, White JD, Johnston JA, Buist AS, Sachs DPL, Rigotti NA, Niaura R, Hays T, Hurt RD. Effects of Gender on Relapse Prevention in Smokers Treated with Bubropion SR. *American Journal of Preventive Medicine*. 2002;22:234-239.

[20] Collins BN, Wileyto EP, Patterson F, Rukstalis M, Audrain/McGovern J, Kaufmann V, Pinto A, Hawk L, Niaura R, Epstein LH, Lerman C. Gender differences in smoking cessation in a placebo/controlled trial of bupropion with behavioral counselling. *Nicotine and Tobacco Research*. 2004,6:27/37

[21] Steinberg MB, Akincigil A, Delveno CD, Crystal S, Garson JL. Gender and Age Disparities for Smoking-Cessation Treatment. *American Journal of Preventive Medicine*. 2006;30(5)405-412.

[22] Sherman SE, Fu SS, Joseph AM, Lanto AB, Yano EM. Gender differences in smoking cessation services received among veterans. *Women's Health Issues*. 2005;15:126-133.

[23] Chernof BA, Sherman SE, Lanto AB, Lee ML, Yano EM, Rubenstein LV. Health habit counselling amidst competing demands: effects of patient health habits and visit characteristics. *Medical Care*. 1999;37:738-747.

[24] Cooper TV, Klesges RC, DeBon MW, Zbikowski SM, Johnson KC, Clemens LH. A placebo controlled randomised trial of the effects of phenylpropanolamine and nicotine gum on cessation rates and post-cessation weight gain in women. *Addictive Behaviours*. 2005;30:61-75.

[25] King A, De Wit H, Riley RC, Cao D, Niaura R, HatsukamiD. Efficacy of naltrexone in smoking cessation: A preliminary study and an examination of sex differences. *Nicotine and Tobacco Research*. 2006;8(5):671-682.

[26] Gratziou C, Roussos Ch.Smoking Prevention and Cessation Policies. In Tumors of the Chest : Biology, Diagnosis and Management. Eds : Syrigos KN, Nutting C, Roussos Ch. Springer-Verlang, New York, 2006, pp 627-639.

[27] Kottke T, Battista R, De Friese G. Attributes of successful smoking cessation interventions in medical prectise. A meta-analysis of 39 controlled trials. *The Journal of the American Medical Association*. 1988;259:2883-2889.

[28] Perkins K, Sexton J, Epstein L, Fonte C, DiMarco A. Thermogenic effects of nicotine plus caffeine during light activity in male and female smokers. *Annals of Behavioural Medicine*. 1994;16:S060.

[29] Perkins KA, Epstein LH, Fonte C,Grobe JE. The reinforcing value of food during brief smoking abstinence in male and female smokers. *Annals of Behavioral Medicine*. 1994;16:S110.

[30] Epstein LH, Dickson BE, McKenzie S, Russel PO. The effects of smoking on perception of mulcle tension. *Psychopharmacology*. 1984;83:107-113.

[31] Knott V. Neurophysiological aspects of smoking behavioural: Aneuroelectric percspective. *Br. J. Addict.* 1991;86:511-515.

[32] Shiffman S. The tobacco withdrawal syndrome. In: Kresnegor NM, ed. Cigarette smoking as a Dependence Process. Rockville, Md: Nationale Institute on Drug Abuse, Unitred States Department of bHealth, Education and Welfare;1979:158-184.

[33] Hatsukami D. Effects of nicotine gum on withdrawal symptoms in females versus males. Paper presented at American Phychological Association, Psychosocial and Behavioral Factors in Women's Health: Creating an Agenda for the 21st Century, Washington, DC,1994.

[34] Repsher LH, Group TTNS. Smoking cessation by women and older persons: Results from the Trandermal Nicotine Study Group. *Mod. Med.* 1994;62:34-38.

[35] Gritz ER, Carr CR, Marcus AC. The tobacco withdrawal syndrome in unaided quitters. *Br. J. Addict.* 1991;86:57-69.

[36] O' Hara P, Poster SA, Anderson BP. The influence of menstrual cycle changes on the tobacco withdrawal syndrome in women. *Addict. Behav.* 1989;14: 595-600.

[37] Pomerlau CS, Zucker AN, Steward AJ. Characterizing concerns about post-cessation weight gain: results from a national survey of women smokers. *Nicotine Tob. Res.* 2001;3: 51-60.

[38] Piri PL, McBride CM, Hellerstedt W et al. Smoking cessation in women concerned about weight . *American Journal of Public Health.* 1992;82:1238-43.

[39] US Department of Health and Human Services.Efforts to Reduce Tobacco Use Among Women and Girls, *A Report of the Surgeon General*. US Public Health Service, Office of the Assistant Secretary for Health, Office on Smoking and Health; 2001.

[40] French SA, Jeffrey RW, Klesges LM, Forster JL. Weight concerns and change in smoking behaviour over two years in a working population. *American Journal of Public Health.* 1995;85: 720-721.

[41] Hall SM, Tunstall CD, Vila KL, Duffy J. Weight ain prevention and smoking cessation: cautionary findings. *American Journal of Public Health.* 1992;82: 799-803.

[42] Pekings KA, Weight gain following smoking cessation. *J. Consult. Clin. Psychol.* 1993;61:768-777.

[43] Kawachi I, Troisi RT, Rotnitzky AG, Coakley EH, Colditz GA. Can Physical Activity Minimize Weight Gain in Women After Smoking Cessation? *Amer. Journal of Public Health.* 1996;86:999-1004.

[44] Pinto BM, Marcus BH, Audrian JE, Taylor ER, Eating habits and weight management in women smokers. Paper presented at American Phychological Association, Psychological and Behavioral Factors in Womens's Health: Creating an Agenda for the 21st Century, Washinton, DC, 1994.

[45] Gritz ER, Nielsen IR, Brooks LA. Smoking Cessation and Gender: The Influence of Physiological, Psychological, and Behaviral Factors. *Journal Amer. Med. Women Assos.* 1996;51: 35-42.

[46] Fisher EB, Auslander WF, Sussman LJ, et al. Community organization and social support among African American women. Paper presented at Workshop on Recruitment and Retention of Women in Clinical Studies, St. Louis, Missuri, 1993.
[47] Walsh PM, Carrili P, Flores G, Masuet C, Morchon S, Ramon JM. Effects of partner smoking status and gender on long term abstinence rates of patients receiving smoking cessation treatment. *Addictive Behaviors.* 2006;xx:xxx-xxx.
[48] Fiore MC, Novotny TE, Pierce JP, et al. Methods used to quit smoking in *the USA. JAMA. 1990;263:2760-2765.*
[49] Owen N, Davies MJ. Smokers' preferences for assistance with cessation. *Preventive Medicine* .1990;19: 424-431.
[50] Lacey LP, Manfredi C, Balch G, Warnecke RB, Allen K, Edwards C. Social support in smoking cessation among black women in Chicago public housing. *Public Health Rep.* 1993;108: 387-394.
[51] McKee SA, Maciejewski PK, Falba T, Mazure CM. Sex differences in the effects of stressful life events on changes in smoking status. *Addiction.* 2003; 98: 847-855.
[52] Brandon TH, Baker TB. The smoking consequences questionnaire: the subjective expected utility of smoking in college students. *Psychological Assessments.* 1991; 3: 484-491.
[53] Borland R. Slip-ups and relapse in attempts to quit smoking. *Addictive Behaviours.* 1990;15: 235-245.
[54] Glassman A, Helzer JE, Covey LS, et al. Smoking, smoking cessation and major depression. *JAMA.* 1990;264: 1546-1549.
[55] Breslau N, Kilbey MM, Andreski P, Nicotine dependence major depression and anxiety in young adults. *Arch. Gen Psychiatry.* 1991; 48: 1069-1074.
[56] Hall SM, Munoz RF, Reus VI,. Cognitive-behavioral intervention increases abstinence rates for depressive-history smokers. *J. Consult. Clin. Psychol.* 1994;62: 141-146.
[57] Weden MM, Astone NM, Bishai D. Racial, ethnic and gender differences in smoking cessation associated with employment and joblessness through young adulthood in the US. *Social Science and Medicine.* 2006;62: 303-316
[58] Sorenson G, Pechacek TF. Attitudes toward smoking cessation among men and women. *J Behav Medicine* 1987;10: 129-137.
[59] Orleans CT, Melvin CL, Marx JF, Maibach E, Vose KK. National action plan to reduce smoking during pregnancy: *The National Partnership to Help Pregnant Smokers Quit. Nicotine and Tobacco Research.* 2004; 6: S269-S277.
[60] Coleman T. ABC of smoking cessation. *BMJ.* 2004; 328: 575-576.
[61] ASPECT Consortium. *Tobacco or Health in the European Union: Past, Present and Future.* Luxembourg: Office for Official Publications of the European Communities, 2004.
[62] Currie C, Roberts C, Morgan A et al. Young People's Health in Context, Health Behaviour in School-aged Children Study: International Report from the 2001/2002 Survey. Copenhagen: WHO Regional Office for Europe, 2004.
[63] INWAT Europe. Part of the Solution? Tobacco Control Policies and Women. London: Health Development Agency, 2000.

[64] Bostock Y. Searching for the Solution: Women, Smoking and Inequalities in Europe. London: Health Development Agency/INWAT, 2003.
[65] Samet JM, Yoon S-Y. Women and the Tobacco Epidemic, Challenges for the 21st Century. Geneva: WHO, 2001.
[66] WHO. WHO Framework Convention on Tobacco Control. Geneva: WHO, 2003.
[67] Kobus K. Peers and adolescent smoking. Addiction 2003; 98 (Suppl. 1):s37-55.
[68] Pierce JP, Distefan JM, Hill D. Adolescent smoking. In: Boyle P et al. (eds). *Tobacco and Public Health: Science and Policy*. Oxford: Oxford University Press, 2004, 315-328.
[69] Lambert M, Hublet A, Verduyckt et al. *Gender Differences in Smoking in Young People*. Belgium: Flemish Institute for Health Promotion, 2002.
[70] Michell L, Amos A. Girls, pecking order and smoking. *Soc. Sci. Med.* 1997;44: 1861-1869.
[71] Amos A, Bostck Y. Young people, smoking and gender-a qualitative exploration Health Education Research Theory and Practice 2006;August:1-12.
[72] US Department of Health and Human Services. *Marketing Cigarettes to Womenl*. US Public Health Service, Office of the Assistant Secretary for Health, Office on Smoking and Health; 2001.
[73] Department of Gender, Women and Health Family and Community Health. *Gender in Lung Cancer and Smoking Research*. World Health Organization; 2004.

In: Progress in Smoking and Health Research
Editor: T. C. Jeffries, pp. 157-176

ISBN: 978-1-60021-686-2

Chapter VII

The Impact of Intrauterine Tobacco Exposure on Childhood Obesity on Population Level

***Simon Rückinger*[1] *and André Michael Toschke*[2†]**
[1]Ludwig-Maximilians-University of Munich, Germany
[2] King's College London, UK

Abstract

Overweight and obesity are the most common nutritional disorders in industrialized countries which continue to increase in their prevalences and, in particular, in the US. Childhood obesity predicts obesity in adulthood and later cardiovascular disease. Effective prevention strategies against childhood obesity are needed because therapeutic interventions are expensive and tend to have poor long term results. However, for primary prevention of childhood obesity potential modifiable risk factors have to be identified. Nowadays we know that more than energy intake alone regulates our body mass index. In fact, there are hormone-modulating risk factors that might promote obesity. A number of such new risk factors like intrauterine tobacco exposure were recently identified. The individual association of this risk factor to childhood obesity is estimated in a large population with respect to potential confounders and its impact population level is estimated by using adjusted attributable risk fractions and preventable potentials.

† Correspondence to: Priv.Doz. Dr André Michael Toschke, MD, MSc, MPH, Clinical Senior Lecturer in Health Services Research, King's College London, Division of Health and Social Care Research, Department of Public Health Sciences, Floor 7 Capital House, 42 Weston St, London SE1 3QD, UK, email: +44 (0)207 848 6620, url: http://www.kcl.ac.uk/schools/medicine/research/hscr

Introduction

Overweight and obesity are the most common nutritional disorders in industrialized countries. They continue to increase in their prevalences, in particular, in the US and other Western countries [1-4]. This trend is remarkable, as several studies suggest. Ritchie et al. report a three-fold increase in pediatric overweight in the U.S. in recent decades [5]. In Central-Europe the obesity prevalence for German recruits increased from 3.4% for recruits born in 1970 to 5.7% for recruits born in 1979 [1].

Childhood obesity predicts obesity in adulthood. Overweight or obese children have a higher risk to become overweight or obese adults [6]. This comes along with an increased risk for associated diseases such as atherosclerosis and cardiovascular diseases [7]. Remarkably, overweight and obesity in adolescence seems to be a predictor for these diseases independent from overweight or obesity in adulthood [8].

Effective prevention strategies against childhood obesity are needed because therapeutic interventions are expensive and tend to have poor long term results [9, 10]. Secondary prevention is defined as identification of asymptomatic individuals in an early state of disease. Such an early diagnosis could improve disease prognosis. Thus, early identification of children at high risk for overweight and obesity might offer a chance for early effective preventive measures.

Primary prevention is defined as prophylactic measures to decrease disease probability and is desired for every disease. However, for primary prevention modifiable risk factors have to be known or identified.

Identification of Risk Factors

Odds Ratios and Logistic Regression in the Context of Epidemiological Studies

Odds ratios are useful to describe, to measure and to interpret effects of explaining variables on dichotomous outcomes (overweight/obesity – yes/no). Since overweight and obesity are the most common nutritional diseases, the rare disease assumption might not be assumed and the odds ratio as an approximation for the relative risk is probably not possible. An odds ratio of 1.0 describes no (unity) effect, while an odds ratio above 1 describes a risk factor, and an odds ratio below 1 describes a protective factor.

Given a 2x2 cross table

Exposure	Disease		sum
	yes	no	
yes	a	b	a+b
no	c	d	c+d
sum	a+c	b+d	n

michael.toschke@kcl.ac.uk, phone: +44 (0)207 848 6261, fax: +44 (0)207 848 6620, url: http://www.kcl.ac.uk/schools/medicine/research/hscr

the odds ratio is calculated by

$$OR = \frac{a \cdot c}{b \cdot d}$$

To adjust for possible confounding factors in an analysis with a dichotomous outcome variable a multiple logistic regression represents a suitable model [11].

The logistic regression model tries to explain a dichotomous outcome variable. For a dichotomous outcome the presumptions for linear models are not fulfilled. In a linear model the response variable can take values from $-\infty$ to $+\infty$. A dichotomous variable takes either the value 1 or 0.

Thus, the logistic regression uses a function of the probability (P), that the outcome takes the value 1, given certain values of explanatory variables. This function is called the logit or logg odds transformation and given by

$$\text{logit(P)} = \ln(\text{odds(P)}) = \ln\left(\frac{\text{P}}{\text{1-P}}\right).$$

While P takes values between 0 and 1, logit(P) takes values between $-\infty$ and $+\infty$.

This leads to the following equation

$$\text{logit(P)} = \beta_0 + \beta_1 \cdot x_1 + \beta_2 \cdot x_2 + \ldots + \beta_k \cdot x_k + \varepsilon$$

where β_0 denotes the intercept just like in a linear regression. β_1 to β_k denote the parameters for the explanatory variables, which have to be continuous or coded with dummy or effect coding.

The parameters β_0 to β_k are usually estimated by maximizing the likelihood function. Adjusted odds ratios for an explanatory variable x_i in the model can now easily be calculated by

$$OR_{adjusted} = \mathrm{e}^{\beta_i}.$$

Known Risk Factors for Overweight and Obesity in Childhood

There are numerous studies dealing with risk factors for overweight and obesity.

One of the most evident risk factors is low physical activity [12]. Children who lack physical activity have a higher risk for overweight. This risk factor is hard to quantify, though parental reporting seems quite reliable.

Watching too much TV is highly correlated with less physical activity and is sometimes even seen as a risk factor of its own [13, 14]. However, it might be an adequate surrogate for physical inactivity.

Parental factors such as overweight and education were reported to be related to offspring's overweight. Several studies showed that children of parents with less education have a higher risk for overweight [15, 16] and that there is an inverse association between meal frequency and the prevalence of overweight and obesity in adults [17-20]. Additionally breastfeeding has been reported to prevent children from later overweight [10, 21].

Intrauterine Tobacco Exposure

The long known association between active cigarette smoking and increased mortality due to several subsequent diseases such as cardiovascular disease [22] or bronchial carcinoma [23] is well documented and there is no doubt about the evidence of smoking as a multiple risk factor for human health nowadays. Nevertheless a high prevalence of active smoking with approximately 46.5 million U.S. smoking residents in 1999 [24] reflects its unbroken popularity. Smoking remains the leading cause of death in the US with a total of 442,398 persons who died prematurely each year as a result of smoking from 1995—1999 [24] and approximately 435,000 deaths (18.1% of total US deaths) in 2000 [25]. While active smoking remains an own decision of everybody, passive smoking does not. Although some associations between passive smoking and diseases such as childhood asthma could be observed [26, 27], the majority of multiple possible risks of passive smoking could not be described yet. This might be due to either the difficulty of measuring the exposure of passive smoking or to the long time lag until possible chronic diseases are diagnosed or both. A particular form of passive smoking is intrauterine exposure to tobacco inhaled products by the mother.

Previous studies demonstrated an association between maternal smoking (MS) in pregnancy and offspring's obesity. Simpson already described an association between maternal smoking during pregnancy and low infant birth weight in 1957 [28], which was confirmed by Yerushalmy et al. and Butler et al. in 1971/1972 [29, 30]. The reduction in birth weight was about 100 to 300g in different studies. Simultaneously the risks for perinatal mortality and for sudden unexpected death are increased among offspring of smoking mothers [31, 32].

In a previous study we analyzed data of 4,974 children aged 5-6 years [33]. Never smoking was reported by 3,564 mothers of these children, while 1,028 mothers smoked prior to pregnancy of whom 406 smoked throughout pregnancy. A total of 513 mothers smoked during the first trimester and 223 mothers had not smoked before or during pregnancy but started afterwards.

The focus of this study was to assess the impact on obesity in offspring of smoking in the 1st trimester only, throughout pregnancy and starting smoking after pregnancy. Other patterns of smoking were not analysed due to lack of sample power in the subgroups.

Within this study the prevalence of overweight and obesity in offspring was significantly increased if the mother smoked in the first trimester only or throughout pregnancy (table 1) compared with offspring of mothers who never smoked. Maternal smoking throughout pregnancy was associated with a low educational level, lower prevalence of breastfeeding and increased prevalence of parental obesity, low birthweight, prematurity, single parenthood, high infant weight gain and watching TV/playing electronic games. Whereas, smoking in the first trimester only was only associated with a lower educational level, less breastfeeding and single parenthood (table 1).

Table 1. Prevalences of overweight, obesity and several potential confounders with respect to time period of fetal tobacco exposure. Covariates were dichotomized for better understanding

	% covariate present (95%CI)			
	time period of maternal smoking[1]			
	never (n=3,564)	early pregnancy (n=513)	throughout (n=406)	after pregnancy (n=223)
Outcome				
overweight	9.2 (8.3-10.2)	14.4*** (11.5-17.8)	15.8*** (12.4-19.7)	11.2 (7.4-16.1)
obesity	1.9 (1.5-2.4)	4.5*** (2.9-6.7)	5.9*** (3.8-8.7)	4.5* (2.2-8.1)
Covariates				
birthweight≤10th percentile at respective gestation week [34]	7.0 (6.2-7.9)	9.0 (6.6-11.8)	15.0*** (11.7-18.9)	10.3 (6.7-15.1)
prematurity (<37th gestation week)	4.7 (4.1-5.5)	5.1 (3.3-7.3)	8.9*** (6.3-12.1)	6.7 (3.8-10.9)
breastfeeding up to one month	16.5 (15.3-17.8)	14.8 (11.9-18.2)	21.7** (17.8-26.0)	17.0 (12.3-22.6)
breastfeeding more than one month	63.6 (62.0-65.2)	54.8*** (50.4-59.1)	27.1*** (22.8-31.7)	51.1* (44.4-57.9)
watching TV ≥1h daily	32.9 (31.4-34.5)	43.9*** (39.5-48.3)	58.4*** (53.4-63.2)	44.4*** (37.8-51.2)
playing electronic games occasionally	38.4 (36.8-40.0)	40.2 (35.9-44.5)	46.3*** (41.4-51.3)	42.6** (36.0-49.4)
high educational level (≥10 years)	75.2 (73.8-76.6)	70.0* (65.8-73.9)	48.3*** (43.3-53.3)	64.1*** (57.5-70.4)
BMI of either parent ≥30 kg/m²	13.1 (12.0-14.2)	13.5 (10.6-16.7)	18.5** (14.8-22.6)	20.2*** (15.1-26.1)
single parenthood(2,1%missings)	5.8 (5.0-6.6)	13.8*** (11.0-17.1)	22.7*** (18.7-27.0)	19.3*** (14.3-25.1)
infant weight gain>7.5kg in first year of life	12.0 (11.0-13.1)	12.9 (10.1-16.9)	18.0*** (14.4-22.1)	15.7 (11.2-21.1)
physical activity (never or sometimes lethargic versus often lethargic)	21.5 (20.2-22.8)	20.7 (17.2-24.4)	26.6* (22.4-31.2)	21.1 (15.9-27.0)
population density >500 inhabitants/km²	13.8 (12.7-15.0)	14.4 (11.5-17.8)	16.7 (13.2-20.7)	12.6 (8.5-17.6)

[1] (reference group offspring of never smoking mothers)
* $p<0.05$, ** $p<0.01$, *** $p<0.001$.

Maternal smoking throughout pregnancy accounted for higher unadjusted odds ratios for offspring's obesity compared with maternal smoking in the first trimester only. However, after adjustment for breastfeeding and educational level the odds ratios for obesity associated with smoking in first trimester only and in later pregnancy were almost identical (table 2). The final regression model adjusted for breastfeeding, educational level, parental obesity, TV watching, playing electronic games, physical activity and high infant weight gain.

Stratification by sex did not change the results (data not shown). Adjustment for the same confounders used in the final model (table 2) resulted in an odds ratio of 1.03 (95%CI 0.65-1.61) for maternal smoking only *after* pregnancy and overweight among offspring. The association of maternal smoking only after pregnancy and offspring's obesity is not reported, as there were too few observations (n=10 obese children of mothers who started smoking after pregnancy).

Table 2. Crude and adjusted odds ratios for maternal smoking: early in pregnancy only vs. throughout pregnancy. All potential confounding and independent risk factors were modeled in their ordinal or continuous forms

	Odds ratio for maternal smoking in early pregnancy (95%CI)		Odds ratio for maternal smoking throughout pregnancy (95%CI)	
	overweight	obesity	overweight	Obesity
maternal smoking in specific time period (unadjusted)	1.66 (1.27-2.18)	2.41 (1.49-3.91)	1.85 (1.38-2.47)	3.23 (2.00-5.21)
adjusted for breastfeeding*	1.59 (1.21-2.09)	2.22 (1.37-3.61)	1.62 (1.20-2.19)	2.49 (1.50-4.11)
+ educational level	1.56 (1.19-2.06)	2.16 (1.33-3.52)	1.50 (1.10-2.03)	2.14 (1.29-3.55)
+ parental obesity	1.58 (1.20-2.09)	2.17 (1.32-3.56)	1.47 (1.08-2.01)	2.09 (1.24-3.51)
+ TV watching, playing electronic games occasionally, physical activity, high infant weight gain	1.52 (1.14-2.01)	2.22 (1.33-3.69)	1.23 (0.89-1.70)	1.70 (1.02-2.87)

* confounder (accounted for more than 10%change in estimate)

The odds ratios are all for the association of maternal smoking in pregnancy with overweight and obesity in offspring. These odds ratios are successively adjusted for the cumulative influence of the listed variables.

To further examine differences in the associations of maternal smoking in 1st trimester only and throughout pregnancy with risk of overweight and obesity, both exposures were compared in the same logistic regression model with smoking throughout pregnancy as reference. The adjusted odds ratio for overweight in offspring associated with having a mother who smoked only in the first trimester compared with mothers who smoked throughout pregnancy is 1.10 (0.75-1.59). The adjusted odds ratio for obesity associated with maternal smoking in the first trimester, compared with throughout pregnancy, was 1.03 (0.56-1.91). This analysis revealed no statistically significant difference in the associations with overweight and obesity for maternal smoking only in the first trimester of pregnancy compared with smoking throughout pregnancy, although the odds ratios are slightly (non-statistically significantly) greater for smoking in the first trimester only.

These data suggest that intrauterine exposures associated with maternal inhaled tobacco products increase the risk of childhood overweight or obesity in offspring. This is consistent with earlier research and a wide range of potential confounding factors could not explain this association. The first trimester of pregnancy seems to be instrumental for the association between intrauterine tobacco exposure and obesity. Our analysis also suggests that continuing smoking beyond the first trimester may not independently further increase offspring's obesity risk since adjustment for breastfeeding and other potential confounding factors yielded similar odds ratios compared to intrauterine tobacco exposure in the first trimester only.

The results of this study are in accordance with other studies in direction and strength of observed effects for obesity risks. As in other studies poor educational level [35, 36], high weight gain [37, 38], high birthweight [35], parental obesity [15, 16], watching TV and playing electronic games [13, 14] were associated with childhood obesity whereas physical activity [12, 39] and breastfeeding were apparently protective [40-43].

The aim of this study was to assess the association of maternal smoking with childhood obesity and to differentiate the effects of smoking only in the 1st trimester from those of smoking throughout pregnancy. Underreporting of smoking in pregnancy could be important. Results from other studies suggest that self reported smoking is accurate in general, [44] although digit preference appears to be a problem for establishing the precise number of cigarettes smoked [45]. Since the authors compared smoking with non-smoking, this is unlikely an issue.

In this study 21% of mothers said they had smoked at the beginning of pregnancy as compared with 19% in Sweden in 1999 [46]. Non-differential denial of smoking in any period would result in classification of smokers as never-smokers (reference group) and thus in bias towards unity. Since low educational level was associated with obesity [35], denial of any smoking in pregnancy by highly educated mothers could result in spurious increased odds ratios for maternal smoking and stratification by parental education would result in different odds ratios by strata. This could not be observed (data not shown). If mothers who claimed to have stopped smoking in pregnancy continued throughout pregnancy this should be reflected in lower birth weights as the risk of low birthweight and prematurity is mainly determined by smoking in the last trimester [47, 48]. The observed low birth weight rates among offspring of mothers who smoked only in the 1st trimester (9%) are almost identical to those in non-smoking mothers (7%) but higher for those smoking throughout pregnancy (15%). This indicated that the self-reported smoking data are broadly accurate.

Other potential sources of bias include confounding by parental obesity. We observed that obese mothers were more likely to smoke in pregnancy. It is also known that obese mothers often have obese partners [49] which could result in selection of genetic mechanisms increasing obesity risk among their children. Since adjustment for parental obesity could not explain the association between intrauterine tobacco exposure and obesity a genetic explanation seems to be unlikely. Selection bias by restriction to children with complete information on potential confounders seems to be unlikely since additional analysis using multiple imputation resulted in similar adjusted odds ratios (data not shown).

There are some biological mechanisms which might explain the observed association between smoking early in pregnancy and childhood obesity. Smoking in the 1st trimester could mimic fetal malnutrition by reduced food intake of the mother or reduced blood supply by vasoconstrictive effects on maternal and uteroplacental vessels [50]. Thus smoking would reflect a surrogate for hunger in the 1st trimester similar to famine in early pregnancy that accounted for higher proportions of obese offspring in the Dutch Famine Study [51, 52]. Nutritional deprivation may affect the differentiation of hypothalamic centers regulating food intake, growth and number of filled adipocytes [53]. Additionally, agents of inhaled tobacco might have a potentiating effect on hypothalamic structures resulting in impaired insulin signaling and metabolism. Some animal and human studies indicate an effect of intrauterine nicotine exposure on neurobehavioral impulse control [54-57].

Breastfeeding is the most important confounding factor in our study and was responsible for the most marked reduction of risk estimates for maternal smoking throughout pregnancy and offspring's obesity. This might be due to insufficient milk production among smokers [58-60] although other studies suggest psychological rather than physiological reasons for lower breastfeeding rates in smoking mothers [61]. Since the interaction of breastfeeding with maternal smoking was not significantly associated with obesity in offspring ($p > 0.6$ for both outcomes (overweight/obesity) and two different exposures (smoking in the first trimester only/smoking throughout pregnancy)), breastfeeding appears to be a confounder rather than an effect modifier. Therefore some of the association of maternal smoking in *later* pregnancy might be due to a deficit in breastfeeding, as well as other associated characteristics.

We hypothesized that maternal smoking in the first trimester of pregnancy has a more profound influence on the risk of obesity in offspring due to neuroendocrine or other metabolic dysregulation than maternal smoking in later pregnancy. It seems to be likely that the apparently greater influence of smoking in later pregnancy is largely due to confounding, such that children of mothers who smoke throughout pregnancy are more likely to accumulate further risks for obesity that are not caused directly by maternal smoking during pregnancy. This is demonstrated by the analysis described in table 3 and by the comparisons of smoking in the 1st trimester only with smoking throughout pregnancy for risk of overweight or obesity in the same logistic regression model. The statistically significantly raised odds ratios for obesity and overweight in offspring associated with maternal smoking in the first trimester of pregnancy are only marginally affected by multiple adjustments for other risks associated with obesity. In contrast with this, the odds ratios associated with smoking throughout pregnancy are notably reduced by adjustment for the other obesity risks. This is consistent with the hypothesis that smoking in the first trimester of pregnancy has a direct metabolic effect on offspring, while smoking in later pregnancy is a marker of familial cultural and material circumstances that influence obesity risk through other mechanisms.

Smoking throughout pregnancy might even dilute the effect of smoking in the first trimester, as smoking-related fetal malnutrition may have a similar influence to nutritional deprivation in the last trimester of pregnancy as observed in the Dutch famine study, which was associated with a *decreased* risk of obesity [62].

The effects of confounding (that may vary with time of exposure) and potentially contradictory influences of smoking in early and late pregnancy are likely to result in inconsistent associations of smoking during pregnancy and offspring's obesity. To disentangle these various influences, research into this subject should identify the period during pregnancy when the mother smoked, as well as quantifying the potential confounding influences of breastfeeding and other exposures that occur after birth.

The observed association of early fetal tobacco-related exposure and subsequent obesity underlines the importance of advising women on smoking cessation in contexts such as gynecology and obstetric outpatient clinics. Like folic acid supplementation, smoking cessation is another challenge which must be aimed for stopping prior to conception. Women of reproductive age should be advised that they should stop smoking before attempting to become pregnant, as cessation after they find out that they are pregnant may be too late to protect their baby from potential obesity and other associated risks with intrauterine tobacco exposure.

In order to identify potential confounders we assessed the associations a) between meal frequency and other explanatory variables and b) between explanatory variables and overweight/obesity (table 3). Frequent daily meals were associated with a high educational level, decreased prevalence of having main meals alone, daily TV watching not more than 1 hour, no regular snacking in front of TV, having siblings, non-smoking in pregnancy and breastfeeding > 1 months (data not shown).

Table 3. Description of study sample (n=4,370). Prevalences of overweight and obesity with respect to explanatory variables

covariate (no. of exposed subjects to covariate)	Prevalence			
	overweight (%)		obesity (%)	
	exposed to covariate	non–Exposed to covariate	Exposed to covariate	non–Exposed to ovariate
parental education (≥ 10 school years)* (n=3,207)	9.1	13.5	2.0	3.8
parental obesity (either parent BMI≥30 kg/m²) *(n=594)	22.1	8.5	8.6	1.6
male sex (n=2,300)	9.3	11.5	2.1	3.0
having at least one main meal/week alone (n=185)	15.1	10.1	4.3	2.5
daily watching TV > 1h*(n=1,571)	14.8	7.8	4.7	1.4
child's consumption of instant food at least once a week (n=982)	11.2	10.1	3.2	2.4
breastfed > 1months*(n=2,637)	8.8	12.7	1.8	3.8
little physical activity at school entry*(n=953)	17.1	8.4	5.9	1.6
having siblings (n=3,568)	9.9	13.0	2.5	2.9
birth order: first child (n=1,850)	11.4	9.1	2.8	2.3
smoking in pregnancy*(n=905)	14.7	9.2	5.0	1.9
regular snacking while watching TV *(n=1,686)	12.0	9.2	3.4	2.0

*significantly ($p<0.05$) associated with outcome (overweight and obesity).

A higher meal frequency reduced the odds ratio for child's overweight and obesity with a clear dose response effect (table 4). Adjustment for parental education, parental obesity, watching TV, breastfeeding, little physical activity, smoking in pregnancy and snacking in front of TV could not explain the effect of meal frequency on overweight/obesity (table 4).

The highest variance inflation factor (1.3 for snacking in front of TV) was clearly lower than 2.5 suggesting absence of multicollinearity.

Table 4. Results of multiple regression analysis including main exposure and confirmed confounders (associated to both, meal frequency and childhood overweight/obesity)

explanatory variable	odds ratio for meal frequency (95%CI)			
	overweight		obesity	
	crude	adjusted	crude	adjusted
4 daily meals*	0.70 (0.54-0.90)	0.73 (0.56-0.96)	0.67 (0.42-1.07)	0.73 (0.44-1.21)
5 or more daily meals*	0.50 (0.38-0.66)	0.56 (0.42-0.75)	0.39 (0.23-0.66)	0.51 (0.29-0.89)
parental education (≥ 10 school years)	0.65 (0.53-0.80)	0.85 (0.68-1.06)	0.51 (0.34-0.75)	0.82 (0.54-1.25)
parental obesity (either parent BMI≥30 kg/m^2)	3.06 (2.44-3.83)	2.65 (2.09-3.35)	5.72 (3.90-8.39)	4.40 (2.93-6.60)
daily watching TV > 1h	2.04 (1.68-2.48)	1.63 (1.31-2.03)	3.45 (2.33-5.11)	2.34 (1.50-3.65)
breastfed > 1months	0.66 (0.54-0.80)	0.85 (0.69-1.06)	0.47 (0.32-0.68)	0.73 (0.48-1.11)
little physical activity at school entry	2.24 (1.82-2.76)	2.05 (1.66-2.55)	3.75 (2.57-5.47)	3.11 (2.10-4.63)
smoking in pregnancy	1.70 (1.37-2.12)	1.38 (1.10-1.74)	2.65 (1.81-3.90)	1.86 (1.22-2.84)
regular snacking while watching TV	1.34 (1.10-1.64)	0.94 (0.75-1.17)	1.74 (1.19-2.53)	0.93 (0.61-1.43)

* 3 or less daily meals as reference group.

Shift of the Entire BMI Distribution or the Upper Tail Only?

If all exposed individuals in a population under study were exposed to a similar dose of a certain risk factor for obesity a shift of the entire BMI distribution among the exposed would be expected. However, a risk factor for obesity might affect only a proportion of those exposed. This proportion of exposed individuals is probably more susceptible to this risk factor. The susceptibility can be interpreted as an interaction between a certain predisposition and exposure. The genetic disposition might account for such a predisposition or other known or unknown risk factors.

Tukey Mean-Difference Plots

To assess the shift of the BMI distribution for intrauterine tobacco exposure and meal frequency cumulative distribution and Tukey mean-difference plots were used. Tukey mean-difference plots are an adaption of quantile-quantile plots. A quantile-quantile plot (or q-q plot) is a graphical data analysis technique for comparing the distributions of 2 data sets. The quantile-quantile plot is a graphical alternative for the various classical 2-sample tests (e.g., t for location, F for dispersion). The "quantiles" of a distribution are the distribution's "percent points" (e.g., .5 quantile = 50% point = median). The advantage of the quantile-quantile plot is 2-fold: 1) the sample sizes do not need to be identical and 2) many distributional aspects can be simultaneously tested. For example, shifts in location, shifts in dispersion, changes in symmetry/skewness, outliers, etc. Given a q-q plot, assume its y coordinates are in T_i and its x coordinates are in D_i, then the Tukey mean-difference is defined as:

$$\text{Vertical axis} = T_i - D_i;$$
$$\text{Horizontal axis} = (T_i + D_i)/2.$$

The Tukey mean-difference plot also plots a horizontal reference line at zero. That is, it plots the difference of the quantiles against their average. The advantage of the Tukey mean-difference compared to the q-q plot is that it converts interpretation of the differences around a 45 degree diagonal line to interpretation of differences around a horizontal zero line. However, the Tukey mean-difference plot should only be applied if the two variables are on a common scale.

It is typical for the response points to be represented as some character with no connecting line, and the reference line as a connected line with no character.

Shift of Upper Tail of the BMI Distribution among Exposed Individuals Only

Both exposures yielded a shift of upper BMI percentiles only. The cumulative distribution plot was only shifted among upper percentiles. This finding can also be seen in the mean difference plots, in which upper percentiles accounted for a larger difference between distributions of exposed and unexposed individuals (figure 1).

Such a shift in the upper part of the distribution only may be an indicator of an effect modification of the exposure confined to a subpopulation of the exposed. The effect modifier may be another environmental exposure or genetic predisposition. Such a gene environmental exposure interaction was recently demonstrated for passive smoking and asthma in children: a genetically determined deficiency of glutathione S transferase (GST) enzymes involved in the detoxification of environmental tobacco smoke (ETS) accounted for a massive increase in the risk for current asthma and asthma symptoms such as wheeze and shortness of breath [63].

It might well be possible that susceptibility to the known effects of risk factors for childhood obesity is confined to children with hitherto unknown genetic polymorphisms.

Population Attributable Risk Fractions (PARF) and Preventable Potential of Identified Risk Factors

After identifying modifiable risk factors, the population attributable risk fractions are important in decision making on preventive measures. For example, if strong risk factors like some genetic predispositions are present in only few individuals, such risk factors probably account only for few disease cases on population level. On the other side a moderate risk factor with high exposure prevalence might account for many cases on population level. To assess population attributable risk fractions and preventable potentials of modifiable risk factors the following study was performed.

Study Population, Data Sources and Measures

Children in the year before school entry have to attend the mandatory school entry health examination in local public health offices. The purpose of this compulsory examination is to assess deficits which might influence school performance (i.e. impaired visual acuity) but can easily be corrected (i.e. prescription of glasses). Most of the children are at age 5 and 6 when examined. Parents of 8,741 children were invited to participate in a voluntary self-completion questionnaire study as part of their child's obligatory school entry examination in six Bavarian communities (Germany) from September 2001 to August 2002. Questionnaires were mailed together with the invitations for the school entry health examination. About 80% (n=7,026) completed questionnaires were returned. Data on a number of sociodemographic and potential risk factors for childhood obesity were linked with children's stature and weight measures. The study was approved by the Bavarian State Office for Data Protection.

Stature and weight were measured in light clothing and without shoes by trained nurses of respective public health offices. Stadiometers and balances are periodically calibrated by respective public gauging offices. Overweight and obesity were defined according to sex- and age-specific BMI cutpoints proposed by the International Obesity Task Force [64] which are equivalent to the widely used cut points of 25 and 30 kg/m^2 for adult overweight and obesity.

The parental questionnaire was self-administered. The question on child's daily frequency of meals was: How many meals per day does your child consume? Possible answers were 1/2/3/4/5/'more than 5' and 'do not know'. In order to define a meal examples were given (i.e. breakfast, lunch, tea, dinner). These examples represent meals, which are conventionally served on a plate.

The quality of the external data entry company was controlled at our institute. A 1% random sample of collected questionnaires was compared to the dataset delivered by the data entry company. Entry errors were clearly below 1%/ variable and 0.0023%/ variable for this survey reflecting a valid data entry.

The following variables were a priori considered as potential confounding factors for the association between main meal frequency and respectively intrauterine tobacco exposure and childhood obesity due to their reported or possible associations with childhood overweight/obesity:

- Parental education: highest level attained by either parent, ordinal in 5 levels (self-reported by parents) [35]
- Parental obesity: metric self-reporting, height in cm and weight in 0.1 kg steps [15, 16]
- Watching TV or playing video games: daily hours at school entry (self-reported by parents) [13, 14]
- Children's temperament based on parental report
- Breastfeeding: in categories of none, up to 1 month and >1 month [40]
- Low physical activity as reported by parents

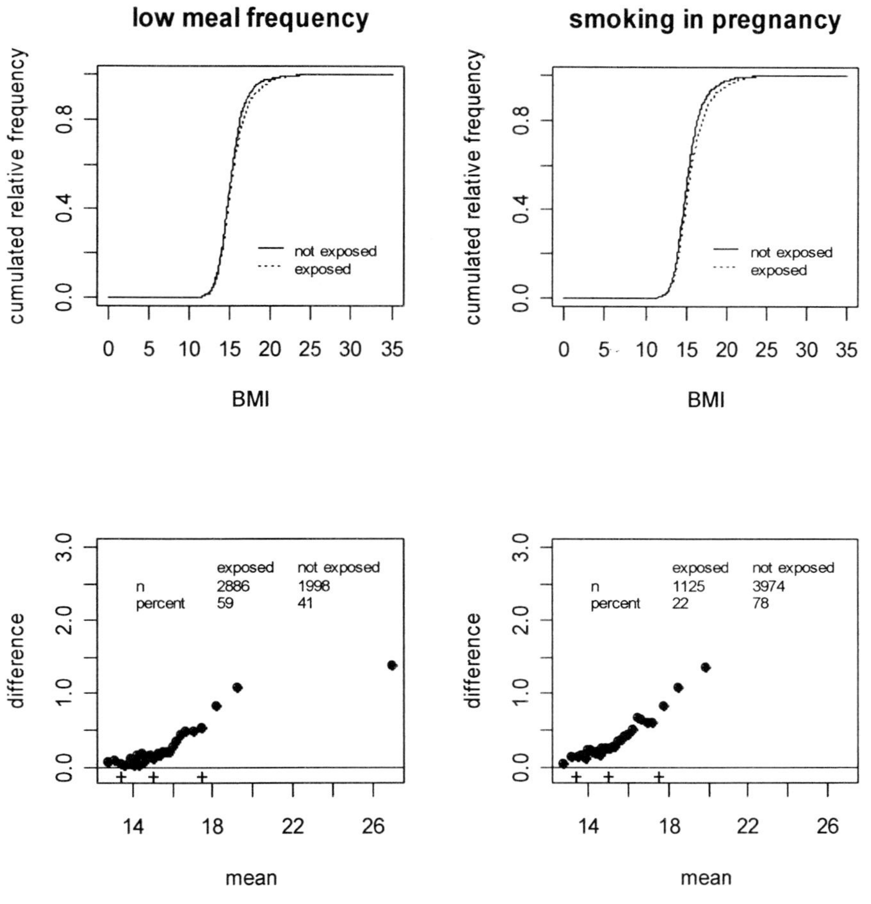

Figure 1. Cumulative distribution function and mean difference plots for risk factors low meal frequency and smoking in pregnancy. Both risk factors mainly affect upper percentiles; 10th, 50th and 90th percentile are marked by a '+'.

Statistical Methods

The prevalence of overweight/obesity and 95% exact confidence limits associated with meal frequency was calculated based on the binomial distribution [65]. Dose response effects were estimated with the Cochran-Armitage test for trend ($p < 0.05$). Crude and adjusted odds ratios and their respective 95% confidence limits for maternal smoking and overweight/obesity were calculated using logistic regression analysis. All covariates associated both with meal frequency and overweight/obesity ($p<0.2$ [66]) were considered as potential confounders. Multicollinearity of respective covariates was identified by a variance inflation factor (VIF) > 2.5 [67]. A number of possible interactions (parental education, child's sex, parental obesity, breastfeeding) with meal frequency and their influence on offspring's obesity were considered. All potential confounding and independent risk factors ($p<0.05$) were included in multiple logistic regression analysis. The potential confounders had been dichotomized for the sake of better comprehensibility.

Adjusted Population Attributable Fractions

A high odds ratio for a risk factor means that an individual with present exposure is more likely to get overweight or even obese. However, this gives no information on the number of cases that can be ascribed to that certain risk factor on population level. However, especially this information is important for recommendations, which have to be made in order to decrease the prevalence of overweight and obesity. Population attributable fractions express the proportion of cases ascribed to a certain risk factor.

The formula for unadjusted attributable fractions is given by:

$$AF = \frac{P(\text{disease}) - P(\text{disease} \mid \text{no exposure})}{P(\text{disease})}$$

or as

$$\frac{\text{Observed cases - expected cases on removal of the exposure}}{\text{Observed cases}}$$

The problem about crude attributable fractions is that they might be biased in the same way as crude effect estimates of associations [68]. In addition, adjusting for possible confounding factors is not possible for such crude attributable fraction estimates.

Model based adjusted attributable fractions are a remedy for these problems. The basic idea is to fit a logistic regression model, in which the occurrence of the disease is the response. Calculating the predicted probability of disease for each individual and then summing over all individuals, gives the number of cases predicted by the model. This is equal to the observed number of cases in the study.

After that the corresponding exposure covariate is set to zero for all individuals and the cases predicted by the model are calculated again. This gives the number of cases one would expect if the exposure was removed from the entire population.

An adjusted attributable fraction can now be calculated with the formula given above. In a recent study, the risk factors regarded as preventable were calculated given the factors which were seen as unpreventable [69]. This approach gives the unpreventable risk factors a higher weight but has two decisive benefits. Firstly, the estimates are much more realistic and secondly the PARFs are additive.

A simple way to get more stable estimates for the PARF is to remove covariates sequentially from the model and calculate the corresponding PARFs. This procedure gives covariates which are firstly removed from the model a higher weight. This, however, can be corrected by repeating the procedure for all possible orders of the covariates and calculate the PARF as the mean over all PARFs for the permutations. The maximal achievable reduction of prevalence was calculated by multiplying the adjusted population attributable fractions by the prevalence of overweight/obesity.

Table 5. Adjusted population attributable fractions (PARF) for respective risk factors concerning overweight/obesity and the corresponding maximal achievable reduction of prevalence

Risk factor	Overweight		Obesity	
	PARF adjusted	Max. achievable reduction of prevalence (obs. prevalence 10.6%)	PARF adjusted	Max. achievable reduction of prevalence (obs. prevalence 2.9%)
Low physical activity	13.4	1.4	19.9	0.6
At least one parent obese	11.0	1.2	16.5	0.5
Low educational level of parents	4.1	0.4	3.8	0.1
Watching TV >1h/day	11.4	1.2	16.2	0.5
Less than 5 meals a day	15.6	1.7	14.6	0.4
Formula feeding	2.9	0.3	5.8	0.2
Smoking during pregnancy	4.3	0.5	7.8	0.2
Overall adjusted PARF	62.8		84.6	

Results

Low physical activity had the highest PARF when regarding obesity. Although meal frequency had one of the lowest adjusted odds ratios, the corresponding PARF for overweight was highest due to its high exposure prevalence (59.1%). Smoking during pregnancy is estimated to account for 4.3% of cases of overweight and 7.8% of cases of obesity (table 5).

Conclusion

A combination of high TV consumption, maternal smoking in pregnancy, low meal frequency and early postnatal formula feeding could explain a high amount of overweight (32.3%) and obese (36.8%) children due to their respective high combined population attributable risk fractions. This combination is usually amenable for prevention and thus could theoretically decrease the prevalence of overweight children from 10.6% to 7.2% and of obese children from 2.9% to 1.7%.

Smoking during pregnancy, watching too much television, formula feeding and a low frequency of meals are risk factors which are not inevitable at all. If there were a common awareness that a significant proportion of cases of overweight and obesity can be ascribed to these factors, a serious reduction of prevalence would be likely. Especially the risk factor of maternal smoking in pregnancy should be targeted, as this association might be 1) unknown to most fertile women, 2) the association might be difficult to understand and 3) this risk factor has a multiple bad impact on health.

References

[1] Toschke, A.M., et al., *The obesity epidemic in young men is not confined to low social classes--a time series of 18-year-old German men at medical examination for military service with different educational attainment.* Int J Obes (Lond), 2005. 29(7): p. 875-7.

[2] Flegal, K.M., et al., *Prevalence and trends in obesity among US adults, 1999-2000.* Jama, 2002. 288(14): p. 1723-7.

[3] Ebbeling, C.B., D.B. Pawlak, and D.S. Ludwig, *Childhood obesity: public-health crisis, common sense cure.* Lancet, 2002. 360(9331): p. 473-82.

[4] Ogden, C.L., et al., *Prevalence and trends in overweight among US children and adolescents, 1999-2000.* Jama, 2002. 288(14): p. 1728-32.

[5] Ritchie, L.D., et al., *Alarming trends in pediatric overweight in the United States.* Soz Praventivmed, 2003. 48(3): p. 168-77.

[6] Stark, O., et al., *Longitudinal study of obesity in the National Survey of Health and Development.* Bmj, 1981. 283(6283): p. 13-7.

[7] Gunnell, D.J., et al., *Childhood obesity and adult cardiovascular mortality: a 57-y follow-up study based on the Boyd Orr cohort.* Am J Clin Nutr, 1998. 67(6): p. 1111-8.

[8] Must, A., et al., *Long-term morbidity and mortality of overweight adolescents. A follow-up of the Harvard Growth Study of 1922 to 1935.* N Engl J Med, 1992. 327(19): p. 1350-5.

[9] Feldman, W., *Periodic health examination, 1994 update: 1. Obesity in childhood. Canadian Task Force on the Periodic Health Examination.* Can Med Assoc J, 1994. 150(6): p. 871-9.

[10] Koletzko, B., et al., *Obesity in children and adolescents worldwide: current views and future directions--Working Group Report of the First World Congress of Pediatric Gastroenterology, Hepatology, and Nutrition.* J Pediatr Gastroenterol Nutr, 2002. 35(Suppl 2): p. S205-12.

[11] Kleinbaum, D., *Logistic Regression - A Self-Learning Text.* Statistics in the health sciences. 1994, New York, Berlin, Heidelberg: Springer.

[12] Moore, L.L., et al., *Preschool physical activity level and change in body fatness in young children. The Framingham Children's Study.* Am J Epidemiol, 1995. 142(9): p. 982-8.

[13] Dietz, W.H., Jr. and S.L. Gortmaker, *Do we fatten our children at the television set? Obesity and television viewing in children and adolescents.* Pediatrics, 1985. 75(5): p. 807-12.

[14] Robinson, T.N., *Reducing children's television viewing to prevent obesity: a randomized controlled trial.* Jama, 1999. 282(16): p. 1561-7.

[15] Locard, E., et al., *Risk factors of obesity in a five year old population. Parental versus environmental factors.* Int J Obes Relat Metab Disord, 1992. 16(10): p. 721-9.

[16] Stunkard, A.J., et al., *An adoption study of human obesity.* N Engl J Med, 1986. 314(4): p. 193-8.

[17] Fabry, P., et al., *The Frequency of Meals. Its Relation to Overweight, Hypercholesterolaemia, and Decreased Glucose-Tolerance.* Lancet, 1964. 18: p. 614-5.

[18] Edelstein, S.L., et al., *Increased meal frequency associated with decreased cholesterol concentrations; Rancho Bernardo, CA, 1984-1987.* Am J Clin Nutr, 1992. 55(3): p. 664-9.

[19] Kant, A.K., et al., *Frequency of eating occasions and weight change in the NHANES I Epidemiologic Follow-up Study.* Int J Obes Relat Metab Disord, 1995. 19(7): p. 468-74.

[20] Metzner, H.L., et al., *The relationship between frequency of eating and adiposity in adult men and women in the Tecumseh Community Health Study.* Am J Clin Nutr, 1977. 30(5): p. 712-5.

[21] von Kries, R., et al., *Breast feeding and obesity: cross sectional study.* BMJ, 1999. 319: p. 147-150.

[22] Doll, R. and A.B. Hill, *The mortality of doctors in relation to their smoking habits; a preliminary report.* Br Med J, 1954. 4877: p. 1451-5.

[23] Doll, R. and A.B. Hill, *Smoking and carcinoma of the lung; preliminary report.* Br Med J, 1950. 2(4682): p. 739-48.

[24] *Annual smoking-attributable mortality, years of potential life lost, and economic costs--United States, 1995-1999.* MMWR Morb Mortal Wkly Rep, 2002. 51(14): p. 300-3.

[25] Mokdad, A.H., et al., *Actual causes of death in the United States, 2000.* Jama, 2004. 291(10): p. 1238-45.

[26] Hu, F.B., et al., *Prevalence of asthma and wheezing in public schoolchildren: association with maternal smoking during pregnancy.* Ann Allergy Asthma Immunol, 1997. 79(1): p. 80-4.

[27] DiFranza, J.R., C.A. Aligne, and M. Weitzman, *Prenatal and postnatal environmental tobacco smoke exposure and children's health.* Pediatrics, 2004. 113(4 Suppl): p. 1007-15.

[28] Simpson, W.J., *A preliminary report on cigarette smoking and the incidence of prematurity.* Am J Obstet Gynecol, 1957. 73(4): p. 807-15.

[29] Yerushalmy, J., *The relationship of parents' cigarette smoking to outcome of pregnancy -- implications as to the problem of inferring causation from observed associations.* Am J Epidemiol, 1971. 93(6): p. 443-56.

[30] Butler, N.R., H. Goldstein, and E.M. Ross, *Cigarette smoking in pregnancy: Its influence on birth weight and perinatal mortality.* Br Med J, 1972. 1972 ii: p. 127-30.

[31] Schellscheidt, J., G. Jorch, and J. Menke, *Effects of heavy maternal smoking on intrauterine growth patterns in sudden infant death victims and surviving infants.* Eur J Pediatr, 1998. 157(3): p. 246-51.

[32] Schellscheidt, J., N. Oyen, and G. Jorch, *Interactions between maternal smoking and other prenatal risk factors for sudden infant death syndrome (SIDS).* Acta Paediatr, 1997. 86(8): p. 857-63.

[33] Toschke, A.M., et al., *Early intrauterine exposure to tobacco-inhaled products and obesity.* Am J Epidemiol, 2003. 158(11): p. 1068-74.

[34] Voigt, M., K.T.M. Schneider, and K. Jährig, *Analyse des Geburtengutes des Jahrgangs 1992 der Bundesrepublik Deutschland.* Geburtsh u Frauenheilkd, 1996. 56: p. 550-8.

[35] Rasmussen, F. and M. Johansson, *The relation of weight, length and ponderal index at birth to body mass index and overweight among 18-year-old males in Sweden.* Eur J Epidemiol, 1998. 14(4): p. 373-80.

[36] Troiano, R.P. and K.M. Flegal, *Overweight children and adolescents: description, epidemiology, and demographics.* Pediatrics, 1998. 101(3): p. 497-504.

[37] Ong, K.K., et al., *Association between postnatal catch-up growth and obesity in childhood: prospective cohort study.* Bmj, 2000. 320(7240): p. 967-71.

[38] Stettler, N., et al., *Infant weight gain and childhood overweight status in a multicenter, cohort study.* Pediatrics, 2002. 109(2): p. 194-9.

[39] Pate, R.R., M. Dowda, and J.G. Ross, *Associations between physical activity and physical fitness in American children.* Am J Dis Child, 1990. 144(10): p. 1123-9.

[40] von Kries, R.K., B. Sauerwald,T. von Mutius, E. Barnert, D. Grunert, V. von Voss, H., *Breast feeding and obesity: cross sectional study.* BMJ, 1999. 319: p. 147-150.

[41] Armstrong, J. and J.J. Reilly, *Breastfeeding and lowering the risk of childhood obesity.* Lancet, 2002. 359(9322): p. 2003-4.

[42] Gillman, M.W., et al., *Risk of overweight among adolescents who were breastfed as infants.* Jama, 2001. 285(19): p. 2461-7.

[43] Toschke, A.M., et al., *Overweight and obesity in 6- to 14-year-old Czech children in 1991: protective effect of breast-feeding.* J Pediatr, 2002. 141(6): p. 764-9.

[44] Patrick, D.L., et al., *The validity of self-reported smoking: a review and meta-analysis.* Am J Public Health, 1994. 84(7): p. 1086-93.

[45] Klesges, R.C., M. Debon, and J.W. Ray, *Are self-reports of smoking rate biased? Evidence from the Second National Health and Nutrition Examination Survey.* J Clin Epidemiol, 1995. 48(10): p. 1225-33.

[46] Wallskar, H., *Smoke-free cildren - a report. The first ten years.* 2003, Stockholm: The Swedish Cancer Society, the Swedish Heart-Lung Foundation, the Swedish National Institute of Public Health.

[47] Cliver, S.P., et al., *The effect of cigarette smoking on neonatal anthropometric measurements.* Obstet Gynecol, 1995. 85(4): p. 625-30.

[48] Vik, T., et al., *Pre- and post-natal growth in children of women who smoked in pregnancy.* Early Hum Dev, 1996. 45(3): p. 245-55.

[49] Hebebrand, J., et al., *Epidemic obesity: are genetic factors involved via increased rates of assortative mating?* Int J Obes Relat Metab Disord, 2000. 24(3): p. 345-53.

[50] Horta, B.L., et al., *Low birthweight, preterm births and intrauterine growth retardation in relation to maternal smoking.* Paediatr Perinat Epidemiol, 1997. 11: p. 140-51.

[51] Ravelli, G.P. and L. Belmont, *Obesity in nineteen-year-old men: family size and birth order associations.* Am J Epidemiol, 1979. 109(1): p. 66-70.

[52] Ravelli, A.C., et al., *Obesity at the age of 50 y in men and women exposed to famine prenatally.* Am J Clin Nutr, 1999. 70(5): p. 811-6.

[53] Keesey, R.E., *Physiological regulation of body weight and the issue of obesity.* Med Clin North Am, 1989. 73(1): p. 15-27.

[54] Levin, B.E. and V.H. Routh, *Role of the brain in energy balance and obesity.* Am J Physiol, 1996. 271(3 Pt 2): p. R491-500.

[55] Peters, M.A. and L.L. Ngan, *The effects of totigestational exposure to nicotine on pre- and postnatal development in the rat.* Arch Int Pharmacodyn Ther, 1982. 257(1): p. 155-67.

[56] Levin, E.D. and T.A. Slotkin, *Developmental Neurotoxicity of Nicotine*, in *Handbook of Developmental Neurotoxicology*, W. Slikker and L. Chang, Editors. 1998, Academic Press. p. 587-615.

[57] Kandel, D.B., P. Wu, and M. Davies, *Maternal smoking during pregnancy and smoking by adolescent daughters.* Am J Public Health, 1994. 84(9): p. 1407-13.

[58] Haug, K., et al., *Secular trends in breastfeeding and parental smoking.* Acta Paediatr, 1998. 87(10): p. 1023-7.

[59] Vogel, A., B.L. Hutchison, and E.A. Mitchell, *Mastitis in the first year postpartum.* Birth, 1999. 26(4): p. 218-25.

[60] Hill, P.D. and J.C. Aldag, *Smoking and breastfeeding status.* Res Nurs Health, 1996. 19(2): p. 125-32.

[61] Amir, L.H. and S.M. Donath, *Does maternal smoking have a negative physiological effect on breastfeeding? The epidemiological evidence.* Birth, 2002. 29(2): p. 112-23.

[62] Ravelli, G.P., Z.A. Stein, and M.W. Susser, *Obesity in young men after famine exposure in utero and early infancy.* N Engl J Med, 1976. 295(7): p. 349-53.

[63] Kabesch, M., et al., *Glutathione S transferase deficiency and passive smoking increase childhood asthma.* Thorax, 2004. 59(7): p. 569-73.

[64] Cole, T.J., et al., *Establishing a standard definition for child overweight and obesity worldwide: international survey.* Bmj, 2000. 320(7244): p. 1240-3.

[65] Clopper, C.J. and E.S. Pearson, *The use of confidence or fiducial limits illustrated in the case of the binomial.* Biometrika, 1934. 26: p. 404-13.

[66] Altman, D.G. and B.L. De Stavola, *Practical problems in fitting a proportional hazards model to data with updated measurements of the covariates.* Stat Med, 1994. 13(4): p. 301-41.

[67] Allison, P.D., *Logistic Regression Using the SAS System: Theory and Application*, ed. S. Institute. 2001: John Wiley & Sons.

[68] Benichou, J., *A review of adjusted estimators of attributable risk.* Stat Methods Med Res, 2001. 10(3): p. 195-216.

[69] Toschke, A.M., et al., *Adjusted population attributable fractions and preventable potential of risk factors for childhood obesity.* Public Health Nutr, 2007. in print.

In: Progress in Smoking and Health Research
Editor: T. C. Jeffries, pp. 177-192
ISBN: 978-1-60021-686-2

Chapter VIII

Smoking and Schizophrenia

Alain Dervaux **[*]** ***and Xavier Laqueille***
Ste-Anne Hospital. Departement of Substance Abuse Treatment
«Moreau de Tours», 1 Rue Cabanis, 75014 Paris, France

Abstract

Frequency: The prevalence of cigarette smoking is significantly higher among patients with schizophrenia (60-90%) than in the general population (23-30%). While tobacco smoking decreases in general population (from 45% in the 1960's to 23-30% in the 2000's), smoking in patients with schizophrenia remains high. Patients with schizophrenia smoke more deeply, thereby increasing their exposure to harmful elements in tobacco smoke.

Impact of smoking on patients with schizophrenia: As in the general population, smoking contributes to the reduced life expectancy in patients with schizophrenia. Patients with schizophrenia are at elevated risk for cardiovascular disease due to high rates of cigarette smoking. In the Department of Mental Health of the commonwealth of Massachussetts, cardiovascular disease was the factor that most strongly associated with excess mortality.

Improvement of cognitive deficits: Patients with schizophrenia may use nicotine to reduce cognitive deficits and negative symptoms or neuroleptic side effects. Smoking may transiently alleviate negative symptoms in patients with schizophrenia in increasing dopaminergic and glutamatergic neurotransmission in the prefrontal cortex. In patients with schizophrenia, nicotine improves some cognitive deficits : 1) Sensory gating deficits and abnormalities in smooth pursuit eye movements associated with schizophrenia are transiently normalized with the administration of nicotine 2) High-dose nicotine transiently normalizes the abnormality in P50 inhibition in schizophrenic patients and in their relatives 3) In tasks that tax working memory and selective attention, nicotine may

[*] Corresponding author : Dr. A. Dervaux. Service d'addictologie. Moreau de Tours, Centre Hospitalier Ste-Anne. 1 Rue Cabanis, 75014 Paris, France. Tel: + 33 1 45 65 80 64 Fax: + 33 1 45 65 88 32; E-mail: a.dervaux@ch-sainte-anne.fr

improve performance in patients with schizophrenia by enhancing activation of and functional connectivity between brain regions that mediate task performance 4) Cigarette smoking may selectively enhance visuospatial working memory and attentional deficits in smokers with schizophrenia. However, Harris et al. found that nicotine affects only the attention without effects of nicotine on learning, memory or visuospatial/constructional abilities. In addition, smoking could facilitate disinhibition in patients with schizophrenia. Some authors stressed that nicotine does not appear to have a long-lasting therapeutic effect on schizophrenia's symptoms.

Impact of smoking on patients with schizophrenia who are on antipsychotic medications : Smoking increases the metabolism of the antipsychotic medications by inducing the cytochrome P450 1A2 isoform. Smoking lowers the blood levels of typical or atypical antipsychotic medications.

Treatment: Although patients with schizophrenia have low motivations to quit smoking, smoking cessation treatment can be effective for these patients. Atypical antipsychotic medications, in combination with the nicotine transdermal patch, or bupropion significantly enhanced the rate of smoking cessation.

Introduction

It is well established that patients with schizophrenia are markedly prone to smoke tobacco. However, the reasons for the widespread smoking behaviours seen in these patients are not well understood. In this chapter, we will review the epidemiological, clinical and treatment data about the links between smoking and schizophrenia. Evidence suggests that smoking could be a form of self-medication to alleviate psychotic or cognitive symptoms of schizophrenia or to reduce medications side-effects.

Epidemiological Data

Frequency of Tobacco Consumption in Patients with Schizophrenia

Many studies have shown that patients with schizophrenia consume tobacco much more often than the general population (table 1), or than patients with other psychiatric diseases. In the United States, as in other countries, the prevalence of cigarette smoking is significantly higher among patients with schizophrenia (60-90%) than in the general population (23%) [5, 9, 11, 13, 20, 33, 75]. In the meta-analysis of De Leon and Diaz of 42 studies including 7,593 patients with schizophrenia from 20 countries, the prevalence of tobacco consumption was 62% [13]. Moreover, while tobacco smoking decreases in general population (from 45% in the 1960's to 23-30% in the 2000's), smoking in patients with schizophrenia remains high [5, 33].

The figures noted for the general population come from studies on the general population at the time and in the countries in which the studies on tobacco consumption in patients with schizophrenia took place.

Characteristics of Tobacco Consumption in Patients with Schizophrenia

Patients with schizophrenia are heavy smokers: a mean of 22 to 27 cigarettes per day [20, 41, 47, 58, 59, 88, 90]. Patients with schizophrenia smoke more cigarettes: 29 to 46% smoke more than 30 cigarettes per day vs 6 to 29 % in controls [13]. Tobacco consumption is more frequent in men than in women: 71% and 44% respectively in a recent meta-analysis [13]. Ninety per cent of patients with schizophrenia began smoking before the psychotic disorder started [47]. Patients smoke more deeply, thereby increasing their exposure to harmful elements in tobacco smoke [88]. They extract more nicotine from each cigarette than controls, and as a result have higher blood levels of nicotine and cotinine, a nicotine metabolite, and higher urinary levels of cotinine, for the same tobacco consumption [73, 83].

Table 1. Frequency of tobacco consumption in patients with schizophrenia

	N	Lifetime	Current	General population Current
Masterson et O'Shea 1984 (Ireland)	100	83 %	-	56 %
Hughes et al. 1986 (USA)	24	-	88%	30 %
Menza et al. 1991 (USA)	99	-	56%	-
Goff et al. 1992 (USA)	78	86 %	74 %	24 %
El-Guebaly and Hodgins 1992 (Canada)	106	-	61 %	32 %
Ziedonis et al. 1994 (USA)	265	76 %	68 %	22 %
De Leon et al. 1995 (USA)	237	-	85 %	24 %
Diwan et al. 1998 (USA)	63	95 %	86 %	28 %
Taiminen et al. 1998 (Finland)	88	-	56 %	23 %
Kelly and McCreadie 1999 (United Kingdom)	168	73 %	58 %	28 %
Mc Evoy and Brown 1999 (USA)	22	-	77 %	25-30 %
Herran et al. 2000 (Spain)	64	-	64 %	51 %
Itkin et al. 2001 (Israel)	64	55 %	45 %	28 %
Beratis et al. 2001 (Greece)	406	61 %	58 %	42 %
Patkar et al. 2002 (USA)	87	81 %	76 %	24 %
De Leon et al. 2002 (USA)	66	92 %	83 %	26 %
De Leon et al. 2002 (USA)	120	-	75 %	-
Llerena et al. 2002 (Spain)	100	-	70%	37 %
Srinivasan et al. 2002 (India)	286	52 %	38 %	40-45 %
McCreadie et al. 2002 (United Kingdom)	316	79 %	65%	40 %
McCreadie et al. 2003 (United Kingdom)	102	84 %	70 %	-
Poirier et al. 2002 (France)	207	70 %	66%	34 %
Mori et al. 2003 (Japan)	137	-	34 %	37 %
Margolese et al. 2004 (Canada)	207	-	66 %	22 %
Etter et al. 2004 (Switzerland)	151	85 %	70 %	28 %
Himelhoch et al. 2004 (USA)	199	-	61 %	27 %
Dervaux et al. 2004 (France)	100	78 %	67 %	30 %
Aguilar et al. 2005 (Spain)	250	73 %	69 %	27-44 %

The Fagerström Test for Nicotine Dependence is widely used to assess nicotine dependence and to predict success in stopping smoking. High nicotine dependence is defined as a total Fagerström Test for Nicotine Dependence score of 6 or higher [13]. Tobacco addiction, evaluated using the Fagerström scale, is severe in patients with schizophrenia, with a mean score between 6 and 7, according to several studies [13, 17, 20, 44, 74, 82, 88, 91]. However, some authors have recently thrown some doubt on the validity of the Fagerström scale in patients with schizophrenia, since this scale can underestimate tobacco addiction in this population [82]. It should also be noted that in some studies, the level of nicotine dependence in patients with schizophrenia is similar to those found in patients with other serious psychiatric disorders [13].

Impact of Tobacco Consumption on the Physical Health of Patients with Schizophrenia

Mortality

As in the general population, smoking contributes to the reduced life expectancy in patients with schizophrenia [36]. The risk of mortality from cardiovascular disease is 2.2 to 5 times higher in patients with schizophrenia than in the general population, and 3.2 times higher for respiratory disease [27, 36, 88].

Cardiovascular Diseases

The reduction in life expectancy from tobacco in schizophrenic patients is mainly due to an increase in cardiovascular disease risk [36, 68]. In the Department of Mental Health of the commonwealth of Massachussetts, cardiovascular disease was the factor the most strongly associated with excess mortality. Cardiac deaths were elevated more than 6-fold. Tobacco consumption in fact increases inflammation, thrombosis and LDL-cholesterol oxidation, which increase the risk of coronary heart disease and myocardial infarction [4]. Tobacco consumption also increases oxygen consumption by the heart muscle. Weight gain, insulin resistance, metabolic syndrome, and diabetes mellitus are frequent in patients with schizophrenia, and may worsen the risk of cardiovascular diseases [19, 36, 78].

Cancers

Premature death in patients with schizophrenia from tobacco is more often caused by cardiovascular disease than tobacco-related cancer. It has been reported that the risk for lung cancer in patients with schizophrenia is lower from that of the general population, despite increased smoking [12, 38, 68]. However, in a study conducted in Finland, a slightly increased cancer risk was found in 27000 patients with schizophrenia. Half of the excess cases were attributable to lung cancer [52].

Chronic Obstructive Pulmonary Disease

In a study of 200 adults with serious mental illness, the prevalence of chronic obstructive pulmonary disease, in particular chronic bronchitis and emphysema was significantly higher among those with serious mental illness than in comparison subjects [42].

Effect of Tobacco Consumption on Schizophrenic Patients' Symptomatology

Effect of Tobacco Consumption on the Psychotic Symptoms

Positive and Negative Symptoms

Several studies have compared the symptomatology of smoking and non-smoking patients with schizophrenia. These studies looked for correlations between psychotic symptoms and tobacco consumption, rather than studying causality. Most of these studies did not find any difference between the smoking and the non-smoking patients, on the evaluation scales used, such as the PANSS score for positive, negative and general psychopathological symptoms [3, 20, 41, 47, 83]. However, in a study by Paktar et al., the smokers obtained higher scores for negative symptomatology with PANSS than the non-smokers [74]. On the other hand, Ziedonis et al. found lower negative symptomatology scores and higher positive symptomatology scores in the smokers than the non-smokers [91]. In a study by Goff et al., the smokers had higher negative and positive symptoms subscales scores than the non-smokers [37]. Finally, Herran et al. found a link between anxiety and the number of cigarettes smoked per day [41].

Cognitive Symptoms

Several studies have shown that nicotine increases the cognitive capacity of healthy individuals, in particular for attention and working memory [Review: 11, 55, 77, 85, 86]. Many studies have shown that tobacco consumption can improve certain specific cognitive disorders found in schizophrenia. However, some authors stressed that nicotine does not appear to have a long-lasting therapeutic effect on schizophrenia symptoms [39].

- Patients with schizophrenia demonstrate a smooth pursuit eye movement dysfunction, involuntary reflexive saccades to a prepotent stimulus during saccadic tasks, and increased response to the second of two identical auditory stimuli, the P50 evoked potential response [1, 2]. Sensory gating deficits and abnormalities in smooth pursuit eye movements associated with schizophrenia are transiently normalized with the administration of nicotine. High-dose nicotine also transiently normalizes the abnormality in P50 inhibition in patients with schizophrenia and in their relatives [1, 2].
- Nicotine also improves prepulse inhibition abnormalities, another sign of a deficit in processing auditory information, found in patients with schizophrenia [49].

- Nicotine normalizes certain smooth pursuit eye movement abnormalities, found in patients with schizophrenia, which according to Olincy et al., could be a sign of a disorder of the inhibitory capacity of the prefrontal cortex [6, 71, 72].
- Cigarette smoking may selectively enhance visuospatial working memory and attentional deficits, assessed with the Continuous Performance Test, in smokers with schizophrenia [33, 79].
- However, Harris et al. found that nicotine affects only the attention without effects of nicotine on learning, memory or visuospatial/constructional abilities [39]. Another recent study found an improvement in delayed recognition memory in patients with schizophrenia by nicotine, but no effect on the working memory [69].
- A functional MRI study showed that nicotine improved attention and working memory in patients with schizophrenia by enhancing activation of and functional connectivity between brain regions, in particular the anterior cingular cortex, the thalamus, that mediate task performance [45]. Nicotine also modulated thalamocortical functional connectivity to a greater degree in patients with schizophrenia than in control subjects [45].
- In addition, smoking could facilitate disinhibition in schizophrenic patients [20].

The effects of tobacco consumption on cognition are independent of the withdrawal symptoms caused by tobacco consumption [39]. The effects of smoking on cognition in patients with schizophrenia remains slight [1, 39]. These are also transitory, because of desensitization of the nicotinic receptors produced by addiction [1].

Neurobiological Aspects

Nicotine fixes on the nicotinic acetylcholinergic receptors in the brain. It then has a modulating action on the dopaminergic, glutamatergic and serotoninergic receptors [33, 50]. In particular, nicotine increases the dopaminergic activity in the prefrontal cortex, the amygdala, the nucleus accumbens and the cingular gyrus [11, 81].

The alpha-7 et alpha 4-beta 2 nicotinic receptors in the hippocampus, play an important role in cognitive functions [77]. A post-mortem study showed that patients with schizophrenia have fewer nicotinic receptors [32]. Adler et al. made a link between a deficit in filtering auditory sensations in patients with schizophrenia and alteration in the expression and function of the alpha-7 nicotinic receptors, whose gene is coded for on chromosome 15 [1, 31].

A transitory improvement in cognitive abnormalities due to nicotine, and perhaps also in negative symptomatology, may be due to its stimulatory action on presynaptic nicotinic receptors of the glutamatergic and dopaminergic neurones, thus enhancing glutamatergic and dopaminergic transmission in the prefrontal cortex [22, 35, 35].

Impact of Smoking on Antipsychotic Treatments

Patients with schizophrenia who smoke, receive higher doses of antipsychotics than non-smokers [13, 15, 64, 75, 83, 91]. The frequency of tobacco consumption appears to be just as high in patients with other psychiatric disorders treated by antipsychotics, as in treated patients with schizophrenia (75). Smoking increases the metabolism of the antipsychotic medications by inducing the cytochrome P450 1A2 isoform [8, 22, 93]. Hence, smoking lowers the blood levels of typical or atypical antipsychotic medications, in particular haloperidol, chlorpromazine, olanzapine and clozapine [22, 46, 33]. Therefore, abstinence can increase many psychotropics' blood levels. Olanzapine clearance is between 37% and 48% lower in non-smokers than in smokers [22]. Nevertheless, there does not appear to be an interaction between tobacco, Risperidone and Aripirazole, which are metabolized by cytochromes P450 CYP2D6 and CYP3A [14].

In addition, administration of nicotine improves the cognitive disorders caused by Haloperidol, in particular on working memory disorders [37, 51]. Tobacco consumption also increases the metabolism of most benzodiazepines and some antidepressants, like Imipramine and Clomipramine.

Effect of Tobacco Consumption on Extrapyramidal Side Effects from Antipsychotic Treatment

Several studies have shown that tobacco consumption reduces the extra-pyramidal side effects of antipsychotic treatment [33, 37, 48, 51, 75]. This may be due to a reduction in the neuroleptic blood levels, to an increase in subcortical dopaminergic transmission and/or to nicotine acting on the GABAergic and glutamatergic systems [33].

However, tardive dyskinesia was found to be more frequent in smokers treated with antipsychotic medications [22, 46, 70]. Nevertheless, these results were not found in all the studies [47]. The differences between the studies may be due to the fact that tardive dyskinesia occurs more frequently in patients who smoke more than 20 cigarettes per day, in particular in patients with the C-->A) genetic polymorphism in the CYP1A2 gene [47, 7]. No interaction was found between tobacco consumption and anticholinergic treatment [3, 18].

Why is Tobacco Consumption so High in Patients with Schizophrenia ?

Self-Medication Hypothesis

Although it was previously thought that patients with schizophrenia smoke mainly because of boredom or because their lifestyle is not stimulating enough, several authors have suggested that tobacco consumption is a type of self-medication, in particular for the cognitive symptoms in schizophrenia, by encouraging glutamatergic and dopaminergic transmission in the prefrontal cortex [1, 37, 45, 74, 77, 83].

Tobacco consumption may also be encouraged by antipsychotic treatment, since tobacco attenuates some of the extra-pyramidal and cognitive side effects caused by antipsychotics [51]. McEvoy et al. showed that starting treatment with Haloperidol was followed by an increase in tobacco consumption [63]. However, other authors have underlined that tobacco consumption started in 90% of cases before the drug treatment began [18, 17, 60].

Other Hypotheses

Other factors may have a role in encouraging tobacco consumption in patients with schizophrenia. The high frequency of comorbidity may be linked to the low rate of stopping smoking in these patients [17, 13, 53]. This may also be linked to abnormalities in the cerebral reward pathways in schizophrenia, which would encourage tobacco consumption [10, 48]. The complexity of the links between tobacco consumption and schizophrenia is illustrated by the differences found in prospective studies, which evaluated smoking in young people, and the later appearance of schizophrenia. In a cohort study of 50,000 Swedish conscripts followed up for 27 years, Zammit et al. recently found a linear relationship between the number of cigarettes smoked and a reduction in the risk of schizophrenia later on (OR= 0.8 [CI= 0.3-0.9]) [89]. On the other hand, in another prospective study on more than 14,000 adolescents, Weiser et al. found a link between tobacco consumption and an increase in the risk of schizophrenia [87].

Role of Genetic Factors

Some authors have suggested that common genetic factors may make individuals vulnerable both to tobacco addiction and to schizophrenia [13, 54]. Freedman et al., in particular, described a genetic abnormality on the locus of the gene coding for the alpha-7 nicotinic receptor on chromosome 15, which would cause neurophysiological disorders, temporarily corrected by nicotine, in schizophrenic patients and in some members of their family [31].

Role of Personality Factors

Several studies on the general population have shown that certain personality traits encourage tobacco consumption, in particular sensation or novelty seeking, impulsivity and antisocial personality traits [23, 66, 92]. As in the general population, patients with schizophrenia who smoke have higher scores than non-smokers on Zuckerman's Sensation Seeking Scale, in particular on the disinhibition subscale scores [20]. They also have higher scores for novelty-seeking on the Tridimensional Personality Questionnaire [84]. However, impulsivity does not seem to encourage tobacco consumption, as is the case in the abuse of alcohol, cannabis or other drugs in patients with schizophrenia [20, 21].

Role of Cultural Factors

The predominant influence of biological factors is suggested by the fact that the high frequency of the schizophrenia/tobacco consumption comorbidity is found in many cultures [13]. However, the frequency of smoking amongst schizophrenic patients in India and Japan is similar to that found in the general population (table 1), which underlines the influence of cultural factors [67, 80]. The role of cultural factors may be linked to the fact that in some countries, smoking initiation is less widespread, especially in women. Tobacco restriction for economic reasons and family customs seems to be particularly predominant in India [80].

Therapeutic Aspects

The rate of smoking cessation in patients with schizophrenia is about half that of the general population [13, 88]. There is little to motivate patients with schizophrenia to quit smoking [33]. A recent Swiss study did however show that the motivating factors for smoking cessation were similar to those of a control group [28]. The amount of cognitive disorders seems to play a role in succeeding smoking cessation: patients with schizophrenia with the lowest performances on the Wisconsin Card Sorting Test, assessing executive functions in the prefrontal cortex, and on the Visuospatial Working Memory task, assessing the visuospatial working memory, were also those who had the most difficulty in smoking cessation [25]. On the other hand, the Stroop Color Word Test and the Continuous Performance Test, assessing other cognitive functions, did not influence these patients in stopping smoking [25]. Some studies found that there was a temporary worsening of certain disorders linked to schizophrenia after stopping smoking, in particular disorders of the working memory [11, 34]. However, studies assessing psychotic symptomatology after administration of nicotine patches or Bupropion, did not show any worsening of the psychotic symptomatology after smoking cessation [33, 35, 29, 36, 40]. It should be underlined that once patients with schizophrenia have given up smoking, they can remain abstinent for a long time [30].

Strategies for Stopping Smoking

The best time to envisage smoking cessation is a period of stabilization of the psychotic symptoms. Atypical antipsychotic medications associated with Bupropion or nicotine transdermal patch, can help motivated patients to quit smoking (35). The doses of conventional and atypical anti-psychotic medications should be reassessed systematically after stopping smoking. In fact, an increase in the plasma levels of these drugs is frequently observed after smoking cessation, due to removal of the interaction by tobacco with cytochrome P450 CYP1A2. For example, in a study of 11 patients, the mean plasma level of Clozapine increased by 57% after stopping smoking [65]. Clinically, overdosage of anti-psychotic drugs is seen by the appearance of sedation and/or extrapyramidal symptoms [22, 93]. It should however be noted that there are no systematic studies with large numbers of patients, in which plasma levels of anti-psychotic drugs have been measured after smoking cessation [65].

Atypical Antipsychotic Drugs

Several studies have shown that administration of atypical anti-psychotic drugs reduced tobacco consumption in patients with schizophrenia, although administration of conventional neuroleptics increased it [33, 62]. In a study including 45 patients, an association of atypical antipsychotic drugs and nicotine transdermal patches was more effective for reducing tobacco consumption (56% stopped smoking at 12 weeks), than an association of conventional neuroleptics and nicotine transdermal patches (22% stopped smoking at 12 weeks) [35]. Several studies have suggested that Clozapine reduced tobacco consumption, in a dose-dependent manner, especially in heavy smokers [33, 61, 62].

Many reasons have been put forward to explain the effect of atypical antipsychotic drugs on tobacco consumption: these medications may produce fewer anti-pyramidal side effects, they may improve the cognitive disorders of schizophrenia which are improved by consuming tobacco, in particular deficits of the P50 wave, and they can improve the negative symptoms. These effects may be linked to an increase in dopaminergic transmission in the prefrontal cortex [1, 62]. Another hypothesis is the inhibitory action of atypical anti-psychotic drugs on the reward pathways in the brain, which are activated by drug-taking and on the reinforcement produced by drugs of abuse in patients with schizophrenia [90].

Nicotine Substitutes

The use of nicotine transdermal patches can help in giving up smoking [33]. The rate of abstinence at 12 weeks after substitution by nicotine transdermal patches are, however, lower in patients with schizophrenia (36%-56%) than in the general population (50%-70%) [33]. The patients must be told that it could be weakly compatible to continue smoking and to use nicotine transdermal patches. They can be used for 8 to 24 weeks or more.

Bupropion

Administration of Bupropion also seems to be useful in smoking cessation, but the results are not as good, compared to those in general population [29, 33, 34]. Up to date, 2 studies did not find that the positive signs of schizophrenia were worsened by Bupropion, despite its property of enhancing dopaminergic transmission, including at doses of 150 to 300 mg/day [29, 33, 34].

Psychosocial Aspects

In general, medical advice and evaluation of motivation for smoking cessation, even when brief or when the patients with schizophrenia do not ask for it, encourage cessation later on [36]. Psychotherapeutic management is based on evaluation of motivation and prevention of relapsing [76]. The educational aspect is particularly important, because patients with schizophrenia have little knowledge of the dangers of tobacco [33]. The patients can be helped to weigh the advantages and disadvantages of continuing smoking or quitting, in particular the reduction of the cardiovascular and pulmonary risks, as well as the money that can be saved by stopping smoking. The cardiovascular risk is close to that of non-smokers 5 years after stopping smoking [4]. It is important to take into account peer pressure, in particular that of other patients, and especially in institutions.

Conclusion

There is a high frequency of tobacco consumption in patients with schizophrenia. Unlike other addictions, tobacco consumption seems to be linked to self-medication, particularly for certain cognitive abnormalities linked with abnormalities of cholinergic, dopaminergic and glutamatergic transmission. Smoking cessation in stabilized patients with schizophrenia is helped by associating atypical anti-psychotic drugs with nicotine transdermal patches or with Bupropion.

References

[1] Adler L. E., Olincy A., Waldo M. et al. Schizophrenia, sensory gating, and nicotinic receptors. *Schizophrenia Bull.* 1998; 24: 189-202.

[2] Adler L. E., Hoffer L. D., Wiser A., Freedman R. Normalization of auditory physiology by cigarette smoking in schizophrenic patients. *Am. J. Psychiatry.* 1993; 150: 1856-1861.

[3] Aguilar M. C., Gurpegui M., Diaz F. J., De Leon J. Nicotine dependence and symptoms in schizophrenia: naturalistic study of complex interactions. *Br. J. Psychiatry.* 2005 ; 186 : 215-21.

[4] Ambrose J. A., Barua R. S. The pathophysiology of cigarette smoking and cardiovascular disease: an update. *J. Am. Coll. Cardiol.* 2004 ; 43 : 1731-7.

[5] Arwidson P., Leon C., Lydie N. et al. Evolutions récentes de la consommation de tabac en France. *Bulletin Epidémiologique Hebdomadaire* 2004 . 22-23 : 95-96.

[6] Avila M. T., Sherr J. D., Hong E. et al. Effects of nicotine on leading saccades during smooth pursuit eye movements in smokers and nonsmokers with schizophrenia. *Neuropsychopharmacology.* 2003 ; 28 : 2184-2191.

[7] Basile V. S., Ozdemir V., Masellis M. et al. A functional polymorphism of the cytochrome P450 1A2 (CYP1A2) gene: association with tardive dyskinesia in schizophrenia. *Mol. Psychiatry.* 2000 ; 5 : 410-7.

[8] Bozikas V. P., Papakosta M., Niopas I. et al. Smoking impact on CYP1A2 activity in a group of patients with schizophrenia. *Eur. Neuropsychopharmacol.* 2004 ; 14 :39-44.

[9] Breslau N., Johnson E. O., Hivipi E., Kessler R. Nicotine dependence in the United States: prevalence, trends, and smoking persistence. *Arch. Gen. Psychiatry* 2001; 58: 810-816.

[10] Chambers R. A., Krystal J. H., Self D. W. A neurological basis for substance abuse comorbidity in schizophrenia. *Biol. Psychiatry.* 2001; 50 : 71-83.

[11] Dalack G. W., Healy D. J., Meador-Woodruff J. H. Nicotine dependence in schizophrenia : clinical phenomena and laboratory findings. *Am. J. Psychiatry.* 1998; 155: 1490-1501.

[12] Dalton S. O., Mellemkjaer L., Thomassen L. et al. Patient Risk for cancer in a cohort of patients hospitalized for schizophrenia in Denmark, 1969-1993. *Schizophr. Res.* 2005 ; 75 : 315-324.

[13] De Leon J., Diaz F. J. A meta-analysis of worldwide studies demonstrates an association between schizophrenia and tobacco smoking behaviors. *Schizophr. Res.* 2005 ; 76 : 135-57.

[14] De Leon J. Atypical antipsychotic dosing: the effect of smoking and caffeine. *Psychiatr. Serv.* 2004 ;55 : 491-3.

[15] De Leon J., Becona E., Gurpegui M. et al. The association between high nicotine dependence and severe mental illness may be consistent across countries. *J. Clin. Psychiatry.* 2002 ; 63 : 812-816.

[16] De Leon J., Tracy J., Mccann E. et al. Schizophrenia and tobacco smoking: a replication study in another US psychiatric hospital. *Schizophr. Res.* 2002 ; 56 : 55-65.

[17] De Leon J., Diaz F. J., Rogers T. et al. Initiation of daily smoking and nicotine dependence in schizophrenia and mood disorders. *Schizophr. Res.* 2002 ; 56 : 47-54.

[18] De Leon J., Dadvand M., Canuso C. et al. Schizophrenia and smoking: an epidemiological survey in a state hospital. *Am. J. Psychiatry.* 1995; 152, 453-455.

[19] Dervaux A. Le diabète chez les patients schizophrènes traités par neuroleptiques. *L'Information psychiatrique.* 2005, 81 : 65-70.

[20] Dervaux A., Bayle F. J., Laqueille X. et al. Smoking in schizophrenia and dishinibition. *Psychiatry Res ;* 2004 ; 128 : 229-234.

[21] Dervaux A., Bayle F. J., Laqueille X. et al. Is substance abuse in schizophrenia related to impulsivity, sensation seeking or anhedonia ? *Am. J. Psychiatry.* 2001; 158: 492-494.

[22] Desai H. D., Seabolt J., Jann M. W. Smoking in patients receiving psychotropic medications: a pharmacokinetic perspective. *CNS Drugs.* 2001; 15 : 469-94.

[23] Dinn W. M., Aycicegi A., Harris C. L. Cigarette smoking in a student sample: Neurocognitive and clinical correlates. *Addict. Behav.* 2004 ; 29 : 107-126.

[24] Diwan A., Castine M., Pomerleau C. S. et al. Differential prevalence of cigarette smoking in patients with schizophrenic vs mood disorders. *Schizophr. Res.* 1998 ; 33 : 113-8.

[25] Dolan S. L., Sacco K. A., Termine A. et al. Neuropsychological deficits are associated with smoking cessation treatment failure in patients with schizophrenia. *Schizophr. Res.* 2004 ; 70 : 263-75.

[26] El-Guebaly N., Hodgins D. C. Schizophrenia and substance abuse: prevalence issues. *Can. J. Psychiatry.* 1992 ; 37 : 704-10.

[27] Enger C., Weatherby L., Reynolds R. F. et al. Serious cardiovascular events and mortality among patients with schizophrenia. *J. Nerv. Ment. Dis.* 2004 ; 192 : 19-27.

[28] Etter M., Mohr S., Garin C., Etter J. F. Stages of change in smokers with schizophrenia or schizoaffective disorder and in the general population. *Schizophr. Bull.* 2004; 30 : 459-68.

[29] Evins A. E., Cather C., Deckersbach T. et al. A Double-blind Placebo-Controlled Trial of Bupropion Sustained-Release for Smoking Cessation in Schizophrenia. *J. Clin. Psychopharmacol.* 2005 ; 25 : 218-225.

[30] Evins A. E., Cather C., Rigotti N. A. et al. Two-year follow-up of a smoking cessation trial in patients with schizophrenia: increased rates of smoking cessation and reduction. *J. Clin. Psychiatry.* 2004 ; 65 : 307-11.

[31] Freedman R., Coon H., Myles-Worsley M. et al. Linkage of a neurophysiological deficit in schizophrenia to a chromosome 15 locus. Proceedings of the National Academy of Sciences of the USA 1997. 94: 587-592.

[32] Freedman R., Hall M., Adler L. E., Leonard S. Evidence in postmortem brain tissue for decreased numbers of hippocampal nicotinic receptors in schizophrenia. *Biol. Psychiatry.* 1995 ; 38 : 22-33.

[33] George T. P., Vessicchio J. C., Termine A. Nicotine and tobacco use in schizophrenia. In: Medical illness and schizophrenia, JM Meyer and HA Nasrallah eds American Psychiatric Publishing 2003. p 163-183.

[34] George T. P., Vessicchio J. C., Termine A. et al. placebo controlled trial of bupropion for smoking cessation in schizophrenia. *Biol. Psychiatry.* 2002 ; 52 : 53-61.

[35] George T. P., Ziedonis D. M., Feingold A. et al. Nicotine transdermal patch and atypical antipsychotic medications for smoking cessation in schizophrenia. *Am. J. Psychiatry.* 2000 ; 157 : 1835-1842.

[36] Goff D. C., Cather C., Evins A. E. et al. Medical morbidity and mortality in schizophrenia: guidelines for psychiatrists. *J. Clin. Psychiatry.* 2005 ; 66 : 183-94.

[37] Goff D. C., Henderson D. C., Amico E. Cigarette smoking in schizophrenia: relationship to psychopathology and medication side effects. *Am. J. Psychiatry.* 1992 ; 149 : 1189-94.

[38] Gulbinat W., Dupont A., Jablensky A. et al. Cancer incidence of schizophrenic patients. Results of record linkage studies in three countries. *Br. J. Psychiatry Suppl.* 1992 ; 18 : 75-83.

[39] Harris J. G., Kongs S., Allensworth D. et al. Effects of nicotine on cognitive deficits in schizophrenia. *Neuropsychopharmacology.* 2004 ; 29 : 1378-85.

[40] Haustein K. O., Haffner S., Woodcock B. G. A review of the pharmacological and psychopharmacological aspects of smoking and smoking cessation in psychiatric patients. *Int. J. Clin. Pharmacol. Ther.* 2002 ; 40 : 404-418.

[41] Herran A., De Santiago A., Sandoya M. et al. Determinants of smoking behaviour in outpatients with schizophrenia. *Schizophrenia Res* 2000; 41: 373-381.

[42] Himelhoch S., Lehman A., Kreyenbuhl J. et al. Prevalence of chronic obstructive pulmonary disease among those with serious mental illness. *Am. J. Psychiatry.* 2004 ; 161 : 2317-9.

[43] Hughes J. R., Hatsukami D. K., Mitchell J. E., Dahlgren L. A. Prevalence of smoking among psychiatric outpatients. *Am. J. Psychiatry.* 1986 ; 143 : 993-997.

[44] Itkin O., Nemets B., Einat H. Smoking habits in bipolar and schizophrenic outpatients in southern Israel. *J. Clin. Psychiatry. 2001* ; 62 : 269-272.

[45] Jacobsen L. K., D'Souza D. C., Mencl W. E. et al. Nicotine effects on brain function and functional connectivity in schizophrenia. *Biol. Psychiatry.* 2004 ; 55 : 850-858.

[46] Joober R., Moatti C., Attar-Levy D. et al. Tabac et psychotropes : incidences pharmacologiques et pharmacocliniques. Editions techniques. Encycl-Med-Chir (Paris-France), *Psychiatrie,* 37-811-A40.

[47] Kelly C., McCreadie R. G. Smoking habits, current symptoms, and premorbid characteristics of schizophrenic patients in Nithsdale, Scotland. *Am. J. Psychiatry.* 1999; 156 : 1751-7.

[48] Kumari V., Postma P. Nicotine use in schizophrenia: The self medication hypotheses. *Neurosci. Biobehav. Rev.* 2005; 29 : 1021-34.

[49] Kumari V., Soni W., Sharma T. Influence of cigarette smoking on prepulse inhibition of the acoustic startle response in schizophrenia. *Hum. Psychopharmacol.* 2001 ; 16 : 321-326.

[50] Leonard S., Adams A. C., Breese C. R. et al. Nicotinic receptor function in schizophrenia. *Schizophrenia Bull.* 1996; 22: 431-445.

[51] Levin E. D., Wilson W., Rose J., McEvoy J. P. Nicotine-haloperidol interactions and cognitive performances in schizophrenics. *Neuropsychopharmacology.* 1996; 15: 429-436.

[52] Lichtermann D., Ekelund J., Pukkala E. et al. Incidence of cancer among persons with schizophrenia and their relatives. *Arch. Gen. Psychiatry.* 2001 ; 58 : 573-578.

[53] Llerena A., De La Rubia A., Penas-Lledo E. M. et al. Schizophrenia and tobacco smoking in a Spanish psychiatric hospital. *Schizophr. Res.* 2002 ; 58 : 323-327.

[54] Lyons M. J., Bar J. L., Kremen W. S., Toomey R. et al. Nicotine and familial vulnerability to schizophrenia: a discordant twin study. *J. Abnorm. Psychol.* 2002 ; 111 : 687-693.

[55] Mancuso G., Warbuton D. M., Mélen M. et al. Selective effects of nicotine on attentional processes. *Psychopharmacology.* 1999; 146: 199-204.

[56] Margolese H. C., Malchy L., Negrete J. C. et al. Drug and alcohol use among patients with schizophrenia and related psychoses: levels and consequences. *Schizophr. Res.* 2004 ; 67 : 157-66.

[57] Masterson E., O'Shea B. Smoking and malignancy in schizophrenia. *Br. J. Psychiatry.* 1984 ; 145 : 429-432.

[58] McCreadie R. G.; Scottish Schizophrenia Lifestyle Group. Diet, smoking and cardiovascular risk in people with schizophrenia: descriptive study. *Br. J. Psychiatry.* 2003 ; 183 : 534-539.

[59] McCreadie R. G.; Scottish Comorbidity Study Group. Use of drugs, alcohol and tobacco by people with schizophrenia: case-control study. *Br. J. Psychiatry.* 2002 ; 181: 321-5.

[60] McEvoy J. P., Brown S. Smoking in first-episode patients with schizophrenia. *Am. J. Psychiatry.* 1999 ; 156 : 1120-1.

[61] McEvoy J. P., Freudenreich O., Wilson W. H. Smoking and therapeutic response to clozapine in patients with schizophrenia. *Biol. Psychiatry.* 1999; 46: 125-129.

[62] McEvoy J., Freudenreich O., McGee M. et al. Clozapine decreases smoking in patients with chronic schizophrenia. *Biol. Psychiatry.* 1995 ; 37 : 550-552.

[63] McEvoy J. P., Freudenreich O., Levin E. D., Rose J. E. Haloperidol increases smoking in patients with schizophrenia. *Psychopharmacology.* (Berl). 1995 ; 119 : 124-126.

[64] Menza M. A., Grossman N., Van Horn M. et al. Smoking and movement disorders in psychiatric patients. *Biol. Psychiatry.* 1991 ; 30 : 109-115.

[65] Meyer J. M. Individual changes in clozapine levels after smoking cessation: results and a predictive model. *J. Clin. Psychopharmacol.* 2001 ; 21 : 569-74.

[66] Mitchell S. H. Measures of impulsivity in cigarette smokers and non-smokers. *Psychopharmacology.* 1999; 146: 455-464.

[67] Mori T., Sasaki T., Iwanami A. et al. Smoking habits in Japanese patients with schizophrenia. *Psychiatry Res.* 2003 ; 120 : 207-209.

[68] Mortensen P. B., Juel K. Mortality and causes of death in first admitted schizophrenic patients. *Br. J. Psychiatry.* 1993 ; 163 : 183-9.

[69] Myers C. S., Robles O., Kakoyannis A. N. et al. Nicotine improves delayed recognition in schizophrenic patients. *Psychopharmacology.* 2004 ; 174 : 334-40.

[70] Nilsson A., Waller L., Rosengren A. et al. Cigarette smoking is associated with abnormal involuntary movements in the general male population--a study of men born in 1933. *Biol. Psychiatry.* 1997 ; 41 : 717-23.

[71] Olincy A., Johnson L. L., Ross R. G. Differential effects of cigarette smoking on performance of a smooth pursuit and a saccadic eye movement task in schizophrenia. *Psychiatry Res.* 2003; 117: 223-236.

[72] Olincy A., Ross R. G., Young D. A. et al. Improvement in smooth pursuit eye movements after cigarette smoking in schizophrenic patients. *Neuropsychopharmacology.* 1998 ; 18 : 175-85.

[73] Olincy A., Young D. A., Freedman R. Increased levels of the nicotine metabolite cotinine in schizophrenic smokers compared to other smokers. *Biol. Psychiatry.* 1997 ; 42 : 1-5.

[74] Patkar A. A., Gopalakrishnan R., Lundy A. et al. Relationship between tobacco smoking and positive and negative symptoms in schizophrenia. *J. Nerv. Ment. Dis ;* 2002; 190 : 604-610.

[75] Poirier M. F., Canceil O., Bayle F. et al. Prevalence of smoking in psychiatric patients. *Prog. Neuropsychopharmacol. Biol. Psychiatry.* 2002; 26: 529-537.

[76] Prochaska J. J., Gill P., Hall S. M. Treatment of Tobacco Use in an Inpatient Psychiatric Setting. *Psychiatr. Serv.* 2004 ; 55: 1265-1270.

[77] Rezvani A. H., Levin E. D. Cognitive effects of nicotine. *Biol. Psychiatry.* 2001; 49: 258-267.

[78] Saari K., Jokelainen J., Veijola J. et al. Serum lipids in schizophrenia and other functional psychoses: a general population northern Finland 1966 birth cohort survey. *Acta Psychiatr. Scand.* 2004 ; 110 : 279-85.

[79] Sacco K. A., Termine A., Seyal A. et al. Effects of cigarette smoking on spatial working memory and attentional deficits in schizophrenia: involvement of nicotinic receptor mechanisms. *Arch. Gen. Psychiatry.* 2005 ; 62 : 649-59.

[80] Srinivasan T. N., Thara R. Smoking in schizophrenia - all is not biological. *Schizophr. Res.* 2002 ; 56 : 67-74.

[81] Stein E. A., Pankiewicz J., Harsch H. H. et al. Nicotine-induced limbic cortical activation in the human brain: a functional MRI study. *Am. J. Psychiatry.* 1998 ; 155 : 1009-15.

[82] Steinberg M. L., Williams J. M., Steinberg H. R. et al. Applicability of the Fagerstrom Test for Nicotine Dependence in smokers with schizophrenia. *Addict. Behav.* 2005 ; 30 : 49-59.

[83] Taiminen T. J., Salokangas R. K., Saarijarvi S. et al. Smoking and cognitive deficits in schizophrenia: a pilot study. *Addict. Behav.* 1998 ; 23 : 263-6.

[84] Van Ammers E. C., Sellman J. D., Mulder R. T. Temperament and substance abuse in schizophrenia: is there a relationship ? *Journal of Nervous and Mental Disease*. 1997; 185: 283-288.

[85] Warburton D. M., Arnall C. Improvements in performance without nicotine withdrawal. *Psychopharmacology*. 1994; 115: 539-542.

[86] Warburton D. M. Nicotine as a cognitive enhancer. *Prog. Neuropsychopharmacol. Biol. Psychiatry*. 1992; 16: 181-191.

[87] Weiser M., Reichenberg A., Grotto I. et al. Higher rates of cigarette smoking in male adolescents before the onset of schizophrenia: a historical-prospective cohort study. *Am. J. Psychiatry*. 2004 ; 161 : 1219-23.

[88] Williams J. M., Ziedonis D. M., Abanyie F. et al. Increased nicotine and cotinine levels in smokers with schizophrenia and schizoaffective disorder is not a metabolic effect. *Schizophr. Res.* 2005 ; 79 : 323-35.

[89] Zammit S., Allebeck P., Dalman C. et al. Investigating the association between cigarette smoking and schizophrenia in a cohort study. *Am. J. Psychiatry*. 2003; 160: 2216-2221.

[90] Ziedonis D. M., George T. P. Schizophrenia and nicotine use: report of a pilot smoking cessation program and review of neurobiological and clinical issues. *Schizophr. Bull.* 1997; 23 : 247-54.

[91] Ziedonis D. M., Kosten T. R., Glazer W. M., Frances R. J. Nicotine dependence and schizophrenia. *Hosp. Community Psychiatry*. 1994 ; 45 : 204-206.

[92] Zuckerman M., Ball S., Black J. Influences of sensation seeking, gender, risk appraisal, and situational motivation on smoking. *Addictive Behaviors*. 1990; 15: 209-220.

[93] Zullino D. F., Delessert D., Eap C. B. et al. Tobacco and cannabis smoking cessation can lead to intoxication with clozapine or olanzapine. *Int. Clin. Psychopharmacol.* 2002; 17: 141-143.

In: Progress in Smoking and Health Research
Editor: T. C. Jeffries, pp. 193-239
ISBN: 978-1-60021-686-2

Chapter IX

Influence of Active and Passive Smoking During Pregnancy on Newborn Health

***Ewa Florek*[1], *Wojciech Piekoszewski*[2], *Agnieszka Hubert*[1] and *Maria K. Kornacka*[3]**
[1] Laboratory of Environmental Research, Department of Toxicology, University of Medical Sciences, Poznan, Poland,
[2] Institute of Forensic Research, Krakow, Poland
[3] Neonatology Clinic, University of Medical Sciences, Warsaw, Poland

Abstract

The aim of the study was the evaluation of the level of cotinine, socio-economic status of the patients and birth parameters of the newborn as an index for the behaviors of pregnant women in relation to smoking tobacco and ETS.

The research included 115 women delivering at the Gynecological-Obstetric Clinic University of Medical Sciences in Warsaw as well as 115 newborns. The patients were divided into three groups: smokers, exposed to ETS and the nonsmokers.

A questionnaire method concerning the socio-economic status, tobacco smoking/passive exposure and pregnancy was used in the research. Most often women smoking tobacco would have the secondary education and performed a white-collar work. 74.47% of women were inhabitants of Warsaw. Among the women who were inhaling the smoke passively, the highest percentage referred to women aged 25-29. 64% of patients had higher education. 72% of women performed the white-collar work. Among the women smoking tobacco, 46.05% were patients who smoked 1-5 cigarettes a day. In all the groups of the tested women, the consciousness of health consequences connected with tobacco smoking and ETS was almost 100%.

In the group of mothers smoking tobacco, there were 76.6% of newborns born at the right time, whereas 23.4% of newborns were born prematurely. The newborns of the smoking women were lighter by 610.9 g in comparison with the newborns of the nonsmoking mothers, and 280.3 g in relation to the newborn of women who were passively exposed to smoke.

The newborns of smoking mothers were 4.06 cm shorter in comparison to the children of non-smoking mothers and the ones who were not exposed to smoke. These newborns were also 1.72 cm smaller than the newborns of mothers passively exposed to smoke.

The concentration of cotinine in the urine and placenta of smoking mothers as well as the first urine of the newborns was respectively: 898 ng/mg of creatinine, 47 ng/g of placenta and 184 ng/mg of creatinine. For women exposed to ETS the concentrations were 53 ng/mg of creatinine, 19 ng/g and 26 ng/mg of creatinine respectively.

A statistically significant relation between the active and passive exposure to tobacco smoke during pregnancy and the risk of premature delivery, low birth body mass and body length was observed.

The presence of cotinine in the placenta and in the first urine of an newborn speaks volumes of the exposure of the fetus to toxic components of smoke.

Introduction

For over 500 years, tobacco and its consumption, along with other "luxurious" goods such as opium and alcohol have all been subject to development. Tobacco was used as a medicine in religious and ceremonial rites and as a product for consumption by society. In the 20th century a new epidemic emerged and developed – addiction to tobacco. Cigarettes became a part of the lifestyle of many people in countries all over the world. The observed growth in the frequency of tobacco smoking is accompanied by an increasing incidence rate of tobacco-related diseases and mortality.

Tobacco Smoke

The smoke is produced during the incomplete tobacco burning. In the course of this process, many chemical and physico-chemical phenomena take place, including: pyrolysis, pyrosynthesis, distillation, sublimation, condensation, oxidation, reduction, decarboxylation and dehydration, which condition the chemical composition of smoke.

The qualitative composition of tobacco smoke is complex and constant. It is estimated that about 4200 chemical compounds and several hundred unidentified substances constitute the composition of tobacco smoke. In the gas phase of tobacco smoke, 400-600 components have been marked, whereas in the particle phase, more than 3600 have been identified [19, 33].

The gas phase of the main tobacco smoke stream consists, among others, of nitrogen, oxygen, carbon monoxide and carbon dioxide. These components constitute about 85-95% of the total mass of the main stream. The particularly toxic compounds in the gas phase of the tobacco smoke include: carbon monoxide, ammonia, nitrogen oxide, hydrogen cyanide, formaldehyde, acetic aldehyde, pyridine and volatile N-nitrosamines [64].

The particle phase is an aerosol of the diameter of molecules ranging from 0.1 to 0.8 μm. [63, 64]. It is composed of hydrocarbons, polycyclic aromatic hydrocarbons (naphthalene, pyrene, phenanthrene, benzo(a)anthracene, benzo(a)pyrene), phenols, alcohols, inorganic components (potassium, calcium, nickel, lead, selenium, cadmium, zinc), radioactive elements (^{210}Po) and N-nitrosamines characteristic for tobacco. There are 10^{10} of free radicals in the main stream [65].

The particle phase contains also pyridene alkaloids, such as, among others, nicotine, which constitutes about 85-90 % of the overall alkaloid mass [62, 149]. The nicotine in the main smoke stream occurs in the particle phase, whereas in the case of the side stream – in the gas phase.

A cigarette with a mass of 1g produces about 500 mg of smoke, of which 5-10% constitutes the particle phase.

In the process of smoking, two smoke streams are created: main stream (MS) and side stream (SS). The main stream is produced during the process of inhalation on a cigarette and this is inhaled by the smoker, whereas the side stream is produced during the breaks between inhalation. On top of all this, the smoke breathed out by the smoker is also present in the environment [66, 150].

Environmental tobacco smoke (ETS) defined as tobacco smoke in the environment is a sum of the side stream of smoke (80-96%) and the smoke breathed out by the smoker (4-20%). The degree of environmental exposure of nonsmokers to the tobacco smoke, "passive smoking", depends on the number of smokers, the amount of smoked cigarettes, the size of a room, ventilation and the time of exposure [163].

Tobacco Smoking among Women in Poland and in the World

The number of cigarettes smoked in highly developed countries has been lowered by about 20% in the course of the last 20 years, whereas in the case of developing countries, the amount of cigarettes smoked has been increasing by about 3.5% per year [144]. The prevalence of tobacco smoking among women is differentiated geographically. The greatest number of female smokers has been noted in Europe and Central Asia, and the smoking habit is most prevalent among persons between the ages of 30 and 50. There are about 200 million female smokers in the world. In developed countries, about 25% of smokers are female, but only 7% of women smoke tobacco in developing countries. It is predicted that by the year 2025, the number of smokers will increase to 1.64 billion, and the percentage of female smokers will increase from 8% to 20% [4, 99].

In Poland, tobacco smoking is a common phenomenon – 34% of women had smoked tobacco at some point in their life, at present the percentage stands at 23% of which 22% of these women smoke every day. The analyses that have been carried out show that among nonsmoking people, 52% of women are exposed to a tobacco smoke environment at home and 27% of women are exposed to it at work [163]. In research carried out in the Wielkopolska region, among the women in the procreative age, 22% of them declared active tobacco smoking. Passive exposure to tobacco smoke occurred in 66% of cases. The analysis of data indicated that 35% of questioned women are exposed to passive inhalation of tobacco smoke at home, 27% at work and 44% during recreation and social meetings [41].

Data concerning the popularity of smoking in the member states of the European Union in the nineties indicate a drop in the frequency of regular tobacco smoking. For instance in the Netherlands, a drop in the number of female smokers from 34% in 1980 to 32% in 1996 was observed, and in Belgium from 28% in 1982 to 22% in 1997 [73, 115]. The situation is different in Portugal, where the percentage of female smokers grew from 12% to 15%. A similar situation can be noticed among women living in Spain. In the years 1978-1993 the popularity of smoking among women grew from 17 % to 25 % [73]. Tobacco smoking became very popular among young women. In the years 1989-1992, one in five women between the ages of 15 and 39 smoked cigarettes, whereas one in eight women smoked between the ages of 40 and 54.

A particularly dangerous phenomenon is the smoking of tobacco by pregnant women. In Canada, 14-16% of women smokes tobacco during pregnancy, whereas in the U.S. the percentage of women who smoke during pregnancy amounts to 20-23%. A constant drop in the number of female smokers has been observed. Contrary to these countries, tobacco smoking within the group of pregnant women grew in France from 10% in 1972 to 17% in 1981 and reached the level of 25% in 1995. A positive fact is that among these women, 27% smoked less than 5 cigarettes a day, and 43% less than 1 cigarette during the day [164].

There is alarming data concerning the popularity of the smoking habit among girls. In Great Britain, smoking among 11—15-year-olds is frequent. In 1994, about 13% of girls in England smoked at least one cigarette a week. Research carried out in the years 1990, 1994 and 1998 in Poland, showed a dynamic growth in the popularity of smoking among children of school age. In 1999, research carried out by WHO indicated that 58% of boys and 57% of girls in Poland smoked a cigarette at least once in their life, whereas 11% of them tried to smoke their first cigarette before they were even 7 years old.

The Impact of Tobacco Smoking on the Health of Women, Pregnancy, Development of a Fetus and a Newborn

Many clinical tests showed that tobacco smoking has an impact on the lowered fertility of women. On the basis of epidemiological research, it has been stated that the infertility of females who smoke is two or three times higher than those who do not smoke [43, 172].

The nicotine affects the level of estrogens and progesterone as well as adrenal gland hormones and pituitary gland hormones, which may lead to the occurrence of a disorder in the correct menstrual cycle and ovulation. It has also been proved that the nicotine affects the functioning of the Fallopian tube, handicapping above all, the activities involved in the transportation of the egg cell and the zygote, the effect of this may be both a delay in fertilization and incorrect implantation. These irregularities may occur at any stage, covering the gametogenesis, ovulation, fertilisation, tubal transportation, implantation and the creation of placenta [37, 41,150, 151]. The lowering of fertility is also connected with a 1.5–2% increase in the risk of idiopathic miscarriages of genetically well-formed fetuses. An increased risk of the premature separation of the placenta, more frequent occurrences of irregular bleedings during pregnancy and an increased risk of the premature rupture of membranes are observed in the cases of the female smokers [35, 109].

As has been proved through research, nicotine as well as its metabolite – cotinine and the remaining components of the tobacco smoke cause the production of progesterone by granule cells to be stopped, this reaction depends on the nicotine dose. This is probably done in two ways; through a direct blockade of progesterone synthesis and also through the cytotoxic effect, which is not determined entirely and which is triggered by the alkaloids of tobacco smoke on granulocytes. Additionally, it has been proved that cotinine has a significant impact on the activity of the placental phospholipase A2 and prostaglandine E2 [122]. Cotinine causes an increase in the secretion of placental phospholipase A2 and an increase in the contraction activity of prostoglandine E2, which leads to the shrinkage of placental vessels and a decrease in the flow of blood. The effect of cotinine activity is stronger than the one triggered by nicotine. The accumulation of cotinine in the placenta and the secretion of prostaglandine E2 connected with it, may lead to the induction of natural miscarriage or premature delivery [88].

Comstock and Lundin observed that the risk of delivering a stillborn fetus, when the parents are not smokers, is 11.9 per 1000, the risk increases significantly, if even one of the parents is a habitual smoker. When the mother does not smoke and the father smokes tobacco, the risk amounts to 17.2. On the other hand, when both parents are smokers, the risk reaches 26.5 per 1000 deliveries [25]. In research carried out by Ahlborg and Bodin it was proved that the exposure of pregnant women to environmental tobacco smoke in the home does not have a significant effect [5]. On the other hand, in the case of women exposed to ETS at the workplace, the risk increases by 1.2–3.8 [42, 169].

Both passive and active exposure to tobacco by women in the procreative period has far-reaching consequences for their progeny. According to different authors, the birth body weight of the newborns of mothers smoking tobacco is lower by 200-300 g than in the case of the babies of nonsmoking mothers [121]. The smoking of one cigarette a day by a pregnant woman causes a decrease in the birth body weight of a newborn by 7.4–9.2 g [76, 77, 159]. Also, smoking 20 or more cigarettes a day in the presence of a pregnant woman causes a decrease in the birth body weight of the newborns of about 120 g in relation to the newborns of nonsmoking parents [133]. The results of the works of many authors indicate that the smoking of tobacco in the third trimester of pregnancy slowed down the growth of the fetus more than smoking in the initial pregnancy period. On the other hand, a consequence of tobacco smoke on the fetus in the early development stages is the postponement of cellular hyperplasia. It has been observed, that the disturbances in the growth of the body weight of the fetus are not an effect of nutritive shortages in the smoking mother, but disturbances in the synthesis of structural proteins of fetal cells caused by the tobacco smoke. Zaren et al. have shown that the newborns of smoking mothers have a significantly thinner layer of subcutaneous fat tissue accumulated when a fetus, beginning at the 28th week of pregnancy, than the newborns of nonsmoking mothers [177].

The cessation of the growth of a fetus is caused not only by a decrease in the number of cell divisions, but also in the chronic tissue hypoxia of the fetus [77]. The tissue hypoxia is caused by multi-factor disorders of the vaginal-placental circulation caused by the tobacco smoke. The reduction of the surface of the vaginal-placental exchange expressed by the quantity of hypovascular and avascular atrophic villi, is directly proportional to the quantity of cigarettes smoked by a pregnant woman [106].

Through the stimulation of adrenal glands, the nicotine contained in the tobacco smoke causes great quantities of adrenaline, noradrenaline, actylcholine and cortisol to be released into the circulation system of a female smoker. These catecholamines trigger a vasopastic action, which causes an increase in blood pressure and tachycardia of both the pregnant woman and the fetus. The shrinkage of tiny vessels in the placenta significantly increases the vascular resistance leading to a reduction in the vaginal-placental flow. It has been proved that within 10 minutes from the moment of the smoking of two cigarettes by a pregnant women, who is in the third trimester of pregnancy, the concentrations of adrenaline and cortisol in her venous blood increase by 60% and 20% respectively, whereas the blood flow in the intervillous space is reduced to 78% of the initial value. Additionally, the nicotine may pass through the placental barrier to the fetal circulation system and in this way, it may exert a direct impact on the cardiovascular system, digestive system and central nervous system [140]. The nicotine, passing through the placenta, to the circulation system of the fetus causes the intensification of its respiratory movements and an increase in arterial blood pressure. It has been observed that after the smoking of the first cigarette by a pregnant women, the cardiac activity of the fetus is accelerated and the body movement is intensified. After the second cigarette, the movements weaken and episodes of bradycardia occur. These observations are confirmed by the tests carried out on animals, where it has been proved that small doses of nicotine (the first cigarette) cause the stimulation of nicotine receptors in autonomic ganglions, and bigger doses block them [40, 106].

Another component of tobacco smoke leading to the hypoxia of a fetus is carbon monoxide [3, 6, 42].

Apart from this, there is the fact that parental smoke is one of the major risks factors for the occurrence of Sudden Infant Death Syndrome – (SIDS) [1]. The risk of the occurrence of this syndrome is four times more frequent among the newborns of smoking mothers. The degree of risk is directly proportional to the number of cigarettes smoked per day. The most significant factor related to the risk of the occurrence of SIDS is the smoking of tobacco by the parents or family members in the room where the child is present. Then, the risk increases as much as eight times.

In a small number of reports, it has been proved that the smoking of tobacco by parents may increase the risk of the occurrence of some inborn defects [110]. These are, among others, defects of the neural tube, hydrocephalus, organic heart diseases, cleft of the facial skeleton and defects of the urinary-reproductive system. There is also an enhanced risk of neoplasms. As the research carried out by Zenzes et al. has proved, it is possible to observe an increased quantity of DNA adducts produced together with the metabolite of benzo(a)pyrene already among embryos before implantation [179]. According to the data presented by the authors, the transfer of modified DNA is possible mainly owing to the sperm cells. Apart from that, the exposure of a mother to tobacco smoke is related to the occurrence of one of the known tobacco specific carcinogenic compounds in the fetus, that is, 4-(methylonitrosoamino)-1-(3-pyridyl)-1-buthanol - NNK. Its two metabolites occur in the urine of the progeny of women smoking much more than in the control group [48].

Among the children exposed to tobacco smoke, it is possible to observe a body height defect not only at the moment of delivery, but also later on during the development period. Clinical research has proved that during the period of breast feeding, the newborns of smoking parents gain approximately 400 g less in weight than the ones coming from nonsmoking families. If a mother was a nonsmoker, but the father was a regular active smoker, the body weight growth was less by about 200 g [133].

Children, whose mothers inhaled tobacco smoke actively or passively, are characterized by more frequent occurrences of ailments related to the respiratory system (coughs, rattling, pneumonia, bronchitis, bronchial asthma and chronic respiratory tract inflammation). Clinical research has proved that decreased parameters of the lungs at the moment of delivery, occurs also among these children in the later period. The lowering of spirometric values related to the exposure to passive smoking during the development period remains significant even in the mature age [155, 160, 161].

As a consequence of this fact, in children who fall ill with the listed disease entities there is a more frequent incidence in the hospitalization of newborns by about 20-40%. Among the children of smokers, an increase in the risk of the occurrence of acute and chronic otitis media is observed. The above-mentioned diseases occur much more frequently among children exposed to tobacco smoke within the age bracket of 0 to 3yrs [101].

There is a supposition that tobacco smoking may also have an impact on the retardation of the intellectual and emotional development (speech disorders, hyperactivity syndrome, lowering of concentration and worse results at school).

The greater incidence of circulatory system diseases is also related to the passive exposure of children to the tobacco smoke. It is caused by the disruption of oxygen transport, changes in the lipid profile (lowered HDL fraction) and irregularities in the functioning of the endothelium. Thrombosis is developed and the LDL lipoproteins are oxidised (as in the case of persons actively smoking tobacco).

Subjects and Methods

One hundred fifteen pregnant women admitted to the Maternity Department of the Gynecological Obstetric Clinic of the University of Medical Sciences in Warsaw in 2005 participated in the research. The protocol of the research was approved by the Bioethical Commission of the University of Medical Sciences in Warsaw. The conducted study was in compliance with the Helsinki Declaration of 1964, 1975, 1983, 1989 1996. Participation in the research was entirely voluntary.

On the basis of a questionnaire as well as cotinine determination in the women's urine, the tested patients (115 women) were divided into three groups: smokers (47 patients), persons exposed to ETS (25 patients) and nonsmokers and non-exposed (43 patients).

Questionnaire Survey

A questionnaire, which consisted of three parts, was used. The survey was conducted when the women were admitted to the Maternity Department of the Gynecological-Obstetrics Clinic of the University of Medical Sciences in Warsaw.

The first part of the questionnaire contained questions concerning the social-economic status: age, education, nature of performed work, place of residence, marital status and mean income for one family member. The second part contained questions concerning the tobacco smoking habits of the women before getting pregnant and during the pregnancy, as well as the number of cigarettes smoked per day. The next questions concerned exposure to carcinogenic substances at the workplace during the pregnancy period. The third part of the questionnaire concerned the pregnancy (duration, type of delivery) and the health of the newborns. The health of a newborn was evaluated by a physician. It was evaluated on the basis of the following parameters: birth bodies weight and body length.

Toxicological Analysis

Urine samples (100 ml) were collected from the women after admission to the hospital The samples of the first urine (~6 ml) of each newborn were collected in sterile adhesive plastic bags. The urine samples were frozen and stored at a temperature of -20°C for later analysis.

The sample from the placenta (50 g) was collected during the delivery, and was then stored at a temperature of -80°C for later analysis.

Analysis of Cotinine and Creatinine in the Urine

Cotinine in the urine was determined by a previously developed and validated high performance liquid chromatography with norephedrine as an internal standard, after the solid phase extraction. The method was linear - from 5 to 1000 ng/ml, the limit of detection (LOD) and limit of quantification (LOQ) were 5 ng/ml and 10 ng/ml respectively [46].

Creatinine was determined by means of a spectrophotometric method (wavelength - 520-560 nm) on a Synchron Cx Clinical System analyzer (Beckman Instruments Inc.) Bio Merieux reagents.

Analysis of Cotinine in the Placenta

In the case of determination of the cotinine in the placenta, the extraction was preceded by a homogenization of the placenta (5 g) using 10 ml of water. To the homogenate thus prepared, 0.1 ml of 1 M HCl and 0,05 ml of norephedrine (0,20 mg/ml) were added. The sample was placed in an ultrasonic bath for 10-15 minutes, and was then centrifuged for 10 minutes (4000–5000 rpm). 0.5 ml of 5M NaOH was added to the collected supernatant in order to obtain a pH of 10 and 5 ml of dichloromethane. Then it was shaken for 15 minutes. The sample was then centrifuged for a further 10 minutes (4000–5000 rpm), the organic phase was sampled and shaken from 2 ml of 0.5 M NaOH on Vortex for 30 seconds. The sample was centrifuged for 5 minutes, at a speed of 4000 – 5000 rpm. Thereafter, the organic phase was collected and evaporated to dry in a stream of compressed air, at a temperature of 37°C. The chromatographic analysis was conducted in the same way as in the case of the cotinine determination in the urine. The linearity of the method was drawn up covered a range between 5-400 ng/ml, and the validation parameters (LOD, LOQ, and repeatability during the day and between the days) approximated those obtained by the method of cotinine determination in the urine.

Statistical Analysis

The information included in the questionnaire, was collected in a computer database, after it had been encoded. The results of the survey and toxicological study were subjected to statistical analysis. The differences in the distributions of the tested variables were evaluated by means of an analysis of variance (ANOVA) and a t-Student test. The mean values were compared applying the variance analysis.

Results

The research encompassed a group of 115 pregnant women giving birth at the Gynecological-Obstetrics Clinic of the University of Medical Sciences in Warsaw.

In accordance with the assumptions of the paper, the patients were divided into three groups: AS (active smokers), PS (passive smokers) and NS (nonsmokers). This division was assumed on the basis of the following criteria: declaration of the patient and cotinine level in urine.

According to Bramer and Kallungal, a concentration of cotinine in urine that is above 200 ng/ml confirms active tobacco smoking [17]. It was assumed that a level of 5 ng/ml of urine (limit of detection) indicates a lack of active and passive exposure, and the range covering the values from 5 ng/ml of urine to 200 ng/ml of urine signifies exposure to ETS. In the research, in order to standardize the results, the concentration of cotinine was calculated into mg of creatinine due to the fact that the elimination of this connection with urine depends on the efficiency of the functioning of the kidneys, blood flow through the kidneys and the pH of urine.

The newborns of women who smoke tobacco were assigned to the AS-N group, the newborns of the patients passively exposed to tobacco smoke – to the PS-N group, and the newborns of women who do not smoke and who were not passively exposed to ETS – to the NS-N group.

The numbers of women in the respective groups were as follows: 47 – AS group, 25 – PS group and 43 NS group.

The Characteristics of the Socio-Economic Status of the Women Participating in the Research

Within the group of women smoking tobacco, the approximate percentages of the tested patients were; women younger than 25 years old - 27.66%, between the ages of 25 and 29 - 31.91% and 30 – 35 - 27.66%. The women from this group most often claimed to have a secondary education – 46.81%. More than a half of them had a white collar job (53.19%).

74.47% of these women were residents of Warsaw. Married women constituted the greatest percentage of women – 65.96%. The mean gross income for one family member was high in the cases of 40.43% of respondents and amounted to more than PLN 1000 (Polish currency, 1$=3PLN) (table 1).

Table 1. Socio-economical status of studied women

Socio-economical status	*Smokers (n=47) [%]*	*Exposed to ETS (n=25) [%]*	*Nonsmokers (n=43) [%]*
Age [years]:			
below 25	27.66	24.00	4.65
25 – 29	31.91	40.00	48.84
30 – 35	27.66	24.00	34.88
above 35	12.77	12.00	11.63
Education:			
primary	12.77	8.00	4.65
vocational	21.28	4.00	0.00
secondary	46.81	24.00	30.23
university	19.15	64.00	65.12
Occupation:			
white collar workers	53.19	72.00	72.09
blue collar workers	25.53	8.00	16.28
the unemployed	21.28	20.00	11.63
Place of residence:			
Warsaw			
other cities	74.47	50.00	69.77
country-side	19.15	41.67	20.93
	6.38	8.33	9.30
Marital status:			
married	65.96	88.00	88.37
maiden	25.53	12.00	9.30
widow	0.00	0.00	0.00
divorcee	8.51	0.00	2.33
Mean income [PLN]:			
below 500	23.40	4.00	2.33
500 – 1000	36.17	28.00	27.91
above 1000	40.43	68.00	69.77

Among the women who inhale tobacco smoke passively, the ones who were 25-29 years old constituted the greatest percentage (40.00%). The women who were younger than 25 years old and between the ages of 30 and 35 constituted 24.00% of respondents, and the patients older than 35 constituted a half of that number, that is (12.00%). 64% of patients claimed to have a higher education. 72.00% of the women had a white collar job. Half of the persons participating in the research lived in Warsaw. 88.00% of them were married women. The greatest percentage – 68.00% - had an mean gross income of more than PLN 1000 for one family member (table 1).

Almost half of the tested women who did not smoke and who were not exposed to ETS, that is, 48.84% were aged 25–29, and 34.88% of the women were patients aged 30–35. 65.12% of the women belonging to the NS group had a higher education, and 72.09% of them carried out white collar work. More than 2/3 of them (69.77%) lived in Warsaw. Married women constituted the greatest percentage – 88.37%. An mean gross income of more than PLN 1000 was earned by 69.77% of the women (table 1).

As has been mentioned before, in the research which was carried out, the division of women into groups: (AS, PS, NS) was based on the declarations of the patients and the measurement of cotinine in their urine.

Within the group of smoking women (47 patients) tobacco smoking was declared by 37 patients (78.72% of women from this group). Within the group exposed to ETS, 24.35% of women declared exposure, however according to the above-mentioned criteria, there were 21.74% women exposed to ETS. Within the group of non-smokers, the conformance of the declarations with actual exposure was 43.48% to 37.39% (figure 1).

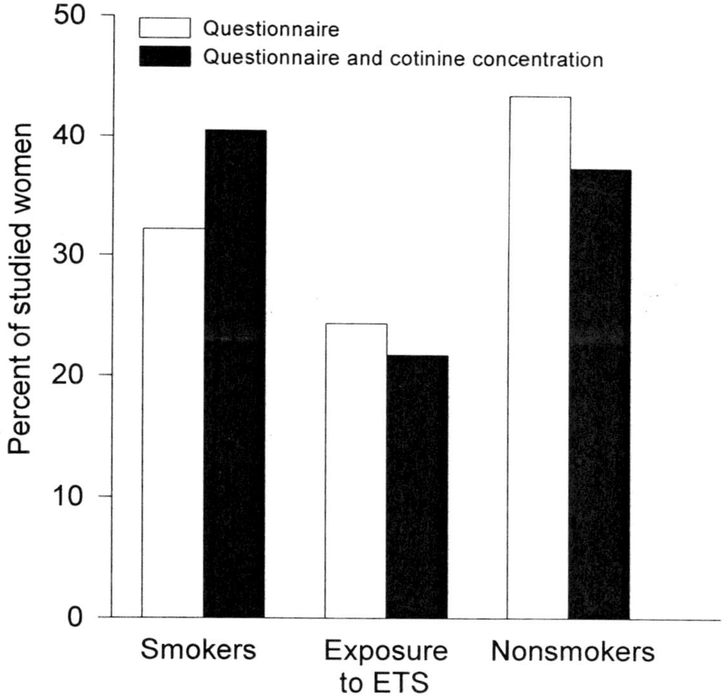

Figure 1. Conformity between the declaration about tobacco smoking and actual exposition.

The AS group consisted of 37 women declaring smoking, and 10 women where smoking was confirmed by the level of cotinine in urine. Among the women smoking tobacco, 45.95% were patients who smoked 1-5 cigarettes a day. A similar percentage of women, that is, 27.03% and 21.62%, smoked from 6 to 10 and from 11 to 15 cigarettes a day respectively. The smallest percentage – 5.41% was represented by women smoking more than 15 cigarettes a day (figure 2).

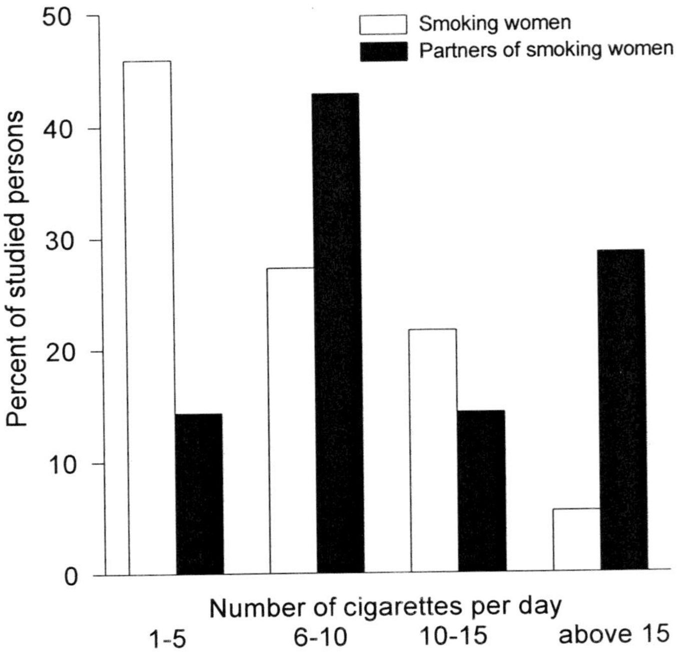

Figure 2. Daily cigarettes intake of women during pregnancy and their partners.

The largest group was represented by women smoking tobacco throughout the pregnancy period, that is, as much as 70.27%. The percentage of women smoking only in the first month of pregnancy (10.81%) as well as pregnant women addicted to tobacco for a period of 7 months was similar (8.11%) (figure 3).

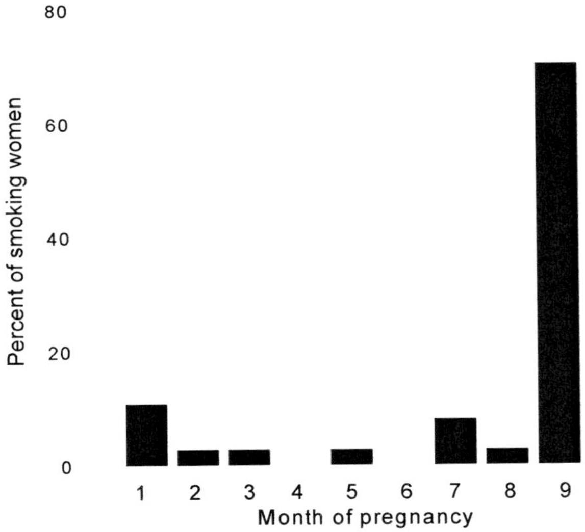

Figure 3. Period of tobacco smoking during pregnancy.

Within the group of women declaring smoking, only 1/3 of the tested patients (29.73%) quit smoking during the ensuing months of pregnancy.

Passive inhalation of tobacco smoke was confirmed in the cases of 25 women. The percentage of women living with a smoking partner within that group amounted to 46.43%. Among the partners, the largest group was formed by persons smoking 6-10 cigarettes a day – 42.86%. On the other hand, the largest number of cigarettes, more than 15, was smoked by 28.56% of partners (figure 2).

The awareness of the health consequences of tobacco smoking and passive exposure to environmental tobacco smoke within all the tested groups – active smokers, passive smokers, and nonsmokers - was almost 100%, however within the group of smokers, it was 11% lower than within the group of nonsmokers.

Information from a physician regarding the harmful effects of tobacco smoking was obtained by 41.74% of the tested women.

Pregnancy and the Characteristics of a Newborn

Within the group of smoking women, 63.83% of the patients planned their pregnancy, the remaining percentage – 36.17% encompassed women who did not plan their pregnancy. Among the women exposed to ETS, the percentage of women who planned their pregnancy was 68.00%, whereas within the group of women who did not smoke and who were not exposed to tobacco smoke, this percentage amounted to 88.37% (figure 4).

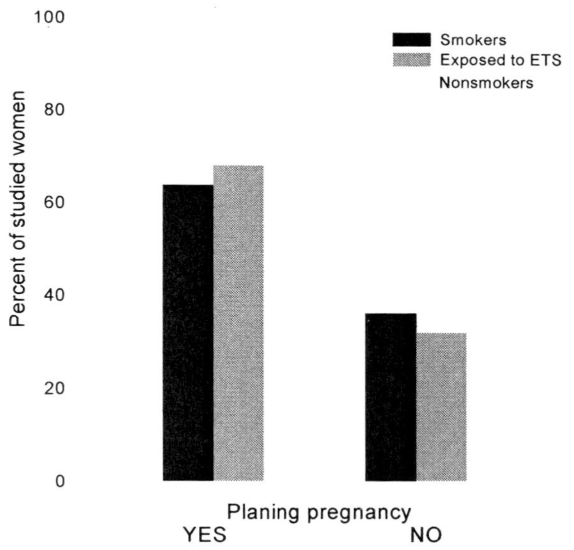

Figure 4. Percent of women planned their pregnancy in studied groups.

The mean duration of pregnancy of the women smoking tobacco was 37.40 weeks (table 2).

Table 2. The duration of pregnancy

Group	The duration of pregnancy [weeks]						
	Mean	Median	Minimum	Maximum	Lower quartile	Upper quartile	Standard deviation
Smokers (n=47)	37.40	38.00	28.00	42.00	37.00	39.00	2.96
Exposed to ETS (n=25)	37.76	38.00	34.00	41.00	36.00	40.00	2.20
Nonsmokers (n=43)	38.58	39.00	31.00	41.00	38.00	39.00	1.64

Within the group of mothers smoking tobacco during the pregnancy period, 76.60% of the newborns were born on time, whereas 23.40% of the newborns were born prematurely (table 3).

Table 3. Percent of women delivered on time and prematurely

Group	Prematurely (< 37 week)	On term (≥ 37 week)
Smokers (n=47)	n=11 23.40%	n=36 76.60%
Exposed to ETS (n=25)	n=7 28.00%	n=18 72.00%
Nonsmokers (n=43)	n=3 6.98%	n=40 93.02%

Within the group of passive smokers, the mean pregnancy period was 37.76 weeks (table 2). Among the newborns of mothers passively exposed to tobacco smoke, the babies born on time constituted 72.00%, and premature babies – 28.00% (table 3).

The mean duration of the pregnancy period in the case of mothers, who did not smoke was the longest and amounted to 38.58 weeks (table 2). The largest percentage of newborns born on time was represented by babies delivered by nonsmoking women – 93.02% and the smallest one concerned the babies born prematurely 6.98% (table 3).

Among the newborns of mothers smoking cigarettes, 53.19% were babies of the female sex, and 46.81% were babies of the male sex. Within the group of women passively inhaling tobacco smoke, the newborns of the female sex constituted 29.17%, and the babies of the male sex constituted 70.83%., Within the group of nonsmoking mothers, this percentage amounted to 44.19% and 53.81% respectively (figure 5).

The mean birth body weight of the newborns of the women smoking tobacco (AS-N) during the pregnancy period amounted to 2919.79±863.82 g (minimal body weight 1220.00 g, maximal body weight 4860.00 g). In the case of the newborns of the female sex it amounted to 2738.00±749.16 g, whereas among the newborns of the male sex, it amounted to 3126.36±953.42 g (table 4).

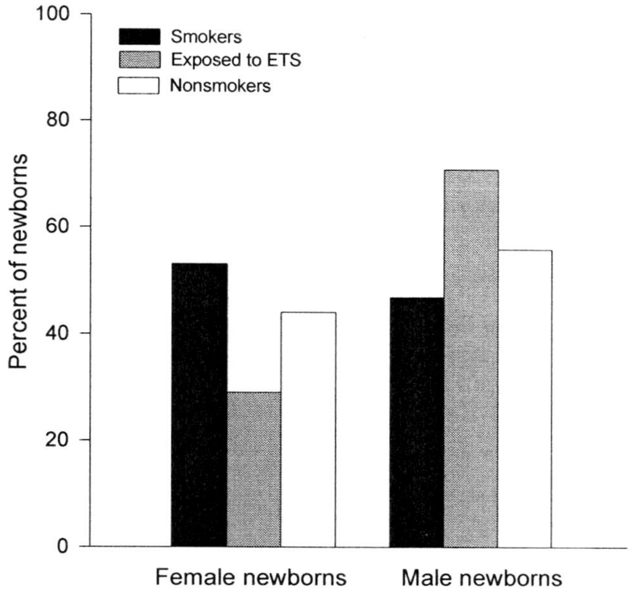

Figure 5. Percent of female and male newborns in studied groups.

Table 4. Mean birth body weight of the female and male newborns

Group	Sex	PARAMETERS						
		Mean	Median	Minimum	Maximum	Lower quartile	Upper quartile	SD
Smokers (n=47)	F	2783.00	2690.00	1220.00	4060.00	2110.00	3230.00	749.16
	M	3126.34	3425.00	1360.00	4860.00	2220.00	3620.00	953.42
		2919.79	2880.00	1220.00	4860.00	2200.00	3550.00	863.82
Exposed to ETS (n=25)	F	3160.00	2810.00	1170.00	5200.00	2290.00	4320.00	1360.34
	M	3279.41	3390.00	2250.00	4190.00	2900.00	3640.00	596.54
		3250.40	3390.00	1170.00	5200.00	2700.00	3700.00	838.85
Nonsmokers (n=43)	F	3328.42	3340.00	2330.00	4220.00	3060.00	3780.00	468.58
	M	3690.83	3655.00	2030.00	5140.00	3350.00	3955.00	700.21
		3530.70	3500.00	2030.00	5140.00	3160.00	3800.00	629.09

The mean birth body weight of the newborns with a body weight below 2500 g amounted to 1930.66±345.53 g (minimal body weight – 1220.00 g, maximal body weight 2460.00 g) (table 5).

Table 5. The mean birth body weight of the newborns with a body weight below 2500g

Group	PARAMETERS						
	Mean	Median	Minimum	Maximum	Lower quartile	Upper quartile	Standard deviation
AS-N (n=15) 31,92%	1930,66	1940,00	1220,00	2460,00	1790,00	2200,00	345,53
PS-N (n=4) 16,00%	2007,50	2270,00	1170,00	2320,00	1710,00	2305,00	559,07
NS-N (n=3) 6,98%	2280,00	2330,00	2030,00	2480,00	2030,00	2480,00	229,13

AS-N - Newborn of smoking mother
PS-N - Newborn of mother exposed to ETS
NS-N - Newborn of nonsmoking mother.

The group of newborns with low birth body weights (below 2500 g) amounted to 31.91%, consisting of 40.00% of those newborns that were born on time and 60.00% of those born prematurely (table 6).

Table 6. Percent of newborns with low birth body weight born in time and prematurely

Group	Week	≥ 2500 g		< 2500 g	
AS-N (n=47)	≥ 37	n=30	93.75%	n=6	40.00%
	< 37	n=2	6.25%	n=9	60.00%
PS-N (n=25)	≥ 37	n=18	85.71%	n=0	0.00%
	< 37	n=3	14.29%	n=4	100%
NS-N (n=43)	≥ 37	n=39	97.50%	n=2	33.33%
	< 37	n=1	2.50%	n=2	66.67%

AS-N - Newborn of smoking mother
PS-N - Newborn of mother exposed to ETS
NS-N - Newborn of nonsmoking mother.

The mean birth body weight of hypotrophic newborns amounted to 2244.16±418.79g (minimal body weight 1360.00 g, maximal body weight 2730.00 g) (table 7).

With the group of newborns of smoking mothers, the eutrophic newborns amounted to 59.58%, including 67.85% of those newborns that were born on time and 32.15% of those born prematurely. The group of hypotrophic newborns amounted to 25.53% of babies, consisting of 91.66% of newborns born prematurely and 8.34% of newborns whose delivery was timely (table 8 and 9).

Table 7. Mean birth body weight of hypotrophic, eutrophic and hypertrophic newborns

Group	Newborn	PARAMETERS						
		Mean	Median	Minimum	Maximum	Lower quartile	Upper quartile	Standard deviation
AS-N	hypotrophic	2244.16	2440.00	1360.00	2730.00	1890.00	2545.00	418.79
	eutrophic	2931.43	3215.00	1220.00	3820.00	2165.00	3215.00	751.88
	hypertrophic	4031.43	4060.00	2640.00	4860.00	3900.00	4580.00	707.07
AP-N	hypotrophic	1860.00	1860.00	1170.00	2550.00	1170.00	2550.00	975.81
	eutrophic	3160.53	3290.00	2250.00	4130.00	2700.00	3290.00	568.02
	hypertrophic	4372.50	4255.00	3780.00	5200.00	3985.00	4760.00	597.74
NS-N	hypotrophic	2660.00	2660.00	2480.00	2840.00	2480.00	2840.00	254.56
	eutrophic	3368.49	3420.00	2030.00	4000.00	3160.00	3420.00	434.59
	hypertrophic	4417.50	4350.00	3780.00	5140.00	3985.00	4875.00	512.33

AS-N - Newborn of smoking mother
PS-N - Newborn of mother exposed to ETS
NS-N Newborn of nonsmoking mot

Table 8. Percent of hypotrophic, eutrophic and hypertrophic newborns

Group	NEWBORNS					
	hypotrophic		eutrophic		hypertrophic	
AS-N (n=47)	n=12	25.53%	n=28	59.58%	n=7	14.89%
PS-N (n=25)	n=2	8.00%	n=19	76.00%	n=4	16.00%
NS-N (n=43)	n=2	4.65%	n=33	76.74%	n=8	18.61%

AS-N - Newborn of smoking mother
PS-N - Newborn of mother exposed to ETS
NS-N - Newborn of nonsmoking mother.

Table 9. Percent of hypotrophic, eutrophic and hypertrophic newborns born in time and prematurely

Group	Week	NEWBORN					
		hypotrophic		eutrophic		hypertrophic	
AS-N (n=47)	≥ 37	n=11	91.66%	n=19	67.95%	n=6	85.71%
	< 37	n=1	8.34%	n=9	32.15%	n=1	14.29%
PS-N (n=25)	≥ 37	n=1	50.00%	n=13	68.42%	n=4	100%
	< 37	n=1	50.00%	n=6	31.58%	n=0	0%
NS-N (n=43)	≥ 37	n=2	100%	n=30	90.90%	n=0	100%
	< 37	n=0	0%	n=3	9.10%	n=0	0%

AS-N - Newborn of smoking mother
PS-N - Newborn of mother exposed to ETS
NS-N - Newborn of nonsmoking mother.

The mean birth body weight of the newborns of women passively exposed to tobacco smoke during the pregnancy period was 3250.40±838.85 g (minimal body weight 1170 g, maximal body weight 5200 g) (table 4). For the female sex it amounted to 3160.0±1360.34 g, whereas for the male sex it amounted to 3279.41±596.54 g (table 4).

The mean birth body weight of the newborns with a body weight below 2500 g was 2007.50±559.07 g (minimal body weight 1170.00 g, maximal body weight 2320.00 g) (table 5). The group of newborns with a birth body weight below 2500 g accounted for 16%, of which all the children were born before the 37th week of pregnancy (table 6).

The mean birth body weight of the hypotrophic newborns was 1860.00g±975.81 g (minimal body weight 1170.00 g, maximal body weight 2550.00) (table 7). The group of hypotrophic newborns amounted to 8% of the babies, including 50.00% of those represented by the newborns who were born prematurely, and 50.00% of those born on time (table 8 and 9). Within the group of newborns of the mothers who were passively exposed to tobacco smoke, 76% were eutrophic newborns, consisting of 68.42% of those born on time and 31.58% of those born before and during the 37th week of pregnancy (table 8 and 9).

Among the nonsmoking women and ones not exposed to tobacco smoke during the pregnancy period, the mean birth body weight of newborns amounted to 35307.0±629.09 g (minimal body weight amounted to 2030.00 g, whereas the maximal one was 5140.00 g) (table 4). The birth body weight of the female newborns amounted to 3328.42±468.58 g, whereas in case of the male newborns, it amounted to 3690.83±700.21 g (table 4). The mean birth body weight of newborns with a body weight below 2500 g was 2280.00±229.13 g (minimal body weight 2030.00 g, maximal body weight 2480.00 g) (table 5). The group of newborns with a body weight below 2500g amounted to 6.98%, consisting of 33.33% of babies born on time and 66.67% of newborns delivered before the 37th week (table 6).

The mean birth body weight of the hypotrophic newborns was 2660.00±254.56 g (minimal body weight 2480.00 g, maximal body weight 2840.00 g) (table 7). The group of hypotrophic newborns amounted to 4.65%, including all whose delivery was timely (table 8 and 9). Within the group of nonsmoking mothers, 76.74% of newborns were hypotrophic, including 90.90% of those whose delivery was timely and 9.10% of those who were born prematurely.

The mean body length of the newborns delivered by tobacco smoking mothers was 50.96±5.31 cm (minimal body length 36.00 cm, maximal body length 59.00 cm).

Among the newborns of the mothers passively exposed to tobacco smoke, the mean body length of the baby was 52.68±4.39 cm (minimal body length 39.00 cm, maximal body length 60.00 cm).

Within the NS-N group – newborns of nonsmoking and ETS non-exposed mothers, the mean body length of the babies was 55,02±3,54 cm (minimal body length 48.00 cm, maximal body length 63.00 cm) (table 10).

Table 10. Newborn body length

Group	Newborn body length [cm]						
	Mean	Median	Minimum	Maximum	Lower quartile	Upper quartile	Standard deviation
AS-N (n=47)	50.96	52.00	36.00	59.00	48.00	55.00	5.31
PS-N (n=25)	52.68	53.00	39.00	60.00	50.00	55.00	4.39
NS-N (n=43)	55.02	55.00	48.00	63.00	53.00	57.00	3.54

AS-N - Newborn of smoking mother
PS-N - Newborn of mother exposed to ETS
NS-N - Newborn of nonsmoking mother.

Cotinine in the Mother's Urine, Placenta and the First Urine of a Newborn

The concentration of cotinine was observed in the urine of the mother, placenta and the first urine of a newborn.

Within the group of tobacco smoking women, in 9 out of 10 cases, the cotinine level in the urine was equal to zero. In the cases of 38 mothers, the mean concentration of this biomarker was 898.53±1254.54 ng/mg of creatinine (figure 6).

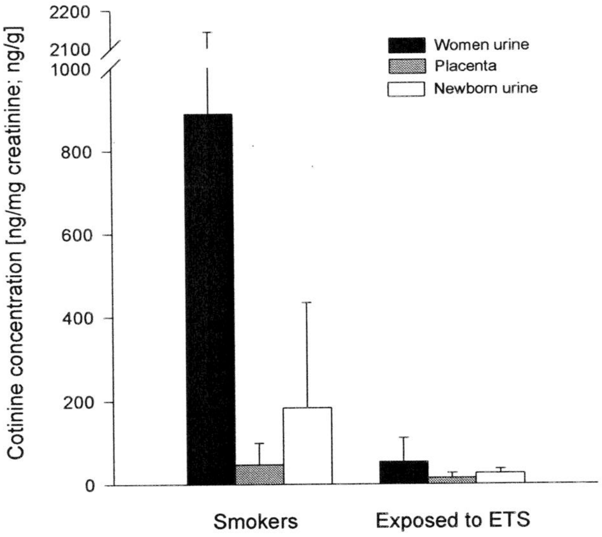

Figure 6. Concentration of cotinine in the urine of mothers their newborns and placenta.

In the placenta of the smoking patients, in 26 samples, the concentration of cotinine amounted to 0, in the remaining 21 placentas a concentration of the value of 46.97±52.59 ng/g of the placenta was noted (figure 7). The presence of cotinine in the first urine of the newborns of smoking mothers was marked in the cases of 25 babies. The mean concentration of the nicotine metabolite was 183.56±251.11 ng/mg of creatinine (figure 6).

In the urine of the women passively inhaling tobacco smoke, the concentration of cotinine in two cases was equal to zero, in the remaining 23 samples, the mean concentration was 53.20±58.02 ng/mg of creatinine was noted (figure 6). In the placenta of women exposed to ETS, in two samples the concentration of cotinine assumed a value above zero and mean amounted to 19.45±12.09 ng/g of placenta (figure 6). The metabolite of nicotine determined in the first urine of the newborns of the passively smoking mothers occurred at the level of 26.03±10.69 ng/mg of creatinine (figure 6).

Within the group of women who did not smoke and who were not exposed to smoke, the presence of cotinine in the urine and placenta of the mother as well as in the first urine of the newborn was not observed. In one case, in the urine of a woman, the concentration of cotinine 3.5 ng/mg creatinine was determined.

On the basis of the research which was carried out, the evaluation of a relation between the concentration of cotinine in the placenta as well as the first urine of a newborn and the metabolite level in the urine of smoking mothers was made.

Figure 7 presents the relation between the concentration of cotinine in the placenta and the level of nicotine metabolite in the urine of smoking mothers. A correlation was shown between the tested parameters, and the correlation coefficient was 0,3300.

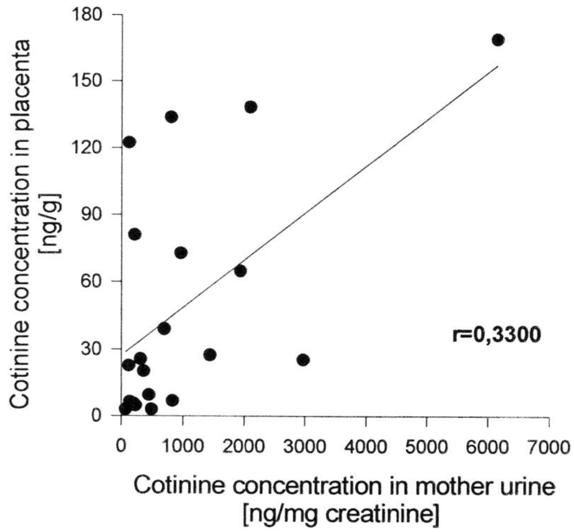

Figure 7. Relationship between concentration of cotinine in urine of smoking women and placenta.

In the research, which was carried out, a correlation between the concentration of cotinine in the first urine of newborns and the level of nicotine metabolite in the urine of the smoking mothers was observed (figure 8).

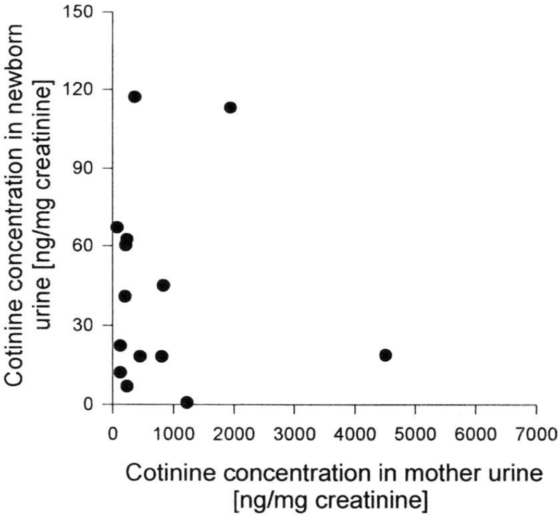

Figure 8. Relationship between concentration of cotinine in the first urine of newborn and urine of their smoking mother.

No correlation was shown between the correlation of cotinine in the placenta and in the first urine of a newborn, and its level in the urine of the mothers passively inhaling the tobacco smoke.

Discussion

Epidemiological research has proved that tobacco smoking is a common phenomenon in the world. It is estimated that every third person who is older than 15, smokes tobacco [99, 171]. Among women, there are 200 million persons who smoke every day.

Tobacco smoking by women, especially of child-bearing age, and in the period of pregnancy, has a negative impact on fertility, procreative ability and progeny. This is achieved, among other ways, by the lowering of the birth body weight and an increase in the risk of the sudden death of a newborn [37, 38, 47, 150, 151, 164]. The exposure of a fetus, newborn to ETS may lead to neuropsychological disorders as well as disorders in the physical development [102, 125, 165, 166, 167]. Tobacco smoking during the pregnancy increases the risk of occurrence of inborn defects among children by 150 per cent [131, 135, 180]. The progeny of smoking mothers falls ill more frequently with the diseases related to the respiratory system [24].

In spite of the fact that the health consequences of active and passive smoking have been well known for a long time, still the behaviour of many women poses a threat to the correct development of a fetus, newborn and even of a baby.

115 pregnant women, who had been divided into three groups, took part in the research. The group of women, who smoked during pregnancy, was represented by 47 mothers. Almost half of them (46.05%) smoked 1-5 cigarettes a day, whereas the percentage of women smoking 6-10 and 11-15 cigarettes was less, that is, 27.03% and 21.62% respectively (figure 2). Women smoking the greatest number of cigarettes, that is, more than 15 per day, constituted the smallest percentage – 5.41% (figure 2). The results of our own research coincide with results obtained by other authors.

In the research carried out by Florek et al. among the patients of the Gynecological-Obstetrics Hospital of the University of Medical Sciences in Warsaw, the greatest number of female smokers smoked from 1 to 5 cigarettes a day (about 40%) [47]. Within a population of 1328 pregnant women living in the Wielkopolska province, Adamek et al. demonstrated that among the female smokers, more than a half (51.1%) were respondents who smoked 1-5 cigarettes/day [2]. Also in other research, about 60% of smoking pregnant women constituted patients smoking occasionally or less than 5 cigarettes a day [49]. In the research of Counsilman et al. it was demonstrated that pregnant women smoking up to 5 cigarettes a day, smoked only for the purpose of socializing [30]. Such a high percentage of women smoking up to 5 cigarettes a day may be a result of the fact that the number of cigarettes smoked by the respondents, who did not quit smoking during pregnancy, went down. Such observations have been noted in research done by many authors [3, 39, 47]. Confirmation that the smallest percentage (5.41%) was represented by pregnant patients, smoking more than 15 cigarettes a day, is the research of Adamek, Adamek et al. and Florek et al. [3, 39,47]. The number of smoked cigarettes has an impact on the course of a pregnancy and perinatal complications. It has been observed that in the case of 1 to 5 cigarettes a day, the risk of extra-uterine pregnancy is 1.6, and in the case of women smoking over 20 cigarettes a day, it increases to 3.5 [128]. The Swedish prospective research of Ahlborg and Bodin carried out among 4701 patients, indicated an increase in the risk of premature delivery OR=2,18 and lower birth weights in the newborns OR=2.38 in the case of women smoking 10-19 cigarettes a day, and a growth to OR=2.30 and OR=2.71 respectively in the case of women smoking >20 cigarettes a day [5]. The smoking of tobacco by a mother is one of the factors contributing to the occurrence of sudden death syndrome in a newborn. The risk of the occurrence of this syndrome was 1.84, when the mother smoked 1-9 cigarettes a day, 2.64 in the case of 10-19 cigarettes a day and as much as 5.06 among the newborns of mothers smoking >20 cigarettes a day [105].

In the present research, the women smoking tobacco during pregnancy represented an approximate percentage in the following age groups: below 25 and within the ages of 25 – 29 and 30 – 35 years, 27.66%, 31.91% and 27.66% respectively. The observations approximate the results of Szamotulska et al. [142]. A higher percentage of smoking pregnant women was noted down by Florek et al. in the age of 30 – 35 years – 42.3% [39]. In research carried out by other authors, the highest percentage of women smoking during pregnancy consisted of, more often than not, young persons aged up to 25. In the research conducted by Adamek et. al. this group was represented by 47.4% of respondents [3].

The group of female smokers was most frequently represented by respondents with the secondary education – 46.81%. More than a half of them – 53.19%, carried out a white collar work. Three quarters of the tested women (74.47%) were inhabitants of Warsaw. The highest percentage, that is, 65.96% encompassed married women. An mean gross income for one member of the family, that is, over PLN 1000 was found in the case of 40.43% of smoking respondents (table 1).

A statistically essential relation has been observed between smoking and the educational level, marital status and an mean gross income assigned to one family member (table 1).

The education of women, who smoked was basic more often than not. Within the group of patients with only a basic education, 12.77% constituted women who smoked during their pregnancy in relation to 4.65% of women who did not smoke and were not exposed to tobacco smoke. The percentage within the groups with vocational and secondary education was 21.28% to 0% and 46.81% to 30.23% respectively. It was observed that among the patients with higher educations, 19.15% smoked in relation to 65.12% of nonsmokers and 64% of persons inhaling smoke passively.

It has been observed that the results of our own research coincide with those of other authors. In the All-Polish research at the beginning of the 90's, carried out by the Institute of Mother and Child in Warsaw, it was proved that about 40% of women with only a basic education smoked tobacco compare to 21% with a higher education [141]. The research carried out by Jaakkola et al. in the 80's and 90's confirmed that pregnant women with only a basic education smoked tobacco more frequently [67]. The research of carried out in Poznan proved that women who smoked more frequently during pregnancy had a vocational education (40.1%), performed physical work (69.8%), were married (78.5%), and the mean gross income per one family member was up to PLN 500 (50.2%) [3].

In our own research, the women smoking tobacco represented different marital statuses – 65.96% of them were married, whereas the unmarried patients constituted 25.53%. The percentage within the group of passively exposed women was 88.00% and 12.00%, respectively, whereas among the nonsmoking women, it was – 88.37% and 9.30% respectively.

A statistically essential dependence concerned also the smoking by women during pregnancy and the mean gross income for one family member. The mean gross income in the case of 23.40% of tested smokers and 4.00% of respondents passively exposed to tobacco as well as 2.33% of non-smokers was below PLN 500. An mean income on the level of over PLN 1000 was declared most frequently by the women who did not smoke and the ones who were passively exposed to tobacco smoke, that is – 69.77% and 68.00% respectively, whereas there were 40,43% of those women, who smoked tobacco with such an income.

In our own research among the women who passively inhaled tobacco smoke (PS group) about 64% encompassed patients who were less than 25 years old (24%) and within the age group of 25 to 29 years old (40%). Patients with a higher education were prevalent among these – 64% and most of them carried out white-collar work (72%). Half of the tested women lived in Warsaw. Married women constituted 88% of them. The highest percentage – 68% had a mean gross income for one family member, that is PLN 1000.

In research concerning the inhabitants of the Wielkopolska province, the percentage of younger women passively smoking tobacco (below the age of 25 and between the ages of 25-29) was slightly higher and amounted to about 80% [1]. A similar percentage (about 75%) to the presented research was noted down by Hanke et al. among the patients of the Lodz region [58]. These women (51.9%) had a basic or vocational education and were not married for the most part. Similar observations were presented by Windham et al. [167]. In Canada and the United States - about a half of pregnant women (49% and 44%) declared a passive inhalation of tobacco smoke. A higher percentage of passively smoking future mothers lives in Sweden (74%) and Japan (81.2%) [58]. Many authors confirm the fact that there is a relation between passive smoking and social-economic status [31, 123, 125]. In Finland, women, who are passively exposed to tobacco smoke, were characterised by a younger age and worse education. They were also unmarried and did not work professionally and, had lower incomes [7].

The presented research demonstrated a statistically important relationship between tobacco smoking by women or passive inhalation of smoke and pregnancy planning. Among the mothers who smoked or were exposed to ETS, the percentage of those who planned their pregnancy was 63.83% and 68%, whereas within the group of non-smokers, there were 88% of the women planned their pregnancy. These results are different from the ones obtained by Adamek et al., where only 15% of the smoking respondents and about 30% of women passively exposed to tobacco smoke planned their pregnancy [3].

In epidemiological research, the evaluation of active or passive exposure is carried out on the basis of surveys conducted within a specified group of respondents. In this type of works, there may be certain irregularities resulting from the fact, for instance, that the tested person evaluates herself, questions are asked incorrectly, the number of questions is limited or the evaluation of tobacco consumption is incorrect, or the answers are incredible. The surveys are very rarely completed with biochemical tests. In the case of evaluation of exposure to tobacco smoke, there are a number of biomarkers of different specificity [9-11, 116]. In the presented research, the division of women into three groups: smokers, passively exposed and nonsmokers was assumed on the basis of the following criteria: the declaration of the patient and the cotinine level – the main nicotine metabolite in the urine, as a verification of the answers of women to the questions concerning smoking (active or passive).

Within the group of smoking women (47 persons), tobacco smoking was declared by 37 patients (78.72%). In the case of 10 "nonsmoking women", the concentration of cotinine in the urine exceeded the value of 200 ng/mg of creatinine, which indicated active tobacco smoking before the delivery. Within the groups of women exposed to ETS and the ones who did not smoke, the compliance with the declarations with the actual exposure was 100%. The obtained results confirmed the results of research carried out by other authors, which indicates the necessity of using biomarkers for the purpose of verification of answers given concerning tobacco smoking or passive exposure to tobacco smoke [32, 53, 113]. The research of Florek et al. carried out among the women delivering at the Gynecological-Obstetrics Clinic of the University of Medical Sciences in Poznan demonstrated that a high level of cotinine in the urine was found in the cases of 15.5% of patients [45]. A lot of research has proved that pregnant women, constituting an enhanced risk group, smoke more frequently than is indicated in the results of a survey, and the discrepancies can markedly affect the results in a misleading way. However, Benowitz et al. pay attention to the fact, that when applying cotinine for the purpose of the validation of results of questionnaire-based research, it is necessary to take into account the differences in the pharmaco-kinetics of nicotine [12].

Within the group of women who confirmed tobacco smoking and the ones who denied it ("non-smokers"), the mean value of cotinine concentration in the urine was 898.53±1254.54 ng/mg of creatinine. In the case of one patient, a very high concentration of cotinine, which amounted to 6153.60 ng/mg of creatinine, was observed. Among the women who declared their smoking habits, there was also a group of tested patients in whom, the cotinine level in the urine suggested nonsmoking or passive inhalation of tobacco smoke. This fact may be explained by a small number of smoked cigarettes or a longer period of time, which expired from the time when the last cigarette was smoked to the time when the urine was sampled for the purpose of carrying out the tests. The observed concentrations of the main metabolite of nicotine in the urine were higher than the ones provided by authors of other research. Among the women delivering at the Gynecological-Obstetric Clinic of the University of Medical Sciences in Poznan, the values of cotinine amounted to 471.7±820.5 ng/mg of creatinine [45].

Among the patients who smoked tobacco, the largest group – 70.27% consisted of women who smoked throughout the whole pregnancy, and only one third of the patients gave up their smoking habit in the consecutive months of pregnancy. The alarming fact is that, although pregnancy and waiting for the delivery of a baby is an ideal moment in a woman's life to quit smoking, it was not taken advantage of by the tested women. It follows from the research of other authors, that a decision regarding the limitation of the number of smoked cigarettes or the quitting of smoking is often made during this period [168, 176]. Therefore, educational actions directed at women in the procreative age should be intensified, particularly in regard to the first weeks of pregnancy.

25 patients were exposed to passive inhalation of smoke, however only 56% of the women in labor declared exposure to environmental tobacco smoke (home and work). The mean concentration of cotinine in the urine of the tested women was 53.20±58.03 ng/mg of creatinine. The percentage of smoking partners was 28% and the largest group of them (42,86%) consisted of men smoking 6 to 10 cigarettes a day.

The period of pregnancy is often a time during which, a woman decides to change her lifestyle. The health-conscious behaviors of pregnant women contribute to the limitation or quitting of smoking, which is connected with the awareness of the negative impact of smoking on pregnancy, development of the fetus and the health of the baby. Among the tested women, the awareness of the health consequences of tobacco smoking as well as passive exposure to tobacco smoke was almost one hundred percent (93.6%). The results of the presented research differ a bit from the results obtained by other authors. The research of Price et al. carried out among American women in the procreative age put the awareness of health consequences at a level of 68-85% [120]. Adamek et al in their research proved that almost 90% of women declared an awareness of health consequences related to tobacco smoke exposure [3]. In the research of Florek et al. carried out among the women in labor, living in a smaller town, Srem, a high percentage of women declaring awareness – 85.2% - was observed [50]. Most frequently these were women aged 25-29, with a higher education and incomes greater than PLN 500 for one family member.

However, the alarming fact is that only 41.74% of women obtained information from a physician regarding the detrimental effects of tobacco smoking to health. In the research carried out among women in the Wielkopolska province, more than a half of them (61%) obtained information from a physician regarding the detrimental effects of smoking and the impact of tobacco smoke on the development of a fetus [3]. Similar results were noted down by Florek et al., where 63.2% of patients were informed by a physician [50].

Many factors such as socio-demographic ones, lifestyle and natural environment as well as harmful factors at the workplace have an impact on the fundamental indices of the health of the children. The babies of women smokers are additionally exposed to toxic and carcinogenic tobacco smoke components. By means of the passive diffusion, these substances go through the placenta. The placental barrier, which separates the blood circulation of a mother and a fetus limits access to the fetus only to a limited extent. The transported amounts depend on the surface of the placenta, blood supply, and speed of blood flow. The components of tobacco smoke of a molecular weight below 600, e.g. nicotine, easily penetrate the placenta [117]. Due to smoking, it is observed that the body weight of 32000-61000 delivered babies is below 2500 g and there are 14000-26000 deliveries of newborns that require treatment at the Intensive Newborn Care Department [54]. The duration of the pregnancy is correlated with the birth body weight. According to the World Health Organization, premature births are defined as births before the 37th week of the fetal life or before the 259th day, starting from the first day of the last menstruation. Timely births are defined as a delivery between the completed 37th, and 42nd, week of pregnancy or between the 259th and 293rd day of pregnancy. The births after that time are considered late after the 42nd week of pregnancy [18]. The complications of pregnancy regarding the placenta praevia, separation of the placenta and premature crushing of the fetal membrane may lead to a premature delivery (< 37 week of pregnancy).

Many authors pay attention to a relation between smoking and the duration of pregnancy [147, 148]. The first report regarding the harmfulness of tobacco smoking during pregnancy presented the results of research carried out by Simpson in 1957. The tested population counted 7499 women, among whom, the percentage of premature deliveries was two times higher in the case of smoking mothers, and was correlated with the number of cigarettes smoked per day [138].

In our own research, a larger percentage of deliveries on time – 93.02% was observed in the group of women, who did not smoke, whereas the premature deliveries constituted 6.98%. Among the mothers, who passively inhaled tobacco smoke, and the ones who smoked during pregnancy, a percentage of deliveries on time were more or less similar and constituted 72% and 76.6% respectively. The premature deliveries constituted 28% and 23.4%. An essential influence of active and passive exposure to tobacco smoke during pregnancy on the occurrence of premature deliveries was proved as one of the factors. The results of our own research confirm the observations of other authors. Similar observations were made by Jozwik and Laudanski [75]. The influence of smoking on the frequency of the occurrence of premature births was proved by Gajewska et al. within the group of smoking women, the percentage of deliveries before the completion of the 37th week of pregnancy was 10%, whereas among the nonsmoking women, it was only 5.93% [55]. It was also demonstrated that the risk of a premature delivery increases together with an increased number of cigarettes smoked daily. Among the factors determining the health of a newborn, it is possible to distinguish the socio-demographic factors, that is, the age of a mother below 18 and above 30, worse education, marital status – unmarried, inappropriate diet, bad housing and economic conditions [85]. Wen et al. proved that the influence of tobacco smoking on the number of premature deliveries of newborns with low birth body weight grows with the age of delivering women [162]. In the research carried out by Karwan-Plonska, most of the premature deliveries occurred among women between ages of 25-35. A six-fold increase in the risk of a premature delivery was observed among women who delivered when they were older than 35 [79]. According to the research of other authors, premature deliveries are more frequent in the case of women smoking during pregnancy (OR=1.7), of an age of more than 30 (OR=2.23), of marital status – unmarried (OR=2.87), or coming from the lower social classes, having lower education and lower incomes [14, 59, 112, 137]. According to the research carried out by the Center for Disease Control and Prevention, tobacco smoking determined premature delivery at 6% [14]. The factor that predisposed to premature delivery was passive smoking, which was demonstrated by Jaakkola et al. in the case of 9.6% of tested women [67]. The statistical growth of risk was also confirmed by Ahluwalia et al. and Windham et al. [6, 165]

In our own research it was demonstrated that, among the women who smoked, 53.19% of children of the female sex and 46.81% of children of the male sex were born. Within the group of women passively exposed to tobacco smoke, the female newborns constituted 29.17%, and the babies of a male sex 70.83%. The nonsmoking women gave birth to boys more frequently – 55.81% than girls – 44.19%. Because the number of groups is too small, it is not possible to analyze the dependence between tobacco smoking by pregnant women and the sex of a baby.

Tobacco smoking and passive exposure to smoke are the causative factors of pregnancy disorders and influence on the progeny. Still, it has not been fully clarified which of the components of smoke plays an essential role in lowering the birth body weight of newborns. A hypothesis presented by Longo concerns, above all, two components: nicotine and carbon monoxide, which are responsible for oxygen deficiency in tissues [94]. The oxygen deficiency in tissues caused by the nicotine appears immediately after a cigarette is smoked, whereas the one caused by carbon monoxide develops more slowly, and when the mother continues to smoke, it may last for a long period. The level of carboxyhemoglobin in the blood of a smoking pregnant woman ranges from 6% to 8% and returns to its initial level only after 12 hours from the moment of quitting smoking.

The growth of a fetus, the birth body weight and the pregnancy age may be disturbed both by the active and passive exposure of women to tobacco smoke [13, 22, 38, 91, 156].

According to different authors, the newborns of mothers who smoke, during pregnancy are lighter by 150 - 300 g than the babies of nonsmoking mothers [35, 38, 44, 47, 49, 92, 121, 172]. The newborns of smoking mothers appear twice as often in the babies with low body birth weight when compared to with the progeny of nonsmoking women, with reference to a delivery which occurs on time. In the cases of premature deliveries (before the 37th, week of pregnancy), the risk of a lowered birth body weight in newborns in relation to the age of pregnancy increases three times among the smoking women [114]. If, however, the mother stops smoking in the first half of the pregnancy period, the birth body weight of a newborn will be comparable to the body weight of babies of nonsmoking women [134].

In our own research, the women smoking tobacco during pregnancy gave birth to babies who were statistically lighter by 610.91 g in comparison with the newborns of mothers, who did not smoke and were not exposed to the passive inhalation of smoke. These babies were also lighter by 330.6 g in relation to the babies of passively smoking women. Within the group of women passively exposed to smoke, the birth body weight of newborns was lower by 280.31 g in comparison with the babies of nonsmoking mothers.

The newborns with a birth body weight below 2500 g are defined as the ones with a low birth body weight, of which 95% are born before the completion of the 37th week of pregnancy. Within this group, it is possible to distinguish newborns of a low birth body weight – below 2500 g, newborns of a very low birth body weight – below 1500 g, newborns of a very, very low birth body weight – below 1000 g and those with extremely low birth body weight – below 500 g [18]. In the evaluation of the health of a newborn in the first hours of life, a 26-parameter scale is applied (SNAP - Score for Neonatal Acute Physiology) [82]. The biochemical parameters connected with oxygen deficiency in the fetus affect significantly the amount of points in the SNAP scale. Analyzing the percentage distribution of newborns with a low birth body weight (< 2500 g) the highest percentage concerned the babies of smoking mothers – 31.92%; among the mothers passively inhaling smoke – 16% and only 6.98% of the newborns of nonsmoking women. Their mean body weight was 1930.66 g, 2007.50 g and 2280.00 g respectively, of whom 60.00%, 100.00% and 66.67% encompassed the newborns delivered prematurely.

At this point in time, standards based on the body weight and the gestational age, expressed in percentile divisions, are introduced. The newborns, whose body weight is between the tenth and ninetieth percentile, are defined as eutrophic newborns. The newborns with a body weight and gestational age above the ninetieth percentile are defined as hypertrophic newborns, and the ones below the tenth percentile are named hypotrophic newborns, and they are the newborns with intrauterine growth retardation [18].

Within the group of smoking mothers, the hypotrophic newborns constituted 25.53%, among the women who passively inhaled the tobacco smoke, they constituted 8.0%, and there were only 4.65% of hypotrophic newborns within the group of nonsmoking mothers. The body weight amounted to 2244.16 g, 1860.00 g and 2660.0 g respectively. The results of our own research coincide with the results of other authors [25, 100, 146,].

The research demonstrating that the newborns of fathers who smoked were lighter by 3 g to 42 g when compared with the ones of nonsmoking parents was confirmation of the influence of passive smoking on birth body weight [25, 146, 175]. The decrease in the birth body weight in the newborns of nonsmoking mothers and their smoking partners in the presence of pregnant women was confirmed by the reports of many authors [15, 97, 125, 126]. The research conducted by Borlea showed that the birth body weight of the newborns of nonsmoking mothers, whose fathers smoked tobacco, was lower by 228 g in comparison with the newborns of nonsmoking parents [15]. However, the results of this research were criticized in view of the fact that there were cases of inborn defects, which also had an influence on the birth body weight [93, 127, 173, 174]

Rubin and co-authors proved that the smoking of 20 cigarettes a day by a father, in the presence of a pregnant woman caused a lowering in the birth body weight of their babies by 120 g [125]. The results of the research indicate that there is dependence - dose-response, with reference to the passive exposure of pregnant women to tobacco smoke.

The reduction in the birth body weight of the newborns of mothers exposed to ETS was from 1 g [60] to 253 g [95]. The research of Saito confirms that the body weight of newborns of tobacco smoking fathers is lower by 33 g, whereas in the case when both parents smoke, it is lower by as much as 100 g [126]. Other scientists point to a drop in the birth body weight of 14 to 100 g, caused by the passive exposure of pregnant women to smoke [21, 58, 97, 111]. In the research carried out by Misra and Ngupyen, the exposure of mothers to ETS caused 1.5 - 4 times as many occurrences of lowered body weight in newborns (by 25-90 g) in comparison with the babies of mothers, who were not exposed to tobacco smoke in the environment [104]. According to Peacock et al. and Eskenazi, mothers exposed to ETS gave birth to babies who were lighter by 31 g and 45 g in comparison with the babies of mothers, who were not exposed to ETS [34, 112].

In the presented research, it is significant that the decrease in the birth body weight of newborns was more frequently observed in the case of women who smoked. The results of our research coincide with the results of many authors. Hjalmarson et al. proved that the body weight of the newborns of mothers smoking during pregnancy was lowered by 328 g in comparison with the ones of the babies of nonsmoking women [61]. In other research, it was observed that the weekly growth of the birth body weight of babies of the smoking mothers was 2.6 g lower in relation to the newborns of nonsmoking women [13]. The results of the next two researches confirm the decrease in the birth body weight in the newborns of smoking mothers [7, 78]. The metaanalysis of Lassen and Oei unambiguously demonstrated the proportional dependence between the number of cigarettes smoked by women during pregnancy and the birth body weight and the length of a newborn's body [91]. According to Schellscheidt et al, there is a dependence between the low birth body weight of the newborns (< 2500 g) and tobacco smoking during pregnancy (>10 cigarettes/day) [132]. On the basis of the research carried out in Westphalia among 227 791 newborns of smoking mothers, the decrease in the body weight by 239 g on in relation to the babies of nonsmoking women was observed. Among the Afro-American women, the risk of occurrence of a low birth body weight in newborns of mothers smoking up to 10 cigarettes/day in relation to the nonsmoking mothers was 1.89 (1.15-3.13) [107]. The increase in the risk up to 3.03 (1.90-4.86) occurred in the case of women smoking more than 10 cigarettes per day.

One of the proofs of an impact of nicotine on the body weight is a decrease in the birth body weight of newborns delivered mothers chewing tobacco [84]. In India, where tobacco chewing is popular among women, research aimed at discovering the effects of the removal of nicotine from the leaves was carried out. The second factor, that is, carbon monoxide, which is responsible for an oxygen deficiency in the tissues of a fetus was excluded [84]. Within the tested population of 1388 women, 15.8% chewed tobacco. A significant increase in spontaneous abortions and a decrease in the birth body weight were observed among the women who chewed tobacco. The index of abortions within the group of mothers chewing tobacco amounted to 50 cases in 1000. The same index within the group of women, who did not take any tobacco, amounted to 17.1 from 1000 deliveries. The lowering of the birth body weight in the newborns of mothers chewing tobacco ranged from 100 g to 200 g when compared to the women who did not chew the tobacco leaves. Excluding all the components of tobacco smoke that are responsible for the increase in the risk of lowering the birth body weight of newborns, with the exception of nicotine, Krishna proved the influence of this alkaloid on the newborn body weight [84].

The lowering of the degree of maturity and intrauterinal development of a fetus, caused by the fact that mothers smoke during pregnancy or are passively exposed to tobacco smoke, has been defined by scientists (since 1985) as Fetal Tobacco Syndrome) [87]. The factors detrimental to health (such as e.g. tobacco smoke) may lead to intrauterinal hypotrophy which has a symmetrical character (proportional decrease in all dimensions of a body and organs of a fetus/newborn) or an asymmetrical one (low birth body weight, correct circumference of the head and length of the body) [18].

The measurement of the birth body weight, as well as biometrical parameters allows us to evaluate the relative risk (expressed by the odds ratio – OR) of harmful effects of tobacco on the fetus and the newborn.

Many authors proved that the active and passive exposure of pregnant women to tobacco smoke has an impact on the decrease in the birth body weight, and body length of a newborn and also a decrease in the head circumference [23, 26, 28, 72, 83, 98, 101, 108, 139].

In our own research, the babies of smoking mothers were born 4.06 cm shorter in comparison to the babies of mothers, who did not smoke and were not exposed to tobacco smoke, and 1.72 cm smaller than the babies of mothers passively exposed to smoke during the pregnancy. These differences were statistically significant. Similar research by other authors demonstrated a significant decrease in the newborn's body length [72, 132]. The research of Fried and O'Connell as well as Wang et al. proved that the newborns of smoking mothers were 1.2 cm smaller than the babies of nonsmoking mothers [52, 159]. According to the authors, smoking in the third trimester of pregnancy had the greatest influence on the inhibition of intrauterinal growth, whereas smoking in the first trimester of pregnancy had the smallest influence. In the tests of 227 791 newborns carried out in Westphalia, the decrease in the body length of babies of smoking mothers in relation to the ones of the nonsmoking mothers was 1.41 cm [159]. According to Wojculewicz et al. the mean body length of the newborns delivered by smoking mothers was shorter by 0.9 cm than the body length of the babies of nonsmoking mothers [170]. The research of Lach et al. carried out in the year's 1995 and 1996 indicated a relationship between the period of smoking during pregnancy and the birth parameters of newborns. The body lengths of the newborns of the nonsmoking women during pregnancy (56.84 cm) or the women smoking tobacco during only the first trimester of pregnancy (57.19 cm) was greater than that within the group of babies of smoking women. The newborns of mothers smoking in the I and II trimester were shorter by 1.03 cm, and the babies of mothers smoking throughout the whole pregnancy period were shorter by 1.62 cm [87]. The research of Kukla et al. proved that the body lengths of the newborns of the mothers smoking more than 10 cigarettes per day were shorter by 1.22 cm [86]. The results of the consecutive research, apart from the fact that the birth body weights of the newborns of smoking mothers was lower, confirmed that the body lengths of the newborns were shorter by 1 cm in relation to the babies of nonsmoking mothers. The difference in the body lengths of the newborns of mothers smoking less than 10 cigarettes per day amounted to 0.6 cm, whereas to the nonsmoking women – 0.9 cm [91].

Tobacco smoking and exposure to tobacco smoke affects the level of the main alkaloid of tobacco leaves, that is, nicotine and its metabolite – cotinine - in the biological liquids (e.g. in blood, saliva, urine) and tissues. Many authors use cotinine for the purpose of evaluating the active tobacco smoking or exposure to tobacco smoke [3, 32, 38, 39, 44, 48, 70, 71, 74, 116, 143].

According to Guerin et al., in the case of nonsmokers and persons who are not exposed to smoke, the level of cotinine in serum or saliva may be 15 ng/ml, and in the case of urine its concentration may even amount to 50 ng/ml [56]. In the research of other authors, the concentration of cotinine in the urine of nonsmokers amounted to 8.84 ng/ml (within the scope of 0-85 ng/ml). Coultas et al. carried out some population research among non-smokers in New Mexico, in the case of whom, the concentration of cotinine in saliva ranged from 0 to 6 ng/ml [29]. In our own research, the measurement of the concentration of cotinine in urine of the women in labor lead to an unambiguous differentiation between the smoking patients and the ones passively exposed to smoke or the nonsmoking ones. It also served the purpose of verifying the data from the questionnaire. In the research carried out by Jarvis et al., the distribution of cotinine concentrations among the non-smokers was bimodal, which speaks volumes for the fact that the answers given in the survey were not true [70]. Apart from this, research by other authors confirms the non-compliance's between the declaration of the patients and tobacco smoking or nonsmoking [7, 16, 29, 32 , 57, 68, 113, 118, 124, 157].

In the conducted research, 47 women smoked tobacco during pregnancy. In the cases of 38 patients, the mean concentration of an alkaloid amounted to 898.53±1254.55 ng/ml of creatinine (figure 6). According to Bramer and Kallungal, a concentration of cotinine above 200 ng /ml of urine, confirms active tobacco smoking [17]. Among the positive results of cotinine in the cases of 8 women, the level of the alkaloid was below 200 ng/ml of urine. The obtained lower values of cotinine within the tested group said a lot about the length of time that had to expire from the moment of the smoking of the last cigarette to the moment of taking a sample of urine for testing, which was considerable. The biological material – urine for toxicological tests - was collected on the admission of the pregnant women to the Maternity Department of the Gynecological-Obstetric Clinic of the University of Medical Sciences in Warsaw. This could have also have been caused by an increase in the consciousness of the young women and the smoking of a smaller number of cigarettes before the delivery. Also Barlow et al. observed low concentrations of cotinine in urine during the pregnancy of smoking women. These authors suggest that the metabolism of nicotine and cotinine during pregnancy is intensified [8].

The concentration of cotinine in urine depends on the dose of nicotine (the number of cigarettes smoked per day), activity of metabolic changes, as well as diuresis and pH of urine [9]. In research by other authors, the measurements of nicotine and cotinine in the serum of the women who smoke in the first trimester of pregnancy demonstrated that the values are lower than the concentrations in the population in general. According to the research of Selb et al., the cotinine concentration after smoking one cigarette amounted to 19.1 ng/ml in the group of pregnant women, whereas in the general population it amounted to 13.0 ng/ml, which speaks volumes for a faster biotransformation of nicotine during pregnancy [136]. Also, the results of analysis of the urine of nine smoking women, in the cases of whom, the presence of cotinine was not detected, speak volumes for the extended time that had passed by since the moment of admission to the Maternity Department. Probably these patients quit smoking before delivery in spite of the fact that they declared smoking during pregnancy. Such cases are described also by other authors. The biological period of semi-duration of cotinine is long and ranges from 10 to 27 hours [90]. The presence of this biomarker in systemic fluids may be confirmed even after 78 hours from the moment of quitting smoking. From the research carried out at the Institute of Mother and Child in Warsaw, it follows that the mean level of cotinine in the urine of pregnant women in all three trimesters amounted to 2000 μg/g of creatinine, and depended on its concentration in the serum [90]. However, these values were lower than the ones stated for the smokers in general (more than 3000 μg/g of creatinine) [124]. In research by Jordanov, the level of cotinine in the urine of the pregnant women amounted to 20-127 μmol/l [74].

The paper also presented the measurements of cotinine in the placenta and in the first urine of a newborn, which was aimed at the evaluation of his/her exposure to the toxic components of smoke.

In the placenta of smoking women, in 26 samples, the cotinine concentration amounted to 0, in the remaining ones – 21 placentas, a concentration amounting to 46.98±52.59 ng/g of placenta was determined (figure 6).

The presence of cotinine in the amniotic fluid, cord blood and first urine of a newborn speaks volumes for the exposure of the developing fetus to the toxic components of tobacco smoke. The toxic components of tobacco smoke, including nicotine, penetrate the placental barrier and enter into the fetal circulation, thereby the concentrations of nicotine in the organism of a fetus are at least 15% higher than in the organism of a mother [80, 81]. The research of Luck et al. proved that the ratio of nicotine concentration in the plasma of the cord blood at the moment of delivery, and the level of nicotine in the plasma of the mother's blood amounted to 1.12 ± 0.3. The concentration of nicotine in the fetal waters taken during the intra-trimester diagnostic tests of the fetus was 54% higher than the corresponding concentrations in the serum of the mother's blood. These authors demonstrated also the presence of nicotine in the placenta [96]. In placenta, about 1% of nicotine is metabolized into cotinine. [129]. Luck et al. determined the nicotine in the placenta – 3.3-28 ng/g, amniotic fluid - 1.5-23 ng/ml, and serum of the cord blood - 0.5-25ng/ml. The cotinine level in the placenta amounted to 10-131 ng/g, in the amniotic fluid - 5-188 ng/ml, in the serum of the fetus - 15-233 ng/ml, and was lower than in the case of the mother [96]. The results of our own research concerning the cotinine level in the placenta coincide with the results presented by Luck et al. Jordanov proved that the concentration of cotinine in the amniotic fluid of nonsmoking women amounted to 15 μmol/l, in the case of women passively exposed to tobacco smoke, it was 37 μmol/l and 111 μmol/l among the patients smoking tobacco [74].

Both nicotine and cotinine affect the physiological maternal-fetal parameters at all stages of the intrauterinal development, causing vaginal and cardiovascular changes as well as changes in the respiratory system, circulation and development of the cerebral cortex. Research conducted by Sastry et al. demonstrated that tobacco smoking stimulates the metabolism of phospholipids in the placenta and increases the synthesis of E_2 (PGE_2) prostaglandines, which are responsible for homeostasia in the maternal-fetal circulation [129, 130]. Nicotine, through the activation of acetylocholine receptors in the placenta, stimulates the secretion of acetylocholine, which, through the muscarine receptors, increases the release of EDRF (Endothelium Derived Relaxing Factor) in the endothelial cells. The main alkaloid of tobacco causes the contraction of circumferential blood vessels and raises the arterial blood pressure through the stimulation of adrenal glands and hypothalamus leading to the release of catecholamines. Operating through the acetylocholine receptors, it increases the level of catecholamines and peptides. The nicotine, penetrating through the placenta, decreases the blood flow in the intervillous space (the inhibition of the transport of amino acids may be a result of this). It may cause the symptoms of metabolic acidosis and oxygen deficiency in tissues of a fetus. The alkaloid damages the placental vessels, causing the overgrowth of cytotrophoblast cells, as well as the necrosis of the deciduous membrane on the circumference of the placenta. It may lead to a fetal-placental insufficiency, and an increase in the risk of an occurrence of delayed fetal growth syndrome. The state of hypoxia in the fetus is an effect not only of nicotine, but also of other toxic components of tobacco smoke, such as carbon monoxide, cadmium and free radicals.

In our own research, the presence of cotinine was observed in 183.56 ± 251.11 ng/mg of creatinine in the first urine of 25 newborns delivered by smoking mothers (figure 6). These results coincide with the results of Jordanov, confirming the presence of cotinine (44 ± 18 μmol/l of urine) in the urine of one-day old newborns of mothers who smoke during pregnancy [74].

Most of the research regarding the non-smokers exposed to ETS that has been carried out so far, demonstrates an enhanced level of nicotine and cotinine in the urine, serum and saliva [27, 32, 68, 69, 119, 124, 143, 145, 158]. The results of the research presented in this paper constitute a confirmation of this observation. In the urine of women, who passively inhale tobacco smoke, the concentration of cotinine in two cases amounted to zero, whereas in the remaining 23 samples, it amounted to 53.20±58.03 ng/mg of creatinine (figure 6). The presence of cotinine in the urine of pregnant women, who inhale tobacco smoke passively, was also demonstrated by other authors [74, 96]. The level of metabolite in the research conducted by Jordanov amounted to 9-26 μmol/l [74].

In the placenta of women exposed to ETS, the concentration of cotinine in two samples was above zero and its mean value amounted to 19.45±12.09 ng/g of the placenta (figure 6). The determination of cotinine in the placenta of mothers, who were passively exposed to tobacco smoke only in two cases, may be a result of an extended time that had expired from the exposure to the tobacco smoke to the collection of the sample of urine for a test, or an insignificant exposure to ETS.

The metabolite of nicotine was marked in the first urine of five newborns of passively smoking mothers. The mean concentration of cotinine amounted to 26.03 ± 10.69 ng/mg creatinine (figure 7). The research carried out by Jordanov demonstrated that the levels of cotinine in the urine of one-day old newborns of mothers exposed to ETS ranged from 13 to 25 μmol/l [74].

The conducted research proves that the active and passive exposure of a future mother to tobacco smoke has an impact on the development of a fetus. It follows from the reports of many authors that there is a relationship between the number of cigarettes smoked per day and the degree of retardation in the development of the fetus and its birth body weight [35, 51, 89]. The nicotine, contracting the maternal vessels, causes the placental hypoperfusion. Additionally, penetrating the placental barrier, it gets into the fetal circulation, exerting an influence on the cardiovascular, digestive and central nervous systems of the fetus [140], and lowers its respiratory movements. This effect was apparent after 30 minutes since the moment of starting to smoke a cigarette by a mother, and lasted for 90 minutes [129]. According to Jauniaux et al. tobacco smoke components may freely penetrate the placental barrier, at least from the start of the twelfth week of pregnancy [71]. The index of penetration through the placental barrier for nicotine amounts 1.0 after 60 - 80 minutes, whereas for cotinine, the value of 1.0 is reached already after 40 minutes [129]. This has a significant impact on the activity of the placental cells, the developing fetus, the metabolism of fetal proteins, and even the activity of enzymes. Tobacco smoke contains more than 4300 chemical substances of which each may affect the fetus that is developing itself within the mother's womb. The morphological changes in placentas caused by the fact that women smoke tobacco during pregnancy indicate significant disturbances with regard to the exchange surface between the mother and the fetus. [20]. Bush et al., in spite of the fact that their morphometric research concerning the placentas of smoking women demonstrated an increase in the relative volume of maternal intervillous space and relative surface of capillaries in the fetal part, however also observed a statistical lowering of the relative and absolute capacity of the capillaries in the fetal part [20]. The authors proved that the basement membranes of villous vessels become thickened significantly. In this group of newborns, an increase in the quantity of haematocrite in blood was observed, which might be a result of the compensatory mechanism for minimizing the effects of retardation of gas exchange through the changed vessels. The experimental research proved that the exposure of proliferating vessels to tobacco smoke causes disorders in their structure [103]. Apart from the fact that the creation of new branches of proliferating vessels is inhibited, the authors observed changes in the structure of basement membranes. The increase in the quantity of collagen of Ist and IIIrd type, as well as fibronectin was demonstrated, whereas the level of hyaluronic acid was lower.

Conclusion

The results of the research indicate that cotinine may, on the one hand, be used for the purpose of confirming the credibility of answers given by mothers in a survey, in regard to active or passive smoking, and on the other hand, it may be used to evaluate the exposure of a baby in the fetal period to tobacco smoke. It seems that the urine of a woman in labor and a newborn should be the material from selection, the research did not indicate that the cotinine markings in the placenta could be useful to evaluate the exposure of a fetus to the components of tobacco smoke.

Tobacco smoking is one of the factors affecting reproduction and perinatal results. The results of scientific research carried out all over the world emphasize the impact of tobacco smoke on fertility, reproductive ability, development of a fetus, birth body weight, abortions, perinatal mortality and inborn defects. The interest in tobacco smoke in the environment and so called passive smoking of women, particularly during pregnancy is relatively recent. The report of the Surgeon General of the United States – *Women and Smoking* published in 2001 summed up the results of research concerning the impact of tobacco smoke on a woman, pregnancy and a fetus [152] Research concerning the health consequences of active smoking in mothers during pregnancy were comprehensively reviewed in the Report of the Surgeon General of the USA in 2004 [153]. In 2006, a new Report of the Surgeon General was published. It indicated the possible effects of passive exposure to smoke in the activity of man's reproduction [154]. The estimation of active and passive exposure to tobacco in research concerning fertility, development of a fetus, a newborn as well as health and development of a baby should be treated in a complex manner. For each of the three biologically significant periods – before a pregnancy, during a pregnancy and the period after the delivery of a baby, there are many potentially different biological mechanisms in tobacco smoke, which damage the organism. Even in the course of nine months of pregnancy, the vulnerability to the effects of tobacco smoke may be changed, taking into consideration the different mechanisms that damage the developing organs of a fetus and its growth. The results of our research allowed this phenomenon to be compared with the data from other countries. In spite of various actions taken for the purpose of increasing the awareness and educational programs, the passive exposure to tobacco smoke and active exposure of women in the procreative age constitute an important problem in Poland. The research provided reliable information on the subject of the negative impacts of chemical substances of tobacco smoke on the mother and the newborn, which will allow preventive actions to be taken. Any individual or group counseling, educational programs, information and raising of the awareness on the detrimental effects of smoking and passive exposure to tobacco smoke should be directed above all at girls and women. This is of particular significance in the period of procreation. The growth in awareness and changes in behaviors are connected with the health and economic benefits of the society. Raising the general health of society is the priority of not only the World Health Organization and the World Bank, but also the statutory activity of the state. The preparation and introduction of anti-tobacco policy at a national and international level will eliminate one of the causes of premature deaths triggered by tobacco use.

References

[1] Adamek, R;. Adamek, AM. Environmental tobacco exposure and the risk of Sudden Infant Death Syndrome – a review (Polish). In Florek, E; Piekoszewski, W; Wrzosek, J. Woman and Tobacco – Current Research in Poland. Poznan: Department of Toxicology University of Medical Sciences; 2002; 136-137.

[2] Adamek, R; Florek, E; Beborowicz, GH; Anholcer, A; Kaczmarek, E. Relationship between tobacco smoking by pregnant women and birth body weight of their newborns (Polish). In: Florek, E; Piekoszewski, W. Tobacco and Health. Poznan: Department of Toxicology University of Medical Sciences; 2003, 83-91.

[3] Adamek, R; Florek, E; Beborowicz, GH; Anholcer, A; Karczmarek, E. The awareness of health consequences of active and passive smoking and access to the information of these consequences in the population of pregnant women (Polish). *Przeglad Lekarski,* 2004, 61, 1012-1015.

[4] Adamek, R; Florek, E; Piekoszewski, W; Beborowicz; GH. The socio-economical status of women smoking during pregnancy and birth weight of their newborn (Polish). *Przeglad Lekarski,* 2004, 61, 1006-1011.

[5] Ahlborg, G; Bodin, L. Tobacco smoke exposure and pregnancy outcome among working women. A prospective study at prenatal care centers in Orebro County Sweden. *American Journal of Epidemiology,* 1991, 133, 338-347.

[6] Ahluwalia, IB; Grummer-Strawn, L; Scanlon, KS. Exposure to environmental tobacco smoke and birth outcome: Increased effects on pregnant women aged 30 years or older. *American Journal of Epidemiology,* 1997, 146, 42-47.

[7] Bardy, AH; Seppala, T; Lillsunde, P; Kataja, JM; Koskela, P; Pikkarainen, J; Hiilesmaa, VK. Objectively measured tobacco exposure during pregnancy: neonatal effects and relation to maternal smoking. *British Journal of Obstetrics and Gynaecology,* 1993, 100, 721-726.

[8] Barlow, RD; Wald, NJ. Use of urinary cotinine to estimate exposure to tobacco smoke. *JAMA,* 1988, 259, 1808-9.

[9] Benowitz, NL. Cotinine as a biomarker of environmental tobacco exposure. *Epidemiological Review,* 1996, 18, 188-204.

[10] Benowitz, NL. Biomarkers of cigarette smoking. In. U.S. Department of Health and Human Services. Public Health Service. Monograph 7. The FTC cigarette test method for determining tar, nicotine, and carbon monoxide yield of U.S. cigarettes: Report of the NCI Expert Committee. Bethesda: National Institutes of Health; 1996.

[11] Benowitz, NL. Biomarkers of environmental tobacco exposure. *Environmental Health Perspectives,* 1999, 107, 349-354.

[12] Benowitz, NL; Jacob, P; Jones, RT; Rosenberg, J. Inter-individual variability in the metabolism and cardiovascular effects of nicotine in man. *Journal of Pharmacology and Experimental Therapeutics,* 1982, 221, 368-372.

[13] Bernstein, IM; Mongeon, JA; Badger, GJ; Solomon, L; Heil, SH; Higgins, ST. Maternal smoking and its association with birth weight. *Obstetrics and Gynecology,* 2005, 106, 986-991.

[14] Blackmore, ChA; Rowley; DL; Kiely, JL. Preterm birth. *CDC's Public Health Surveillance for Women, Infants and Children,* 2003, 10, 179-183.

[15] Borlee, I; Bouckaert, A; Lecha, MF; Misson, CB. Smoking patterns during and before pregnancy: Weight, length and head circumference of progeny. *European Journal of Obstetrics, Gynecology and Reproduction Bioliology,* 1978, 8, 171-177.

[16] Boyd, NR; Windsor, RA; Perkins, LL; Lowe, JB. Quality of measurement of smoking status by self-report and saliva cotinine among pregnant women. *Maternal and Child Health Journal,* 1998, 2, 77-83.

[17] Bramer, SL; Kallungal, BA. Clinical considerations in study design that use cotinine as biomarker. *Biomarkers,* 2003, 8, 187-203.

[18] Breborowicz, GH. Pregnancy of high risk (Polish). Osrodek Wydawnictw Naukowych. Poznan: 2000.

[19] Brunnemann, KD; Hoffmann, D. The pH of tobacco smoke. *Food and Cosmetics Toxicology,* 1974, 12, 115-124.

[20] Bush, PG; Mayhew, TM; Abramovich DR; Aggett, PJ; Burke, MD; Page, KR. A quantitative study on the effects of maternal smoking on placental morphology and cadmium concentration. *Placenta,* 2000, 21, 247-256.

[21] Campbell, MJ; Lewry, J; Wailoo, M. Future evidence for the effect of passive smoking on neonates. *Postgraduate Medical Journal,* 1988, 64, 663-665.

[22] Chiolero, A; Bovet, P; Paccaud, F. Association between maternal smoking and low birth weight in Switzerland: the EDEN study. *Swiss Medical Weekly,* 2005, 135, 525-530.

[23] Cnattingius, S. Maternal age modifies the effect of maternal smoking on intrauterine growth retardation but not on late fetal death and placental abruption. *American Journal of Epidemiology,* 1997, 145,319-323.

[24] Colley, JRT; Holland, WW; Corkhill, RT. Influence of passive smoking on parental phlegm on pneumonia and bronchitis in early childhood. *Lancet,* 1974, 2, 1031-1034.

[25] Comstock, GW; Lundin, FE. Parental smoking and prenatal mortality. American Journal of Obstetrics and. *Gynecology,* 1967, 98, 708-718.

[26] Conter, V; Ccortnovis, I; Rogari, P; Riva, L. Weight growth in infants born to mothers who smoked during pregnancy. *British Medical Journal,* 1995, 310, 768-771.

[27] Cook, DG; Whincup, PH; Jarvis, MJ. Passive exposure to tobacco smoke in children age 5-7 years; individual family, and community factors. *British Medical Journal,* 1994, 308, 384-389.

[28] Cornelius, MD; Taylor, PM; Geva, D; Day, NL. Prenatal tobacco and marijuana use among adolescents: effects on offspring gestational age, growth and morphology. *Pediatrics,* 1995, 95, 738-743.

[29] Coultas, DB; Howard, CA; Peake, GT; Skipper, BJ; Samet, JM. Salivary cotinine levels and involuntary tobacco smoke exposure in children and adults in New Mexico. *American Review on Respiratory Disease,* 1987, 136, 305-309.

[30] Counsilman, JJ; Macka, EV. Smoking habits of pregnant women in Brisbane, Australia. *Australian and New Zealand Journal of Obstetrics and Gynaecology,* 1985, 25, 244-247.

[31] Crone, MR; Hirasing, RA; Burgmeijer, RIF. Prevalence of passive smoking in infancy in The Netherlands. *Pathology Education Council.* 2000, 39, 149-153.

[32] Cummings, KM; Markello, SJ; Mahoney, M; Bhargava, AK; McElroy, PD; Marshall, JR. Measurement of current exposures to environmental tobacco smoke. *Archive of Environmental Health,* 1990, 45, 74-79.

[33] Dube, MF; Green, CR. Methods of collection of smoke for analytical purposes. In Recent Advances in Tobacco Science: *Formation, Analysis and Composition of Tobacco Smoke,* 1982, 8, 42-102.

[34] Eskenazi, B. Association of prenatal maternal or postnatal child environmental tobacco smokes exposure and neurodevelopment and behavioral problems in children. *Environmental Health Perspective,* 1999, 107, 991-1000.

[35] Fielding, JE. Smoking and women. Tragedy of the majority. *New England Journal of Medicine,* 1987, 317, 1343-1345.

[36] Florek, E. Biological activity of tobacco smoke (Polish). In. Zatonski, W; Przewozniak, K. Tobacco smoking in Poland. The base, health consequences and prophylactics. Warsaw: *Center of Oncology;* 1996; 65-88.

[37] Florek, E; Adamek, R; Adamek, AM; Anholcer, A; Breborowicz, GH. Active and passive exposure of pregnant women to tobacco smoke and health condition of their newborns – awareness of the risk (Polish). *Nowiny Lekarskie,* 2001, 70, 133-143.

[38] Florek, E; Breborowicz, GH; Lechowicz, W; Basior, A;, Wolna, M;, Ṣenczuk, M. Cotinine in urine of mother and their newborn and in cord serum and placenta as a biomarker of foetal exposure to tobacco smoke (Polish). *Przeglad Lekarski,* 2006, 63, 900-906.

[39] Florek, E; Kornacka, MK; Hubert, A; Wilimowska, J; Basior, A. The level of cotinine in urine and placenta of women smoking or exposure to tobacco smoke during pregnancy (Polish). *Przeglad Lekarski, 2004,* 61, 1090-1093.

[40] Florek, E; Marszalek, A. An experimental study of the influences of tobacco smoke on fertility and reproduction. *Human and Experimental Toxicology,* 1999, 18, 272-278.

[41] Florek, E; Marszalek, A. Health consequence of exposure of women to enviromental tobacco smoke (Polish). *Ginekologia Praktyczna,* 2001, 9, 28-30.

[42] Florek, E; Marszalek, A; Biczysko, W; Szymanowski, K. The experimental investigations of the tonic influence of tobacco smoke affecting progeny during pregnancy. *Human and Experimental Toxicology,* 1999, 18, 245-251.

[43] Florek, E; Marszalek, A; Piekoszewski, W; Wrzosek, J; Opala, T; Moczko, J. Occurrence of exposure to tobacco smoke among women in procreative age (Polish). *Ginekologia Praktyczna.* 2001, 60, 16-21.

[44] Florek, E; Piekoszewski, W. Evaluation of exposure of fetus, newborn and small children to tobacco smoke (Polish). *Ginekologia Praktyczna,* 2002, 67, 10-14.

[45] Florek, E; Piekoszewski, W; Breborowicz GH; Pach, D; Pasich A. Application of questionnaire and biochemical testes in evaluation of tobacco smoking by pregnant women (Polish). *Przeglad Lekarski,* 2004, 61, 345-347.

[46] Florek, E; Piekoszewski, W; Kornacka, MK; Szmanko A. Evaluation exposition to policyclic aromatic hydrocarbons of pregnant women who smoke tobacco (Polish). *Przeglad Lekarski,* 2005, 65, 1013-1018.

[47] Florek, E; Piekoszewski, W; Krol, M; Kornacka, MK; Pasich, A. Tobacco smoking and exposure to environmental tobacco smoke women who delivered in the Gynecological Obstetric Clinic of the Academy of Medical Sciences in Warsaw (Polish). In Florek, E; Piekoszewski, W. Tobacco and Health – Tobacco Related Disease. Poznan: Department of Toxicology University of Medical Sciences; 2003; 72-82.

[48] Florek, E; Piekoszewski, W; Lechowicz, W; Szymanska, A; Kornacka, MK. Determination of 4-(metylonitrosamino)-4-(3-pyridyl)-1-butanol (NNAL) in urine of pregnant women by means of LC/MS/MS (Polish). *Przeglad Lekarski,* 2006, 63, 926-931.

[49] Florek, E; Piekoszewski, W; Rybakowski, Ł; Moczko, J. Using the questionnaire and cotinine concentration in urine for study smoking habit and exposure to ETS of pregnant women. *Przeglad Lekarski,* 2004, 61, 993-996.

[50] Florek, E; Rybakowski, L; Karkucinska, M; Slusarska, E; Hubert, A. Evaluation of awareness about harmful effect of tobacco smoking and health consequences of tobacco smoking among pregnant women (Polish). In Florek, E; Piekoszewski. *Tobacco and Health – Tobacco Related Disease.* Poznan: Department of Toxicology University of Medical Sciences. 2003, 190-197.

[51] Fredricsson, B; Gilljam, H. Smoking and reproduction. *Acta Obstetrics and Gynecology Scandinavia,* 1992, 71, 580-592.

[52] Fried, PA; O'Connell, CM. A comparison of the effects of prenatal exposure to tobacco, alcohol, cannabis and caffeine on birth size and subsequent growth. *Neurotoxicology and Teratology,* 1987, 9, 79-85.

[53] Friedman, GD; Perteti, DB; Bawol, RD. Prevalence and correlates of passive smoking. *American Journal of Public Health,* 1983, 73, 401-405.

[54] Gajewska, M; Celinska, A; Domanska-Janczewska, E. Evaluation of birth body weight of newborn born on time (Polish). In: Florek, E; Piekoszewski, W; Wrzosek, *J. Woman and Tobacco – Current Opinions.* Poznan: Department of Toxicology University of Medical Sciences; 2001, 77-83.

[55] Gajewska, M; Celinska, A; Domanska-Janczewska, E. Cigarettes smoking and delivering before time (Polish). In: Florek, E; Piekoszewski, W; Wrzosek, *J. Woman and Tobacco – Tobacco Related Diseases.* Poznan: Department of Toxicology University of Medical Sciences; 2003, 64.

[56] Guerin, MR; Jenkins, RA; Tomkins, BA. The chemistry of environmental tobacco smoke: Composition and measurement. Boca Raton: Lewis Publisher; 1992.

[57] Haddow, JE; Knight, GJ; Palomaki, GE; McCarty, JE. Second-trimester cotinine level in nonsmokers in relation to birth weight. *American Journal of Obstetrics and Gynecology,* 1988, 152, 481-484.

[58] Hanke, W; Kalinka, J; Florek E. Passive smoking and pregnancy outcome in central Poland. *Human and Experimental Toxicology,* 1999, 18, 265-271.

[59] Hanke, W; Sobala. J. Environmental factors of premature delivery and fetus hypotrophy: study in Lodz region (Polish). *Lodz: Oficyna Wydawnicza IMP;* 1998.

[60] Haug, K; Irgens, LM; Skjaerven, R; Markestad, T; Baste, V; Schreuder, P. Maternal smoking and birth weight: effect modification of period, maternal age and paternal smoking. *Acta Obstetrics and Gynecology Scandinavian,* 2000, 79, 485-489.

[61] Hjalmarson, AIM; Hahn, L; Svanberg, B. Stopping smoking in pregnancy: effect of a self-help manual in controlled trial. *British Journal of Obstetrics and Gynecology,* 1991, 98, 260-264.

[62] Hoffmann D., Hecht S.S.: Advances in tobacco carcinogenesis. In Grover, P. Handbook of Experimental Pharmacology: Springer-Verlag, 1989.

[63] Hoffmann, D; Hoffmann, I. The changing cigarette, 1950-1995. *Journal of Toxicology and Environtal Health,* 1997, 50, 307-364.

[64] Hoffmann, D; Wynder, E.L. Aktives und passives Rauchen. In Marquardt, H; Schafer, SG. Lehrbuch der Toxikologie. Mannheim: Leipzig, Wien, Zurich: BJ-Wiss.-Verlag; 1994, 589-605.

[65] Ingebrethsen, BJ. Aerosol studies of cigarette smoke. *Recent Advances in Tobacco Science,* 1986, 12, 54-142.

[66] International Agency for Research on Cancer. IARC Monographs on the evaluation of the carcinogenic risk of chemicals to humans. *Tobacco Smoking.* Lyon: Vol. 38, 1986.

[67] Jaakkola, N; Jaakkola, MS; Gissler, M; Jaakkola, JK. Smoking during pregnancy in Finland: determinants and trends, 1987-1997. *American Journal of Public Health,* 2001, 2, 284-286.

[68] Jarvis, MJ; Russel, MA. Measurement and estimation of smoke dose to non-smokers from environmental tobacco smoke. *European Journal of Respiratory Disease,* 1984, 133, 68-75.

[69] Jarvis, MJ; Russel, MA; Feyerabend, C. Passive exposure to tobacco smoke; saliva cotinine concentration in a representative population sample of nonsmoking schoolchildren. *British Medical Journal,* 1985, 291, 927-929.

[70] Jarvis, MJ; Tunstall-Pedoe, H; Feyerabend, C. Comparison of testes used to distinguish smokers from nonsmokers. *American Journal of Public Health,* 1987, 77, 1435-1438.

[71] Jauniaux, E; Gulbis, B; Acharya, G; Thiry, P; Rodeck, Ch. Maternal tobacco exposure and cotinine levels in fetal fluid in the first half of pregnancy. *Obstetrics and Gynecology,* 1999, 93, 25-29.

[72] Johnston, C. Cigarette smoking and the outcome of human pregnancies: a status report on the consequences. *Clinical Toxicology,* 1981, 18, 189-209.

[73] Joosens, L. Tobacco. In Weil, O; Mekce, M; Brodin, M; Oberle D. Priorities for public health action in the European Union. European Union: 1999, 44-55.

[74] Jordanov, JS. Cotinine concentration in amniotic fluid and urine of smoking, passive smoking and nonsmoking pregnant women at term and in urine of their neonates on 1st day of life. *European Journal of Pediatrics.* 1990, 149, 734-737.

[75] Jozwik, M; Laudanski, T. Premature delivery. Reasons and solving this problem – new approach (Polish). *Ginekologia i Poloznictwo,* 1995, 1, 9-15.

[76] Kalinka, J; Hanke, W. Tobacco smoking as a risk factor of fetus hypotrophy, premature delivery and low birth body weight (Polish). *Ginekologia Polska,* 1996, 67, 75-81.

[77] Kalinka, J; Hanke, W. The role of tobacco smoking in fetus hypotrophy and premature delivery (Polish). *Przeglad Epidemiologiczny,* 1996, 50, 309-313.

[78] Kallen, K. Maternal smoking during pregnancy and infant head circumference at birth. *Early Human,* 2000, 58, 197-204.

[79] Karwan-Plonska A.: Clinical analysis of premature delivery (Polish). *Nowiny Medyczne,* 1999, 6, 21-27.

[80] Koren, G. Fetal toxicology of environmental tobacco smoke. *Current Opinion in Pediatrics,* 1995, 7, 128-131.

[81] Koren, G; Weiss, J; Eckert, A. Cotinine levels in follicular fluid and serum of IVF patients: effect on granulosa – luteal function *in vivo. Human Reproduction,* 1989, 4, 482-485.

[82] Kornacka, MK; Helwich, E. A newborn with birth body weight bellow 1000 g – the first hour of live as a prognostic factors of survive (Polish). In *Medicine in development age.* Warsaw: Instytut Matki i Dziecka, 1999, III, 21-31.

[83] Kramer, MS. Socjoeconomic determinants of intrauterine growth retardation. *European Journal of Clinical Nutrition,* 1998, 52 Suppl 1, 29-32.

[84] Krishna, K. Tobacco chewing in pregnancy. *British Journal of Obstetrics and Gynecology,* 1978, 85, 726-728.

[85] Kubicki, J. Syndrome of interuterine hypotrophy of fetus. Part I. (Polish). *Nowiny Medyczne,* 1999, 6, 17-18.

[86] Kukla, L; Hruba, D; Tyrlik, M. Smoking and damages of reproduction: evidence of ELSPAC. *Central Europe Journal of Public Health,* 2001, 9, 59-63.

[87] Lach, J; Klyszejko, Cz; Ziolkowski, M; Lach, E; Marcinkowski, Z; Szulczynski, J. Birth parameters of newborns in relation to the period of tobacco smoking during pregnancy. In Florek, E; Piekoszewski, W; Wrzosek, *J. Woman and Tobacco – Current Opinions.* Poznan: Department of Toxicology University of Medical Sciences; 2001, 84-91.

[88] Lackmann, GM; Salzberger, U; Tollner, U; Chen, M; Carmella, SG; Hecht, SS. Metabolites of a tobacco-specific carcinogen in urine from newborns. *Journal of National Cancer Institute,* 1999, 91, 459-465.

[89] Lambers, DS; Clark, KE. The maternal and fetal physiologic effects of nicotine. *Seminars in Perinatology,* 1996, 20, 115-126.

[90] Laskowska-Klita, T; Chelchowska, M; Leibschang, J. Concentrations of cotinine in serum and urine of smoking pregnant women and in placenta and umbilical cord blood (Polish). *Przeglad Lekarski,* 2005, 62, 1007-1009.

[91] Lassen, K; Oei, T. Effects of maternal cigarette smoking during pregnancy on long-term physical and cognitive parameters of children development. *Addictive Behaviors,* 1998, 23, 635-653.

[92] Lazaroni, F; Bonassi, S; Manniello, E; Morcaldi, L, Repeto, E; Ruocco, A; Caolvi, A; Cotellessa, G. Effect of passive smoking during pregnancy on selected perinatal parameters. *International Journal of Epidemiology,* 1990, 19, 960-966.

[93] Lin, RX. Maternal, medical and obstetrics complications are major risk factors for law birth weight infant. *Chinese Medical Journal,* 1993, 28, 24-26.

[94] Longo, LD. Some health consequences of maternal smoking: Issues without answers. *Birth Defects,* 1982, 18, 13-31.

[95] Luciano, A; Bolognani, M; Biondani, P; Ghizzi, C; Zoppi, G; Signori E. The influence of maternal passive and light active smoking on intrauterine growth and body

composition of the newborn. *European Journal of Clinical Nutrition,* 1998, 52, 760-763.

[96] Luck, W; Nau, A; Hansen, R; Steldinger, R. Extent of nicotine and cotinine transfer to the human fetus, placenta and amniotic fluid of smoking mothers. *Development Pharmacology and Therapeutics,* 1985, 8, 384-395.

[97] MacArthur, C; Knox, EG. Passive smoking and birth weight. *Lancet,* 1987, 1, 37-38.

[98] McGann, K; Spanler, JG.; Alcohol, tobacco and illicit drug use among women. *Primary Care,* 1997, 24, 113-122.

[99] Mackay, J; Eriksen, M. The Tobacco Atlas. Geneva, Switzerland: World Health Organization; 2002, 24-35.

[100] MacMahon, B; Alpert, M; Salber, E. Infant weight and paternal smoking habits. *American Journal of Epidemiology,* 1966, 82, 247-261.

[101] Marszalek, A; Biczysko, W; Wasowicz, M; Florek, E. Influence of tobacco smoke on gas stabilization in newborn rat lung. In. Lu, R; Mackay, J; Niu, S; Peto, R. Tobacco: *The Growing Epidemic.* London, Berlin, Heidelberg: Springer-Verlag; 2000, 129-130.

[102] Martin, TR; Bracken, MB. Association of low birth weight with passive smoke exposure in pregnancy. *American Journal of Epidemiology,* 1986, 124, 633-642.

[103] Melkonian, G; Le, C; Zheng, W; Talbot, P; Martins-Green, M. Normal patterns of agiogenesis and extracellular matrix deposition in chick chorioallantoic membranes are disrupted by mainstream and side stream cigarette smoke. *Toxicology and Apply Pharmacology,* 2000, 163, 26-37.

[104] Misra, DP; Nguyen, RHN. Environmental tobacco smoke and low birth weight: A hazard in the workplace? *Environmental Health Perspective,* 1999, 107, 879-904.

[105] Mitchell, EA; Scragg, R; Stewart, AW; Becroft, DM; Taylor, BJ; Ford, RP; Hassall, IB; Barry, DM; Allen, EM; Roberts, AP. Results from the first year of the New Zealand cot death study. *New Zealand Medical Journal,* 1991, 104, 71-76.

[106] Mochizuki, M; Maruo, T; Masuko, K. Mechanism of fetal growth retardation caused by smoking during pregnancy. *Acta Physiologica Hungarica,* 1985, 65, 295-304.

[107] Moore, ML; Zaccaro, DJ. Cigarette smoking, low birth weight, and preterm births in low-income African American women. *Journal of Perinatology,* 2000, 20, 176-180.

[108] Naey, RL. Influence of maternal cigarette smoking during pregnancy on fetal and childhood growth. *Obstetrics and Gynecology,* 1981, 57, 18-21.

[109] Narahara, H; Johnston, JM.: Smoking and preterm labor: effect of cigarette smoke extract on the secretion of platelet-activating factor- a-cetylhydrplase by human decidual macrodhages. *American Journal of Obstetrics and Gynecology,* 1993, 169, 1321-1326.

[110] National Health Institute. Health effects of exposure to environmental tobacco smoke: the report of the California Environmental Protection Agency. Bethesda; 1999, 75-119.

[111] Ogawa, H; Tominaga, S; Hori, K; Noguchi, K; Kaniu, I; Matsubara, M. Passive smoking by pregnant women and fetal growth. *Journal of Epidemiology and Community Health,* 1991, 45, 164-168.

[112] Peacock, JL; Bland, JM; Andersen, HR. Preterm delivery: effects of socioeconomics factors, psychological stress, smoking, alcohol, and caffeine. *British Medical Journal,* 1995, 311, 531-535.

[113] Perez-Stable, EJ; Martin, G; Martin, BV; Benowitz, NL. Misclassification of smoking status by self-reported cigarette consumption. *American Review of Respiratory Diseases,* 1992, 145, 53-57.

[114] Perkins, SL; Belcher, JM; Livesey, JF. A Canadian tertiary care centre study of maternal and umbilical cord cotinine levels as a markers of smoking during pregnancy: Relationship to neonatal effects. *Canadian Journal of Public. Health,* 1997, 88, 232-237.

[115] Peto, R Lopez, AD; Boreham, J; Hun, M; Health, C. Jr. Mortality from tobacco in developed countries. Indirect estimates from national vital statistics. *Lancet,* 1992, 339, 1268-1278.

[116] Piekoszewski, W; Florek, E. Biomarkers of exposition to tobacco smoke (Polish). Department of Toxicology University of Medical Sciences. Poznan; 2001.

[117] Piekoszewski, W; Florek, E. Interaction between drugs and tobacco smoke (Polish). Department of Toxicology University of Medical Sciences. Poznan; 2006.

[118] Pierce, JP; Dwyet, T; DiGiusto, E; Carpenter, T; Hannaom, C; Amin, A; Yong, C; Sarfaty, G; Shaw, J; Burke, N. Cotinine validation of self-reported smoking in commercially run community surveys. *Journal of Chronic Disease,* 1987, 40, 689-695.

[119] Pirkle, JL; Flegal, KM; Bernert, JT. Exposure of the US population to environmental tobacco smoke; the Third National Health and Nutrition Examination Survey, 1888-1991. *JAMA,* 1996, 275, 1233-1240.

[120] Price, JH; Krol, RA; Desmond, SM; Losh, DP; Roberts, SM; Snyder, FF. Comparison of three antismoking interventions among pregnant women in an urban setting: a randomized trial. *Psychological Reports,* 1991, 68, 595-604.

[121] Pulkkinen, P. Smoking and pregnancy, with special reference to fetal growth and certain trace element distribution between mother, placenta, and fetus. *Acta Obstetrics and Gynecology Scandinavia,* 1990, 69, 543-545.

[122] Rama-Sastry, BV; Hemontolor, ME; Olenick, M. Prostaglandin E_2 in human placenta: its vascular effects and activation of prostaglandin E_2 formation by nicotine and cotinine. *Pharmacology,* 1999, 58, 70-86.

[123] Rebagliato, M; Bolumer, F; Florey, CV. Assessment of exposure to environmental tobacco smoke in nonsmoking pregnant women in different environments of daily living. *American Journal of Epidemiology,* 1995, 142, 525-530

[124] Riboli, E; Presto-Martin, S; Saracci, R. Exposure of non-smoking women to environmental tobacco smoke; a 10-country collaborative study. *Cancer Causes Control,* 1990, 1, 243-252.

[125] Rubin, DH; Krasilnikoff, PA; Leventhal, JM. Effect of passive smoking on birth-weight. *Lancet,* 1986, 2, 415-417.

[126] Saito, R. The smoking habits of pregnant women and their husbands, and the effect on their infants. *Nippon Koshu Eisei Zasshi,* 1991, 38, 124-131.

[127] Samuelsen, SO; Magnus, P; Bakketeig, L.S. Birth weight and mortality in childhood in Norway. *American Journal of Epidemiology,* 1998, 148, 983-91.

[128] Saraiya, M; Berg, CJ; Kendrick JS; Strauss, LT; Atrash, HK; Ahn, YW. Cigarette smoking as a risk factor for ectopic pregnancy. *American Journal of Obstetrics and Gynecology,* 1998, 178, 493-498.

[129] Sastry, BV; Chance, MB. Hemontolor, ME; Goddijn-Wessel, TA. Formation and retention of cotinine during placental transfer of nicotine in human placental cotyledon. *Pharmacology,* 1998, 57, 104-116.

[130] Sastry, BM; Hementolor, ME; Olecnick, M. Prostaglandin E_2 in human placenta; its vascular effects and activation of prostaglandin E_2 formation by nicotine and cotinine. *Pharmacology,* 1999, 58, 70-86.

[131] Savitz, DA; Schwingl, PJ; Keels, MA. Influence of paternal age, smoking, and alcohol consumption on congenital anomalies. *Teratology,* 1991, 44, 429-440.

[132] Schellscheidta, J; Jorch, G; Menke, J. Effects of heavy maternal smoking of intrauterine growth patterns in sudden infant death victims and surviving infants. *European Journal of Pediatrics,* 1998, 157, 246-251.

[133] Schwartz-Bickenbach, D; Schulte-Hobein, B; Abt, S; Plum, C; Nau, H. Smoking during pregnancy and early infancy: effects on birth weight, lactation period, and cotinine concentrations in mother s milk and infant s urine. *Toxicology Letters,* 1987, 35, 73-81.

[134] Secher, NJ; Hjortdal, J; Hjortdal, V. Smoking effects fetal growth selectively. *Acta Obstetrics and Gynecology Scandinavia,* 1990, 69, 469-471.

[135] Seidman, DS; Eter-Hadani, P; Gale, R. Effect of maternal smoking and age on congenital anomalies. *Obstetrics and Gynecology,* 1990, 76, 1046-1050.

[136] Selby, P; Hackman, R; Kapur, B; Klein, J; Koren, G. Heavily smoking women who cannot quit in pregnancy: evidence of pharmacokinetic predisposition. *Therapeutic Drug Monitoring,* 2001, 23, 189-191.

[137] Shah, N; Bracken, MB. A systematic review and meta-analysis of prospective studies on the association between maternal cigarette smoking and preterm delivery. *American Journal of Obstetrics and Gynecology,* 2000, 182, 465-472.

[138] Simpson, WJ. A preliminary report on cigarette smoking and the incidence of prematurity. *American Journal of Obstetrics and Gynecology,* 1957, 73, 808-815.

[139] Steward, DE; Streiner, DL. Cigarette smoking during pregnancy. *Canadian Journal of Psychiatry,* 1995, 40, 603-607.

[140] Stillman, RJ; Rosenberg, MJ; Sachs, BP. Smoking and reproduction. *Fertility and Sterility,* 1986, 46, 545-566.

[141] Szamotulska, K; Brzezinski, ZJ. Report on smoking among women of reproductive age pregnant women in Poland. WHO Project on Youth and Tobacco: Free Initiative-Draft report on the effects of tobacco smoke on the health of Polish children. Health Promotion Foundation. Warsaw, Poland; 1999, 78-88.

[142] Szamotulska, K; Brzezinski, ZJ. Tobacco smoking by pregnant women. Health condition of newborn in Poland (Polish). *Alkoholizm i Narkomania,* 2000, 13, 389-398.

[143] Thompson, SG; Stone, R. Nanchahal K. Wald, NJ. Relation of urinary cotinine concentrations to cigarette smoking and to exposure to other people's smoke. *Torax,* 1990, 45, 356-361.

[144] Townsend, JL; Roderic, P; Cooper J. Cigarette smoking by socioeconomic group, sex and age: Effect of price, income and health publicity. *British Medical Journal,* 1994, 309, 923-926.

[145] Tunstall-Pedoe, H; Woodward, M; Brown, CA. Tea drinking, passive smoking, smoking deception and serum cotinine in Scottish Heart Health study. *Journal of Clinical Epidemiology,* 1991, 44, 1411-1414.

[146] Underwood, PB; Kesler, KF; O'Lane, JM; Callagan, DA. Parental smoking empirically related to pregnancy outcome. *Obstetrics and Gynecology,* 1967, 29, 1-8.

[147] U.S. Department of Health, Education, and Welfare. Smoking and Health. A Report of the Surgeon General. Washington: U.S. Department of Health, Education, and Welfare, Public Health Service, Office of the Assistant Secretary for Health, Office of Smoking and Health, 1979. DHEW Publication No. (PHS) 79-50066.

[148] U.S. Department of Health and Human Services. The Health Consequences of Smoking for Women. A Report of the Surgeon General. Washington (DC): U.S. Department of Health, and Human Services, Public Health Service, Office of the Assistant Secretary for Health, Office of Smoking and Health; 1980.

[149] U.S. Department of Health and Human Services. The Health Consequences of Smoking: Cancer. A Report of the Surgeon General. Rockville (MD): U.S. DHHS, Public Health Service, Office on Smoking and Health. DHHS Publication No. (PHS) 82-50179; 1982.

[150] U.S. Department of Health and Human Services. Reducing the Health Consequences of Smoking. 25 Years of Progress. A report of the Surgeon General. Washington (DC): US Government Printing Office; 1989.

[151] U.S. Department of Health and Human Services. The Health benefice of smoking cessation. A report of the Surgeon General. Washington DC: US Government Printing Office; 1990

[152] U.S. Department of Health and Human Services. Women and Smoking. A Report of the Surgeon General. Rockville (MD): Department of Health and Human Services, Public Health Service, Office of the Surgeon General; 2001.

[153] U.S. Department of Health and Human Services. The Health Consequences of Smoking. A Report of the Surgeon General. Atlanta (GO): U.S. Department of Health and Human Services, Centers for Disease Control and Prevention, National Center for Chronic Disease Prevention and Health Promotion, Office of the Surgeon General; 2004.

[154] U.S. Department of Health and Human Services. The Health Consequences of Involuntary Exposure to Tobacco Smoke. A Report of the Surgeon General. Atlanta (GO): U.S. Department of Health and Human Services, Centers for Disease Control and Prevention, National Center for Chronic Disease Prevention and Health Promotion, Office of the Surgeon General; 2006.

[155] U.S. Environmental Protection Agency, Office of Health and Environmental Assessment, Office of Research and Development. Respiratory health effects of passive smoking: Lung cancer and other disorders: Washington; 1992.

[156] Valero De Bernabe, J; Soriano, T; Albaladejo, R; Juarranz, M; Calle, ME; Martinez, D; Dominguez-Rojas, V. Risk factors for low birth weight: A review. *Obstetrics and Gynecology,* 2004, 116, 3-15.

[157] Wagerknecht, LE; Burke, GL; Perkins, LI; Haley, NJ; Freidman, GD. Misclassification of smoking status. A comparison of self-reported with serum cotinine level. The CARDIA study. *American Journal of Public Health,* 1992, 82, 33-36.

[158] Wald, NJ; Ritchie, JE. Validation of studies on lung cancer in nonsmokers married to smokers. *Lancet,* 1984; 1, 1067.

[159] Wang, X; Tager, B; Van Vunakis, H; Speizer, FE; Hanrahan, JP. Maternal smoking during pregnancy, urine cotinine concentrations, and birth outcomes. A prospective cohort study. *International Journal of Epidemiology,* 1997, 26, 978-988.

[160] Wasowicz, M, Zurawski, P; Florek, E; Senczuk, W; Biczysko, W. Retardation of lung development after maternal cigarette smoking and low protein diet in animal model. *Polish Journal of Pathology,* 1994, 45, 155-162.

[161] Weibel, FJ. Health affects of passive smoking. In Bolliger, CT; Fagestrom KO. The tobacco epidemic Basel: Karger; 1997, 27, 107-121.

[162] Wen, SW; Goldenberg, RL; Cutter, GR; Hoffmann, HJ; Cliver, SP; Davis, RO, Du Bard, MB. Smoking, maternal age, fetal growth and gestational age at delivery. *American Journal of Obstetrics and Gynecology,* 1990, 162, 53-58.

[163] WHO Air Quality Guidelines for Europe. Environmental Tobacco Smoke. World Health Organization. European Center for Environment and Health: Bilthoven Division; 1998, 1-28.

[164] WHO: Tobacco or Health: A Global status report. Geneva: World Health Organization; 1997.

[165] Windham, GC; Eaton, A; Hopkins, H. Evidence for an association between environmental tobacco smoke exposure and birth weight: a meta-analysis and new data. *Pediatrics and Perinatal Epidemiology,* 2000, 108, 73-82.

[166] Windham, GC; Hopkins, B; Fenster, L; Swan, SH. Prenatal active or passive tobacco smoke exposure and the risk of preterm delivery or low birth weight. *Epidemiology,* 2000, 11, 427-433.

[167] Windham, GC; Swan, SH; Fenster, L. Parental cigarette smoking and the risk of spontaneous abortion. *American Journal of Epidemiology,* 1992, 135, 1394-1403.

[168] Windsor, RA; Boys, NR; Orleans, CT. A meta-evaluation of smoking cessation intervention research among pregnant women: improving the science and art. *Health Education Research,* 1998, 13, 419-438.

[169] Witschi, H; Lundgaardt, SM; Rajini, G; Hendrickx, AG; Last, JA. Effects of exposure to nicotine and to side stream smoke on pregnancy outcome in rats. *Toxicology Letters,* 1994, 71, 279-286

[170] Wojculewicz, J; Kawinska-Kilianczyk, A. Effect of tobacco smoking by pregnant women on somatic condition of newborn. Approach to pro health behaviour of women. In Florek, E; Piekoszewski, W; Wrzosek, J. Woman and Tobacco – Current Research in Poland. Poznan: Department of Toxicology University of Medical Sciences; 2002; 74-84.

[171] World Bank. Development in practice. Curbing the Epidemic. Governments and the Economics of Tobacco Control: World Bank: Washington; 1999, 15.

[172] Wyser, C; Bolliger, CT. Smoking-related disorders. In Bolliger, CT; Fagerstrom KO. The tobacco epidemic. Basel: Karger; 1997, 27, 78-106.

[173] Xiao, KZ. A survey on the constitutional status of perinates in China. *Chinese Medical Journal,* 1989, 69, 185-188

[174] Xu, J. 126 Small gestational age infants: clinical characteristic and long-term observation. *Chinese Medical Journal,* 1992, 72, 459-461.

[175] Yerushalmy, J. The relationship of parents' cigarette smoking to outcome of pregnancy-implications as to the problem of inferring causation from observed associations. *American Journal of Epidemiolgy,* 1971, 93, 443-456.

[176] Zapka, JG; Bert, L; Stoddard, AM; Ockene, JK; Goins, KV; Bonollo. D. Smoking cessation counseling with pregnant and postpartum women: A survey of community health center providers. *American Journal of Public Health,* 2000, 90, 78-84.

[177] Zaren, B; Limdmark, G; Gebre-Medhin, M. Maternal smoking and body composition of the newborn. *Acta Paediatrica,* 1996, 85, 213-219.

[178] Zavos, PM; Zamakoupis-Zavos, PN. Impact of cigarette smoking on human reproduction: its effects on male and female fecundity. *Technology,* 1999, 6, 9-14.

[179] Zenzes, MT; Reed, TE; Kasper, RF. Effects of cigarette smoking and age on maturation on human oocytes. *Human Reproduction,* 1997, 12, 1736-1741.

[180] Zhang, J; Savitz, DA; Schwingl, PJ; Cai, WW. A case-control study of paternal smoking and birth defect. *International Journal of Epidemiology,* 1992, 21, 273-278.

In: Progress in Smoking and Health Research
Editor: T. C. Jeffries, pp. 241-249
ISBN: 978-1-60021-686-2

Chapter X

Parental Awareness of Adolescent Tobacco Use

***Pamela P. Dinapoli*[1] *and Jacquelyn Shelley*[2]**
[1] 247 Hewitt Hall; University of New Hampshire; Durham NH 03824; ppdn@unh.edu
[2] University of New Hampshire; Department of Nursing; Durham NH 03824

Abstract

Tobacco use is the number one cause of preventable death in the United States (U.S. Department of Health and Human Services, 2001). While there has been much research dedicated to adolescents and adolescent health risk activities, there remains a gap in knowledge surrounding parental awareness of these risk behaviors specifically as it relates to the decision to initiate tobacco use. The purpose of this current study is to examine parental awareness of adolescent tobacco use in a population of middle school students. Unique to this study is the dyadic approach to investigation. Twenty-two dyadic pairs of parents and adolescents were surveyed. The results of this study demonstrate that there is a gap in family communication around tobacco use. While parents were generally accurate when reporting that their own child did not smoke, they underestimated the behavior of their child's peers'. Adolescents report rarely having tobacco related conversations with mothers and sometimes talking with fathers about tobacco. There was also concordance between the parents' responses and the adolescents' response around collaborative decision making. The respondents felt that the adolescent within a family is being told exactly what to do by his or her parent; limiting their opportunity to make decisions. Parents must engage their children in conversation about their own behavior and that of their peers. During middle school and high school adolescents are faced with powerful peer influences and decisions about risk behaviors. If these teens are not able to make their own decisions in their home it can be assumed that they will have a difficult time with social decision making, which may lead to detrimental choices. Parents need to be aware of these facts so they can accurately monitor the behaviors of their child and child's peers and potentially health risk decision making.

Keywords: Tobacco, Decision making, parental awareness.

Introduction

Tobacco use is the number one cause of preventable death in New Hampshire as well as the United States (U.S. Department of Health and Human Services, 2001). Every day more than 5,000 young people under the age of 18 make the decision to start smoking by trying their first cigarette. As a public health issue, the current costs of direct medical expenditures attributed to smoking total more than $75 billion per year. In addition, smoking costs an estimated $80 billion per year in lost productivity (http://www.cdc.gov/nccdphp/pe_factsheets/pe_tobacco.htm). Approximately 36 percent of youths who try cigarettes will progress to daily use, most within two years after first trying a cigarette, and three-quarters of them will continue to smoke daily eight years later (Johnston, O'Malley and Bachmann., 1999; U.S. Department of Health and Human Services, 1998). If current trends continue, 6.4 million people currently under the age of 18 will die prematurely from a tobacco-related disease (Thompson, 2003).

While there has been much research dedicated to adolescents and their own perceptions of tobacco and related risk behaviors, there remains a gap in knowledge surrounding parental awareness of these risk behaviors. Parental direction has a powerful effect on the reduction of risk behaviors in young adolescents (Nelson, Patience and MacDonald, 1999). The purpose of this current study is to examine parental awareness of adolescent tobacco use in a population of middle school students. It is known that family attributes, such as consistent open communication around decision making, have a strong persistent effect on adolescent decision making. Unfortunately, it is proposed that parents are not aware of their child's behaviors, including their use of tobacco. If this is true, this may be an important portal for the development of family based interventions designed to decrease engagement and involvement with tobacco.

Literature Review

Parental Awareness and Parental Communication

Parental awareness as defined by both the quantity and quality of parental communication and parental monitoring surrounding decision making and the initiation of adolescent health risk activities, specifically tobacco use, is a topic that has not been widely researched. Studies that exist around parental influence have focused largely on the role of the parent in adolescent smoking emphasizing only the quality of the relationship, operationalized in most studies as family caring (Neumark-Sztainer, 1999). Instead, because of the importance of peer groups in adolescent decision making, the majority of health risk behavior studies consistently demonstrate this relationship rather than the parental relationship (Beal, Ausiello and Perrin, 2001; Chopak, Crockett and Vickary, 1998). There have also been several studies involving adolescents and tobacco use focusing on themes such as access to cigarettes, incidence of initiation, trends in tobacco use, perceived risks, underestimation of use and school based prevention programs (Grandpre, Alvaro, Burgoon,

Miller, Hall, 2002; Panter, 2002; Thakur, Rosenthal, Latta, Robinson, and Diamond, 2003; Williams et al., 2002).

In the study of adolescent risk behaviors in general, it has been shown that parental monitoring has an influence on the behaviors of adolescents. In the limited existing research surrounding parental awareness of tobacco use, a common theme is the underestimation by parents of their child's use. While greater awareness of tobacco use is reported by parents of older adolescents, few studies examine the junior high population (Williams et al., 2002). In order to effectively monitor their children, parents must have knowledge of their child's participation in risk behaviors; unfortunately parents of young adolescents may not have this knowledge.

Studies show that parents significantly underestimated their youth's participation in risk behaviors including tobacco use. Williams, Bertrand, Davis and McDermitt (2002) surveyed 2,118 adolescents and 1,388 parents regarding their knowledge of their child's substance use. The results showed that 23 percent of adolescents reported using 1 to 5 cigarettes per day or more. Of the 1,388 parents surveyed, only 9.8 percent believed their child had used tobacco in the past month. While parents were accurate when reporting their child did not use tobacco, they underestimated when their child was actively smoking. Only 39 percent of parents were aware that their child was using tobacco. Eighty six percent of parents reported that their child did not use tobacco when in fact 48 percent of students reported tobacco use yet, 45.2 percent felt that other children in their own child's class were smoking (Cornick et al, 1999; Deffenbaugh, 2001; Young and Zimmerman, 1998).

The purpose of this study was to explore parental awareness of adolescent tobacco by examining concordance of responses between parent and child relative to family monitoring, family communication and family decision making. The hypothesis of this study was that many parents were not aware of their child's experimentation with tobacco at a young age

Methods

This was a descriptive correlational study using a survey design. Correlational research helps to develop and refine explanatory knowledge for nursing practice (Burns and Grove, 2003). The purpose of this correlational research is to examine relationships between or among family monitoring, family communication, family decision making and the early initiation of tobacco use. A measure of parental awareness of tobacco use reported by parents does not fully illustrate the dynamic of parent communication and parental monitoring. Unique to this study was the dyadic approach to investigation meaning that both the parent and adolescent were participants. The degree of correspondence between parent and child based on parallel measures offers a more dynamic picture of this important social influence.

Theoretical Framework

Socio-Ecological Model of Health Behavior was the conceptual frame for this study measuring parental awareness of adolescent tobacco use. The National Network for Health adapted the Bronfenbrenner (1987) model of health behavior to create a map of influences in adolescent substance abuse. This model views the adolescent substance user as the center unit and is influenced by surroundings such as peer groups, spiritual communities, school, and family. Studies have already shown that peer groups play a large part in adolescent decision-making (Chopak et al., 1998). However, little has been studied surrounding the influence of parents. In this model, family factors that influence adolescents would include communication process, monitoring, and shared activities (The National Network for Health). Parental knowledge or how a child's perception of that knowledge impacts their own decision making process are not included in this model.

Instrumentation

For the purpose of this study a tool was adapted from two previously standardized tools with proven reliability. Questions were extracted from the "Alberta Youth and Family Lifestyle Survey" developed by Williams et al. (2002) and the Youth Risk Behavior Surveillance Survey instrument (http:///www.cdc.gov/nccdphp/dash/yrbs, retrieved April 5, 2005). Confirmatory factor analysis (alpha= .86) was used to confirm the content validity of the new modified tool. The adolescent questionnaire, which was pilot tested for readability and age appropriateness for early adolescents in middle school, was administered on site. The tool consisted of 26 items and included topics such as current tobacco use, influences on making the decision, feelings about parental knowledge, family communication, and the influence of peers. The same questionnaire, was piloted for readability and age appropriateness, was adapted for use as the parental questionnaire and was mailed to parents. The questionnaire included topics such as their knowledge of middle school tobacco use, their own child's tobacco use, their view of family communication, and their own tobacco habits.

Sample

The sampling frame for this study was drawn from a middle school setting, grades 6-8 in a rural New England state. The population of this school is primarily white, other ethnic groups represented a very small percentage of the population and included African American, Hispanic and Asian. There was a wide economic range mirroring the prevalence profile of regular smokers nationally. The gender ratio approached 1:1 male to females. Previous population based assessments revealed that within the school 16% of students report experimenting with or using tobacco regularly before the age of 13, rising to 18% between the ages of 13-14 (http://www.dhhs.state.nh.us/YTS).

Results

Sample Demographics

A total of 60 parental surveys were mailed to randomly selected parents. Twenty-two parental surveys were returned along with adolescent consent (n= 22 dyadic pairs). For a response rate of thirty-six percent. The parent sample was composed of 14 married couples and 8 divorced or separated couples. The mean parental education of participating parents was high school. The parent participants reported most parents either never smoked or no longer use tobacco. The consenting adolescent of the participating parent was then given the adolescent questionnaire. The sample of 22 adolescents was evenly split with 11 students in sixth grade and 11 students in eighth grade. The gender of the adolescent group consisted of 9 females and 13 males. Three adolescents in the sample reported that they were currently using cigarettes. Of these respondents two were in the eighth grade and one was in the sixth grade. Of the total sample of 22 adolescents, 10 participants reported that "a few" to "most" of their friends were currently smoking cigarettes. Among the parents of the 3 adolescents who reported positive smoking behaviors only one parent was aware of their child's behavior.

Data Analysis

Data analysis began with simple measures of central tendency to describe the sample and characteristics of their responses. This was followed by the use of bivariate correlation to examine the concordance between parental and child report of parental awareness variables including parent communication and parental monitoring.

Family Care and Decision Making

Parents and adolescents were asked about their perceptions of how family decisions are made between parent and child. Results of the bivariate correlation indicated that families in this study are not collaborating with their adolescents when making family decisions. Rather the responses demonstrate that the majority of adolescents in this study are being told exactly what to do by his or her parent. Respondents answered questions using a Likert scale rating system of 0 to 4 with 0 being "never" and 4 being "very often". There was concordance between the parents' responses and their adolescents' on this same question (table 1).

Table 1. Perceptions of Family Caring and Decision Making

	Adolescent	Mother	Father
Perceptions of decision making with parents	1.72 (sd=.9)	1.9 (sd=1.1)	1.65 (sd =.7)
Perceptions Index Family Caring (care/support/rule enforcement)	10.0 (sd=1.8)	11.3 (sd=.65)	10.7 (sd 1.8)

In addition to decision making, parents and adolescents were also asked how they viewed parental care, support, and fairness with rule enforcement. Based on the factor analysis, questions were aggregated and used to create an index that was a proxy measure for family caring. An index was used to acknowledge that the concept of family caring is a complex one. The collective responses were totaled to achieve a composite score, therefore the highest score and individual could receive was a 12. There was concordance between parents and children in perceptions of family care, support, and rule enforcement. This finding shows that both adolescents and parents report that parents are "there for them when needed" and are "fair with rule enforcement." Further, both mothers and fathers demonstrate accuracy in their perceptions of their own adolescents' response to these particular questions.

To further understand the quality of family communication around tobacco use in predicting parental awareness, parents and adolescents were asked to report the frequency of tobacco related discussions they had with each other in the past 12 months. On a scale of 1 to 4, adolescents perceived that they rarely had tobacco related conversations with mothers and sometimes talking with fathers about tobacco. Parents reported they sometimes had these conversations while others reported never talking to their adolescent about tobacco in the past year. These results indicate that both adolescents and parents were in agreement that they rarely had family discussions about tobacco (table 2).

Table 2. Tobacco Related Communication

	Frequency of tobacco related conversations with mother	Frequency of tobacco related conversation with father
Adolescent	1.3	2.2
Parent	2.2	1.9

Discussion

Findings in this study revealed that there is a gap in family communication around tobacco use. Perceived parental trust and communication have both previously been shown to protect against the initiation of risk behaviors including tobacco, drug, alcohol and sexual activity (Borawski, Leveres-Landis, Lovegreen, Trapl, 2003). In this study parental perceptions of communication did not correspond with their actual behavior. That is, despite parents feeling like they were communicating well with their children in general, both parent and child agreed they were not having tobacco related conversations. Uncertainty of how to talk to teens about tobacco may be the cause of the gap in family communication of tobacco behaviors. This result is consistent with previous research which suggests that if parents assume their child is not smoking, there is no need for discussions. For example, the perception that "my child would never smoke therefore I do not need to discuss the pros and cons of tobacco use." In fact these discussions are crucial to both adolescent tobacco prevention and cessation.

Despite the small number of current adolescent smokers in this study, the results demonstrate that each of these parents underestimated their child's behavior. While parents were accurate when reporting that their own child did not smoke, they did underestimate the behavior of their child's peers'. These findings have important implications for nursing practice. The literature around peer influence on tobacco use supports the fact that peers have a large influence on adolescent behaviors (Chopak et al., 1998). Another perspective is that parents may feel that if they had one discussion when the child was younger it will endure through adolescence (Deffenbaugh, 2001; Williams et al., 2002). That is, "I talked to my child about tobacco use he would never smoke." In fact these conversations need to be ongoing and context specific. Those adolescents who were not current smokers are vulnerable to the combination of peer influence and lack of parental awareness of peer behavior. These variables, together with a lack of proper parental guidance influencing decision making, have the potential to lead to experimentation with tobacco use leading to nicotine addiction at an early age.

Decision-making is a key factor in adolescent development. A second important theme that emerged in this study was that adolescents were not given the opportunity to make decisions within their families. Rather, adolescents are being told what to do by their parents. These issues around decision making are interesting because not only do the results indicate adolescents are not being allowed to collaborate on family decisions, but there is also evidence that adolescents were aware that they were not being given choices or opportunity by their parents. Without the opportunity to make informed decisions in the home, adolescents have the potential to make poor health behavior decisions when confronted by those behaviors of their peers. Parents need to understand that during adolescence, family communication must involve decision making as an important part of development. A lack of adolescent involvement in decision making can lead to engagement in risk behaviors such as cigarette smoking. It is important for nurses to intervene with families at the vulnerable ages of 12 and 14 because of the pressures faced by this age group.

Nurses have a responsibility to educate parents about the omnipresent danger of tobacco. Parents need to be aware of adolescent behavior so they can begin to have open discussions with their children. Parents need encouragement to both talk to their children at an early age, and they need education on how and when to approach the sensitive topic. Parents also should engage their children in conversation about their own behavior and that of their children's peers. The beginning of middle school and high school presents these adolescents with powerful peer influences and decisions about risk behaviors. If these teens are not able to make their own decisions in their home it can be assumed that they will have a difficult time with social decision making around tobacco use, which may lead to the choice to smoke. Parents need to be aware of these facts so they can effectively monitor their adolescents and prevent their teens from making the decision which is to initiate tobacco use.

The results of this preliminary study indicate that decision making and communication are not occurring within this sample of families. Unfortunately, the response rate in the current study was low. This may have been due to the sampling technique. Consent to participate forms were sent home with middle school students. Parents were then asked to mail their responses. When the responses were received the child was then approached for their assent to participate. This multi step procedure was too cumbersome. In addition, no follow up phone calls or reminder post cards were used in an attempt to increase response rates. While there were identified limitations in this current study, there is a need for further research surrounding adolescents, parents, and tobacco in terms of prevention of initiation for these at risk adolescents.

While the results of this study are limited by the low response rate, there is sufficient evidence to suggest that nurses must alert parents that both quantity and quality make good family communication. Assuming both are occurring within families may lead the practitioner to overlook and important risk factor for the initiation of tobacco use among young adolescents. Simply put, if parents assume there is no risk, they may in fact be putting their children at greater risk for smoking. Parents who learn to incorporate their youth into family decision making, and have frank conversations with their adolescents there may be a better chance of creating a generation who are making healthy decisions when faced with risk behaviors.

References

Borawski, E.A., Leveres-Landis, C.E., Lovegreen, L.D.. and Trapl, E.S. (2003). Parental Monitoring, Negotiated Unsupervised Time and Parental Trust; the Role of Perceived Parenting Practices in Adolescent Health Risk Behaviors. *Journal of Adolescent Health,* 33(2): 60-70.

Burns, N. and Grove, S. (2003). Understanding Nursing Research. (3rd ed.). Philadelphia: W.B. Saunders Company.

CDC. Trends in Cigarette Smoking Among High School Students in the United States, 1991-2001. *MMWR.* 2002;51:409-12.

Chopak, J.S., Crockett, L.J., Vicary, J.R. (1998). Predicting Alcohol and Tobacco Use in a Sample of Rural Adolescents. *American Journal of Health Behavior,* 22(5),334-341.

Cornick, G., Feigelman, S. Galbraith, J., Kaljee, L., Li, X., Stanton, B., Zhou, Y. (1999). Parental Underestimates of Adolescent Risk Behavior: A Randomized, Controlled Trial of a Parental Monitoring Intervention. *Journal of Adolescent Health,* 26,18-26.

Deffenbaugh, K. Hutchinson, R., Blankschen, M. (2001). Substance Use Among Youth (Grades 4-12) in Rural Indiana: Student's Reported Use vs. Parents' Perceptions of Student Use. *Journal of Alcohol and Drug Education,* 39(1). 19-34.

Grandpre, J., Alvaro, E., Burgoon, M., Miller, C., Hall, J. (2003). Adolescent Reactance and Anti-Smoking Campaigns: A Theoretical Approach. *Health Communication,* 15(3), 349-367.

http://www.cdc.gov/nccdphp/pe_factsheets/pe_tobacco.htm accessed March 18, 2005.

http://www.dhhs.state.nh.us/YTS accessed March 18, 2005.

Johnston, L. D., O'Malley, P. M., Bachman, J.G. (1999). National Survey Results on Drug Use, Retrieved September 30, 2003 from www.monitoringthefuture.org.

National Network for Health. (2002). Alcohol, Tobacco, and Other Drugs: Promising Positive Youth Development, Retrieved September 26, 2003 from www.nnh.org/products/pospaper.htm.

Nelson, B. Patience, T., MacDonald, D. (1999). Adolescents Risk Behavior and the Influence of Parents and Education. *Journal of the American Board of Family Practice,* 12(6), 436-443.

New Hampshire Department of Health and Human Services. Tobacco Prevention and Control Program, Retrieved September 26, 2003 from www.dhhs.state.nh.us.

Panter, A.T. (2002). Assessing Tobacco Beliefs Among Youth Using Item Response Theory Models. *Drug Alcohol Dependence,* 68(1), 21-39.

Thakur, N., Rosenthal, M., Latta, P., Robinson, J., Diamond, J. (2003). Cigarettes Sources for Teens by Grade: Implications for Prevention and Intervention. *Internet Journal of Academic Physician Assistants,* 3(1), 35-42.

Thompson, T. (2003). The Burden of Tobacco Use. Retrieved September 26, 2003 from http://www.cdc.gov/nccdphp/aag/aag_osh.htm.

U.S. Department of Health and Human Services. Incidence of Initiation of Cigarette Smoking. *MMWR.* 1998; 47:837-40.

U.S. Department of Health and Human Services. *Women and Smoking: A Report of the Surgeon General.* Atlanta, GA: U.S. Department of Health and Human Services, CDC, National Center for Chronic Disease Prevention and Health Promotion, Office on Smoking and Health; 2001.

Williams, R.J. Bertrand, L. Davis, R. M., McDermitt, D.R. (2002). Parental Awareness of Adolescent Substance Abuse. *Addictive Behaviors,* 28(4),803-809.

Young, T.L., Zimmerman, R. (1998). Clueless: Parental Knowledge of Risk Behaviors of Middle School Students. *Archives of Pediatrics and Adolescent Medicine,* 158(11),1137-1146.

In: Progress in Smoking and Health Research
Editor: T. C. Jeffries, pp. 251-284
ISBN: 978-1-60021-686-2

Chapter XI

Teenage Smoking: Longitudinal vs. Cross-Sectional Modelling

Said Shahtahmasebi
The Good life Research Centre Trust; Principal Consultant,
Research and Development integrated Solutions (RaDiSol);
975A South Eyre Road; RD 1, Rangiora. New Zealand

Abstract

Adolescent behaviour is a dynamic process. Adolescent behaviour outcomes will be due to temporal dependencies, latent variables, feedback effect and other socio-economic and socio-environmental factors most of which are process outcomes themselves. Survey studies, cross-sectional and even some longitudinal studies show very little appreciation for the dynamic nature of the process and often concentrate on the socio-economic variables. Such an approach provides a flat snapshot view of a dynamic and multi dimension process which raises more questions than providing insight. The consequences of failing to account for the dynamic features of the process under study may be erroneous results and misleading conclusions with serious implications for the process of policy development. These issues are illustrated and discussed in this chapter using the behaviour outcome "teenage smoking".

Introduction

Adolescence is considered to be the crucial period during which attitudes and pattern of behaviour are formed[1,2]. The operative phrase is "formation of patterns of behaviour and attitudes"; and the keywords are time, attitudes and behaviour. However, attitudes and behaviour are dynamic processes and are subject to change over time. Thus policy makers, health promotion groups, and counsellors all attempt to apply programmes to change adolescent behaviour by influencing attitudes. There are several problems with this approach. The first is the presumption that a change in attitude would commensurate in a change in behaviour. The second problem is the quality and validity of the evidence used to develop programmes to influence attitudes. Another main issue is the lack of a critical assessment and evaluation of the programmes. The lack of a critical approach will mean that the true effect of any schemes and any consequences whether positive or otherwise would never be known. For example, there is very little evidence to evaluate the global anti-obesity trend; what effect have these trends had on the incidence of anorexia and related issues and conversely, have they actually contributed to a reduction in the prevalence of obesity?

Taken at face value, an initial analysis of the literature may point to a chaos theory to model adolescent behaviour and decision making processes. For example, it is expected that, given the amount of information available to young people via the many formal, informal and unobtrusive sources, young people may modify their behaviour accordingly. However, the expected outcome does not always match real outcomes; policy makers and most adults would like to blame peer pressure, standards of upbringing, personality and individual characteristics, and social class for adolescents' behaviour outcomes. Yet, these outcomes whether smoking, drinking, drugs, teenage sexual behaviour and pregnancy, HIV/AIDS, indulging in dangerous sports, or self harm etc are often the result of a complex decision making process that encompasses not only the above factors but also social policy, the role of the media, and society. Without a point of reference, or social guidelines and framework, adolescence is a period of more volatility and experimentation exacerbating the process of decision making. It is more appropriate to emphasise that past behaviour and learning as more influential.

In an environment that encourages practising evidence-based decision making, policies and decisions are only as good as the evidence that informs the process of decision making. The first issue to consider is the quality and relevance of the evidence. The possibility exists that at any stage during the process of gathering evidence, the integrity of evidence may be compromised e.g. design problems, analytical methods, and interpretation of results. Due to the dynamics of human behaviour, most study limitations are related to translating the available data into information and possible evidence. One major limitation in gathering evidence is from using cross-sectional data. There are complex statistical methods (e.g. structural equation models) for analysing cross-sectional data. However, these methods are computationally intensive and do not alter the fact that we are attempting inference from cross-sectional data. The remedy is, of course, to increase complexities in the study design and methodology[3]. For example, studying dynamic processes require longitudinally designed studies and appropriate longitudinal modelling methods for analysis.

On the other hand, being dynamic means that adolescent behaviour is subject to change, not only due to its own parameters (e.g. individual characteristics) but also due to parameters outside the process (e.g. preventional and interventional policies). Although studies investigating the net effect of preventional/interventional policies is unheard of, it is not difficult to imagine the adverse effects of policies based on intuition, poor or no research, or a gut feeling by a 'youth minister' or policy units – as is often the case - where an attempt to obtain evidence to support and promote a particular policy is made after its implementation. It is not too difficult to recognise this 'elective' model[4] of decision making through a study of available policy documents on changes in the education, social, health systems and other preventional/interventional policies such as youth suicide, obesity and alcohol and drug abuse.

It is rather ironic that, having approved and convincingly promoted the notion of "evidence" based decision making, by adopting an elective model, most decision makers and their associated Policy Units appear to have placed the emphasis on the order of where and when evidence is collected. Consider the educational outcome of "writing". The advancement in communication technologies in particular email and more recently text messaging using cellular phones, young people have created a culture in which "text" language is the common form of communicating. The noticeable consequence of such a culture has been to attenuate the traditional comprehension, reading and writing skills. Ironically, in New Zealand, a recent announcement[5] a few weeks before the final school exams hinted that the use of "text" language would be acceptable and would be marked in the exam. Such an announcement tends to validate the new skills as a replacement for the skills that the curricula was devised to teach. To be evaluated in a formal setting as the final school exams using informal language at the end of the *learning* period which incidentally includes reading, writing and comprehension would lead to an attenuation in educational standards. This is no way to increase the success rates of school leavers. It is noteworthy that "texting" language is not part of the curricula, more importantly; allowing an "exclusive" emphasis on other skills may lead to the erosion of previously learnt skills[6]. This example serves to illustrate some issues of dynamics: the feedback effect on a process outcome through society's behaviour and exogenous factors.

Therefore, this chapter aims to highlight some of the relevant issues associated with the collection and interpretation of evidence which are intended to inform the process of policy formation. These substantive and methodological (research and modelling) issues are illustrated using teenage smoking as an adolescent behaviour outcome.

The smoking literature suggests a large number of variables associated with teenage smoking including demographic, social, environmental, economic, emotional and psychological variables[7-13]. Specifically, smoking behaviour has been associated with the psycho-social effect of wishing to belong to a peer social group[14], self-esteem and parental smoking behaviour[15], the psychological process of risk assessment and risk taking[16-18]. Others suggest smoking behaviour is likely to be influenced through the family environment, which affects psychological well-being, adjustment and problem behaviour, perceived academic performance and school conduct[19,20]. This ambiguity in interpreting the results is further exacerbated by the subjective effect of smoking e.g. feelings of higher self-esteem and being in control[15,21]; a perceived 'benefit' effect as utilised in risk models[16,17].

Most studies of teenage smoking have relied on observational or survey questionnaire data. Most surveys include variables that are subjectively measured, e.g. self-reported health, perceptions and attitudes, and anxiety such as worrying about family or school matters. The inclusion of subjective variables exacerbates the problem twofold; (i) because of the measurement error associated with subjective variables, and, (ii) by adding confusion to the direction of causality. For example, the relationship between high self-esteem and smoking could be working in either direction. The consequences of including such variables in the analysis could lead to an over inflated relationship with the outcome variable and a possible mis-specification error[22].

The reported relationship between high self-esteem and smoking serves to demonstrate these difficulties. For example, Murphy et al [15] reported low self-esteem among the female group who indicated an intention to smoke. This means that the association between higher self-esteem and smoking [23] may become untenable, as it is likely that the individuals had lower self-esteem prior to taking up smoking. It is not surprising that researchers [24,25] applying a cross-sectional statistical technique to longitudinal data, reported a high correlation between smoking status in adolescence and in adulthood - as a cessation will often be accompanied by feelings of unease and anxiety[21,26].

It is not intended to provide a literature review on smoking behaviour - the interested reader is referred to the literature [7,8,27-29] - but rather to be concerned with an examination of evidence from analyses of the relationship between social characteristics and teenage smoking. The analyses seek to identify any effect of social circumstances over and above the better-understood effects of age and sex. Social circumstances are broadly defined and cover behavioural, attitudinal, emotional and self-esteem. In this chapter, the relevant issues are demonstrated, firstly using a typical bivariate analysis followed by a straightforward statistical modelling of a set of cross-sectional data. The cross-sectional modelling approach is further modified to illustrate pitfalls leading to misleading conclusions from cross-sectional analysis. In the final section of this chapter a longitudinal modelling of the same data set is presented and discussed.

Methods

Data

Around 60 secondary schools in the former Yorkshire Regional Health Authority geographical boundary agreed to take part in the survey. Years 9 and 11 (age range 11-16 years) in the 60 schools were surveyed using a health related behaviour questionnaire [30]. The survey was self-administered in classrooms during a normal lesson session. For complete anonymity; names, addresses and area postcodes were not collected. Furthermore, pupils were required to place the completed questionnaire in an unmarked envelope and drop it into a postbag themselves. The postbag was then returned to survey administrators.

The questionnaire covered topics related to the attitudes and behaviour of pupils with regard to health, e.g. physical exercise and out of school activities, nutrition, social contacts, dealing with problems, attitudes to and the use of drugs (including smoking and drinking). Relevant variables which are reported in the literature including self- esteem, worrying about a number of issues, e.g. family, friends and school, were extracted from the data set and are shown in table 2 (see also appendix I). The outcome variable "smoking" is a dichotomous dummy variable and takes the value "0" if a non-smoker (those who claimed they have never smoked or have given up smoking) and the value "1" if a smoker (those who claimed they smoked either regularly/occasionally).

Just over 10,000 pupils responded to the survey. Out of these, 9,230 cases were with a valid response on the smoking variable. Preliminary results suggested roughly equal numbers of boys and girls in the total sample and quite close to the ratio in the Regional population:

Eighteen percent of the 11-16 year olds smoked either occasionally or regularly; 60% of the smokers were girls and 40% were boys; and around 22% of the girls and 14% of the boys were smokers.

The 1994 survey was modified to include a form to be filled in by those who were in their final school year (16+ year olds). The form merely invited the pupils to indicate their interest to participate in a follow-up survey in two years time requiring them to fill in their contact details. Organisational changes within the NHS (National Health Service) during 1994 saw the abolition of the Regional Health Authorities in England and by 1996 the Yorkshire Regional Health Authority had ceased to exist. However, the survey was conducted as planned and 627 young adults were traced and re-interviewed using the same questionnaire instrument with slight modifications to some questions to suit the 18+ age category. This data set provided the linked 2 phase data on teenage smoking for the longitudinal modelling reported later in this chapter.

Statistical Modelling

Cross-Sectional Analysis

For this project we were interested in the prevalence of smoking. For this purpose smokers are defined as those occasional and regular smokers and coded "1". Non-smokers are all the others and coded "0" i.e. those who never smoked, had tried it once or twice, or had given up smoking.

Commonly, proportions on the basis of a bivariate analysis such as those shown in table 1 and sometimes proportions may be reported as a cross-classification with an associated probability as shown in table 2.

Table 1. Smoking status by gender

1994		*Sex*		*Total*
Freqs (Col %s)		*Male*	*Female*	
Smoker	No	188 (81.0%)	296 (76.5%)	484 (78.2%)
	Yes	44 (19.0%)	91 (23.5%)	135 (21.8%)
Total		232 (100%)	387 (100%)	619 (100%)

However, as discussed in the introduction one of the major issues in dealing with survey data is multicollinearity where several variables may be measuring the same effect in relation to an outcome variable. For example, in table 2, the variables "worrying about money" and "being happy with one's weight" appear to be strongly related to smoking. On the other hand as shown in table 3, there is sufficient evidence to suggest that both variables "worrying about money" and "being happy with one's weight" themselves are correlated. Therefore the questions to be asked may be; what is the net effect of each variable on smoking? And, are the net effects on smoking statistically significant? Do both variables measure similar effects (e.g. a personality trait) in relation to smoking?

Table 2. Selected variables from the Health Related Behaviour Questionnaire thought to be associated with smoking habits of young people. Bi-variate cross-classification;

Explanatory variables	Smoking
Socio-demographic	p
1- Age	***
2- Gender	***
3- Which parents live with	***
4- Where live	***
5- Social class (see §3)	*
Socio-environment	
6- Whether smoker	-
7- Whether drinks	***
8- Whether at least one in family smokes	***
9- Whether relative smokes	***
10- Whether best friend smokes	***
Socio-psychological	
11- Self-esteem	**
12- Whether happy with weight	***
13- Whether happy with body shape	***
14- Whether considers health when choosing food	**
14- Whether have a steady partner	***
15- How feels when meeting opposite sex	***
16- How feels when meeting own sex	***
17- Have a drink when have problem	***
How much worry about:	
18- school problems	***
19- money problems	***
20- health problems	***
21- career problems	***
22- problems with friend	***
23- family problem	***
24- the way you look	***

N=9230, *$p<.05$, **$p<0.001$, ***$p<0.00001$.

Table 3. Example of multi-collinearity in data: Cross-classification of selected explanatory variables from the 1994 wave: frequencies (column percentages)

	Happy with weight		Total
Worry about money	put on/lose	happy	
never	149 (44.3%)	151 (53.4%)	300 (49%)
a little	109 (32.4%)	91 (32.2%)	200 (32%)
a lot	78 (23.2%)	41 (14.5%)	119 (19%)
Total	336 (100%)	283 (100%)	619 (100%)
Pearson Chi-sq	8.66	(p=0.013)	
	Best friend smokes		Total
Worry about money	yes	no	
Never	125 (42.1%)	175 (54.3%)	300 (49%)
a little	102 (34.3%)	98 (30.4%)	200 (32%)
a lot	70 (23.6%)	49 (15.2%)	119 (19%)
Total	297 (100%)	322 (100%)	619 (100%)
Pearson Chi-sq	11.13	(p=0.004)	
	At ease with opposite sex		Total
Worry about money	yes	no	
never	240 (47.3%)	60 (53.6%)	300 (49%)
a little	177 (34.9%)	23 (20.6%)	200 (32%)
a lot	90 (17.8%)	29 (25.9%)	119 (19%)
Total	507 (100%)	112 (100%)	619 (100%)
Pearson Chi-sq	9.77	(p=0.008)	

Clearly, there are two major additional problems need to resolve when dealing with survey data; namely multicollinearity and the type of variables. The former can be dealt with within the statistical modelling framework by accounting for other variables when a new variable is fitted in the model. The latter refers to the method of measurement as to whether the variable may be defined as an objective or subjective measurement. In this case worrying about money and being happy with one's weight are both expressions of one's state of mind at a particular point in time and it is very difficult to quantify them objectively. As will be noticed through the remainder of this chapter and as reported in the introduction, subjective measures are responsible for model mis-specification, erroneous results and thus misleading conclusions.

With a binary dependent variable (smoker/non-smoker) and many independent variables, the common statistical approach is to fit a logistic regression model to the data. A logistic regression model (see Appendix II) was fitted to the data with the smoking variable (smoker/non-smoker) as response variable. For model fitting, the computer software package GLIM[31] was used. The method of "forward substitution" successive model fitting was adopted with the "best" additional variable added to the model at each stage. Improvement in the model as a result of adding in each variable in turn was assessed by the likelihood ratio test statistic and the process ceased when no additional variable was significant at 5% level. This approach can be very instructive in an exploratory study. In particular, a marked change in the significance of a remaining variable when a new variable is added to the model is indicative of a spurious relationship arising from statistical association with the added variable. On the other hand, with high multicollinearity in the data, the final model may be heavily dependent upon a marginal choice between two variables at some stage in the model fitting process. It is important to detect when this is occurring to prevent undue emphasis being given to one variable where others are practically indistinguishable in their explanatory power. Moreover, identification of nearly interchangeable variables may guide further research in reducing multicollinearity problems by combining variables in composite indices[32]. The results of this model fitting are shown in table 4.

Table 4. Standard logistic regression: odds ratios for the model of smoking prevalence with their appropriate 95% Confidence Limits after controlling for other factors

Explanatory variables	Lower	Odds Ratio	Upper
Age			
12-13	1.00	1.00	1.00
14-15	1.59	1.84	2.13
Sex			
male	1.00	1.00	1.00
female	1.68	1.96	2.30
Which parent live with			
both parents	1.00	1.00	1.00
mother only	0.92	1.13	1.40
father only	0.92	1.45	2.31
mother and step-father	1.18	1.48	1.84
father and step-mother	0.78	1.31	2.19
foster parents	1.78	3.74	7.87
other	0.79	1.31	2.14
Whether drinks			
no	1.00	1.00	1.00
yes	2.19	2.56	3.00
Whether at least one family smokes			
no	1.00	1.00	1.00
yes	1.40	1.62	1.89
Best friend smokes			
no	1.00	1.00	1.00
yes	12.23	14.16	16.36
Have partner			
never had one	1.00	1.00	1.00
not at the moment	1.44	2.02	2.85
yes, few weeks	2.25	3.25	4.71
yes, up to 6 months	3.21	4.77	7.09
yes, up to a year	1.72	2.80	4.53
yes, > 1 year	2.10	3.17	4.78

Table 4. (Continued.)

Explanatory variables	Lower	Odds Ratio	Upper
How feel with opposite sex			
very uneasy	1.00	1.00	1.00
a little uneasy	1.01	1.32	1.74
at ease	1.43	1.89	2.49
Happy with body shape			
no	1.00	1.00	1.00
yes	0.69	0.80	0.93
Considers health when choosing food			
never	1.00	1.00	1.00
sometimes	0.50	0.62	0.77
quite often	0.38	0.48	0.62
very often	0.23	0.32	0.43
always	0.30	0.44	0.63
Worry about money problems			
never/hardly ever	1.00	1.00	1.00
a little	1.12	1.33	1.58
quite a lot/a lot	1.43	1.71	2.05
Worry about family problems			
never/hardly ever	1.00	1.00	1.00
a little	0.97	1.17	1.42
quite a lot/a lot	1.15	1.37	1.62

Results from the Cross-Sectional Study

First, consider results from the standard logistic model shown in table 4. It can be seen that, from these results, it is quite easy to conclude that "best friend" has the largest effect on smoking followed by the variables "have partner"; "how feel with opposite sex"; "which parent live with"; and the two "worrying" variables. Results in table 4 also suggest that compared to a reference group the odds of being a smoker increased for those who claimed their best friend smokes (OR 14.58, 95% CI 12.63-16.83), for those who claimed to have a partner (OR 3.41, 95% CI 2.36-4.92), those who claimed to be at ease with the opposite sex (OR 1.80, 95% CI 1.37 to 2.36), those who claimed to worry a lot about money problems (OR 1.71, 95% CI 1.43-2.05) and those who claimed to worry a lot about family problems (OR 1.37, 95% CI 1.15-162). On the other hand, the odds of being a smoker decreased for those who claimed to be happy with their body shape (OR 0.75, 95% CI 0.65-0.87) and those who claimed to consider health often when choosing food (OR 0.50, 95% CI 0.39-0.63). Pupils who lived with foster parents appear to have an increased risk of nearly four times that of pupils who lived with both parents.

The result for "which parent live with" can be explained as past behaviour leading to a selection bias; it is plausible that smoking may well have started while in care prior to placement with foster parents[33].

However, as noted earlier, a problem arises, over the inclusion of subjectively measured social and emotional factors (arbitrarily headed socio-environmental and socio-psychological respectively) in the analysis. Social circumstances will have an impact on the prevalence of teenage smoking, in part, by affecting emotional variables e.g. the desire to belong to a peer group[14]. Controlling for these variables may therefore result in an over conservative attenuated estimate of the effects of social circumstances. Reverse causality is also possible, with emotional circumstances influencing social circumstances. Excluding these variables may therefore exaggerate the effect of social circumstances. As emphasized earlier, we cannot unravel completely the complex causal relationships likely between social circumstances, emotional, and teenage smoking. However, the analysis could be improved to get an idea of the role of socio-environmental and socio-psychological variables as independent effects on smoking or as intervening variables between the objective (arbitrarily headed socio-demographic) variables and smoking. We can assess the role of subjective variables by forcing the direction of causality from objective variables to the outcome (smoking). Therefore, models were fitted with and without socio-environment and socio-psychological variables[3,32-34]. Three models were fitted to the data; firstly a model of objective variables was constructed based on demographic variables. Secondly, social variables were introduced to this model, and, thirdly socio-psychological variables were then added to the second model. The results of this modelling process are shown in table 5. Note that the final model is the same as that in table 4.

The role different variables play in smoking can be examined by comparing results from the three models in table 5. The inclusion of socio-environmental factors (model 2) has a major impact on model 1 (table 5): there are significant changes in parameter estimates of the variables "gender", "age", "which parent live with" - and variables reflecting social status "where live" and "social class" are no longer significant and drop out of the model. While some increases in parameter estimates are to be expected when adding new significant variables to the logistic regression model, the large decrease in parameter estimates confirms that the effect of the variables "age" and "which parent live with" have substantially reduced. This is consistent with socio-environmental variables having an intervening effect between age, parent(s) and smoking. Similarly, when socio-psychological variables are added to model 2 (see model 2 to model 3, table 5), a modest decrease in parameter estimates of demographic and socio-environmental variables can be noted. This decrease is consistent with socio-psychological variables having an intervening effect between demographic and socio-environmental variables and smoking.

It is interesting to note that the variables self-esteem, worrying about school and whether happy with weight, significant on their own (table 2) failed to remain in the final model after controlling for other variables. On the other hand, the variable "being happy with body shape" remains significant and enters the final model. It is therefore plausible that the variable "being happy with body shape" may reflect the respondents' state of mind at the time of the interview regardless of actual body shape and weight. This means that, in addition to body shape, the variable "happy with body shape" may well be an indication of this group's insensitivity to social pressures; social influences that may lead to smoking (e.g. see also [35]). In particular, individuals with similar body shape may have different outcomes; some become smokers and some do not.

Table 5. Model fitting results for the model of smoking - N=9230

	Model 1		*Model 2*		*Model 3*	
Explanatory variables	Parameter estimate	Standard error	Parameter estimate	Standard error	Parameter estimate	Standard error
Demographic factors						
Age						
12-13	0.00		0.00		0.00	
14-15	1.06	0.06	0.68	0.07	0.61	0.08
Gender						
male	0.00		0.00		0.00	
Female	0.52	0.06	0.68	0.07	0.67	0.08
Which parent live with						
both parents	0.00		0.00		0.00	
mother only	0.47	0.08	0.23	0.10	0.12	0.11
father only	0.69	0.18	0.49	0.23	0.37	0.24
mother and step-father	0.80	0.09	0.53	0.11	0.39	0.11
father and step-mother	0.77	0.20	0.44	0.25	0.27	0.26
foster parents	1.63	0.29	1.56	0.37	1.32	0.38
Other	0.73	0.19	0.38	0.24	0.28	0.25
Where live						
town/city centre	0.00					
town/city suburb	-0.30	0.13				
small town/city centre	-0.08	0.11				
small town/city sub.	-0.26	0.11				
in village	0.10	0.10				
outside town/village	0.20	0.13				
Social class(see Appendix I)						
high	0.00					
medium	0.15	0.10				
Low	0.25	0.09				
Socio-environmental factors						
Whether drinks						
no			0.00		0.00	
Yes			1.11	0.08	0.94	0.08
Whether at least one family smokes						
no			0.00		0.00	
Yes			0.60	0.08	0.47	0.08
Best friend smokes						
no			0.00		0.00	
Yes			2.81	0.07	2.65	0.07
Socio-psychological factors						
Have partner						
never had one					0.00	
not at the moment					0.70	0.17
yes, few weeks					1.18	0.19
yes, up to 6 months					1.56	0.20
yes, up to a year					1.03	0.25
yes, > 1 year					1.15	0.21

Table 5. (Continued).

	Model 1		Model 2		Model 3	
Explanatory variables	Parameter estimate	Standard error	Parameter estimate	Standard error	Parameter estimate	Standard error
How feel with opposite sex						
very uneasy					0.00	
a little uneasy					0.28	0.14
at ease					0.64	0.14
Happy with body shape						
no					0.00	
Yes					-0.22	0.08
Considers health when choosing food						
never					0.00	
sometimes					-0.48	0.11
quite often					-0.73	0.12
very often					-1.15	0.15
Always					-0.83	0.19
Worry about money problems						
never/hardly ever					0.00	
a little					0.29	0.09
quite a lot/a lot					0.54	0.09
Worry about family problems						
never/hardly ever					0.00	
a little					0.16	0.10
quite a lot/a lot					0.31	0.09

It can be seen that change in the parameter estimate variable "best friend smokes" from model 2 to model 3 (table 5) is over two times its standard error. This change is consistent with variable "best friend" having an intervening effect between smoking and demographic variables. If there is a 'true' best friend effect it is too complex to distinguish with cross-sectional data. As discussed in the introduction, it is plausible that prior to taking up smoking such pupils may have had a lower self-esteem, a wish to gain confidence, a desire to belong to a peer group and possibly lacked social and parental guidance. There is some evidence to suggest that parental influence indirectly predicts lower levels of smoking [36-38]. The "best friend" effect may not be straightforward to interpret with these data because we have no knowledge of these pupil's previous smoking habits; they may have been a smoker prior to the friendship. Furthermore, the high odds ratio for 'best friend' may well be inflated due to a pragmatic sampling strategy. Surveying of all pupils within classrooms in selected schools may have achieved maximum response, but has added complexities to the data, e.g (i) the clustering effect where pupils with similar outcome characteristics tend to form clusters (or social groups), and (ii) the possibility of double counting where pupils in the same classroom cite each other as best friend (e.g., see Stuart[39]). Cross-sectional analysis of such data will lead to an artificially inflated effect of 'best friend" on smoking (e.g., see[40]). Therefore, it is unwise to interpret "best friend" directly as peer pressure effect.

The result for the variable "how feels with opposite sex" in table 4 suggests that feeling at ease with the opposite sex increases the likelihood of being a smoker which may imply that "more confident" pupils are likely to smoke. On the other hand, table 5 suggests the possibility of a more dynamic social process (notice changes in the parameter estimates of model 3 compared with model 2). Once again we have no knowledge either of the pupils' past smoking behaviour or past patterns of their social interactions with the opposite sex. Therefore, it would be unwise to interpret the result for this variable simply as is, and certainly it should not be confused with any causal relationship between confidence and smoking.

From the results in table 4 and 5 similar conclusions can be made for the variables "considers health when choosing food", "worry about money problems" and "worry about family problems". These three variables were statistically significant and remained in the final model. As most pupils have been made aware of the dangers of smoking, these variables may be a proxy for the underlying effect of attitudes to health and smoking. The choice of food represents the health consciousness of pupils suggesting that those who attach importance to health related behaviour have a reduced risk of being a smoker. While the worrying variables serve to demonstrate the subjective effect of smoking where smoking leads to the maintenance of smoking [21,26]. Again without prior information on the pupils smoking behaviour these results do not constitute evidence for worrying leading to smoking. This association between smoking and worrying/health may help explain the prevalence but not incidence of smoking.

It appears that those pupils who have or had a partner (boyfriend or girl friend) are more likely to be a smoker than those who never had a partner. It is not clear whether having a partner is the reason for pupils' smoking habits, or whether young people smoke to be sociable. However, from the results shown in table 5, while there is a small change in the parameter estimate of the objective variables from model 2 to 3, the change in the parameter estimates of the socio-environmental variables are around twice their standard error. It is, therefore plausible that the variable "have a partner" may be reflecting a "best friend" effect or a "foster parent" effect, which were discussed earlier.

Although the incidence and prevalence of smoking has been associated with social deprivation [41] and social class [42,43], our data suggested that there is no supportive evidence that such a link may be through social class.

Longitudinal Approach

Another major problem with survey type studies is that they do not allow an assessment of past behaviour (e.g. state dependence) and do not handle residual heterogeneity due to omitted variables (e.g. personality, the feel good factor and resilience). Residual heterogeneity results when systematic but unmeasured characteristics of individuals contribute to the response pattern over time (e.g. see[44]). In survey studies some individual characteristics are often omitted from the study because they are either unobserved or difficult to measure. Omitted characteristics, such as resilience, could lead to spurious relationships between the observed characteristics and the outcome variable; often leading to overestimation of the relationships between the response (in this case, smoking) and the explanatory variables. In this context, within the literature, residual heterogeneity due to omitted variables is commonly referred to as heterogeneity. In this chapter, the terms residual heterogeneity, omitted variables and heterogeneity are used interchangeably to refer to inherent individual-specific variability (e.g. personality, resilience). Conventional statistical models such as regression models subsume the individual-specific heterogeneity into the structural error term, thus violating the independence assumption and leading to a well-known specification error[22,40]. On the other hand, the traditional methods of analysing longitudinal data, such as analysis of end-points or analysis of variance, do not fully utilise the properties of the data, in particular, such methods exclude the heterogeneity effect[44,45]. A more appropriate method is the application of mixture models in which the error is specified by a "variance component". In such a model, heterogeneity is implicitly defined in the equation as a time-constant term which is separate from the regression error term (see statistical analysis and appendix III). The recent interest in the application of mixture models has led to the inclusion of options for mixture modelling in most major statistical packages such as SAS and GenStat. However, we are particularly interested in the method of estimating mixture models with the specification operationalised by Davies[46-50] and applied within the social sciences (e.g. see[3,50]). This method of estimation uses integrated likelihood and takes into account the fact that some individuals will never (or have a very low probability of) change (see statistical analysis). The adequacy of a model is tested formally using analysis of deviance; in other words, to test the significance of an explanatory variable (e.g. gender), the change in deviance upon adding that variable to the model is compared to the chi-squared distribution on the corresponding number of degrees of freedom (e.g. 1 in the case of gender).

A past behaviour effect exists when the experience of a particular outcome itself changes the probability of experiencing that event on subsequent occasions. It is also important to have measures of past behaviour on smoking and explanatory variables in order to gain some insight into the direction of causality e.g. the confidence-smoking relationship. For example, Murphy et al[15] reported low self-esteem among the female group who indicated an intention to smoke. This means that the assertion that the more confident individuals are more likely to be a smoker[23] may become untenable, as it is likely that the individuals had lower self-esteem prior to taking up smoking. It is not surprising that researchers[24,25] applying a cross-sectional statistical technique to longitudinal data, reported a high correlation between smoking status in adolescence and in adulthood - as a cessation will often be accompanied by feelings of unease and anxiety[21,26].

Most studies of teenage smoking have relied on cross-sectional observational or survey questionnaire data. Although multicollinearity can be addressed with cross-sectional data, to address the omitted variables and past behaviour effects, longitudinal data are required. However, inappropriate analytical methodologies or researchers have employed methods that do not fully utilise the longitudinal nature of data such as the ability to account for heterogeneity will render longitudinal data useless as in[24,25,51-55]. Although, one study[55] had accounted for the past behaviour effect, unfortunately this had been achieved within a cross-sectional analysis framework. The possibility exist that the past behaviour effect owe its significance to a well known mis-specification error where the included explanatory variable (in this case past behaviour), through omitted variables, may be correlated with the structural error, see[3] chapters 6 and 8.

In this section we demonstrate the application of a longitudinal statistical modelling approach to the two-time point smoking data from a health related behaviour survey. For this purpose, we have adopted the same definition of smoking and fitted the cross-sectional model reported above to the longitudinal data. The main reason for this decision is to illustrate changes in moving from the cross-sectional model to a longitudinal model. As mentioned earlier, data for the longitudinal analyses came from 627 school leavers who had given consent to a follow up interview.

The descriptive analysis shown in table 6 suggests that out of the 627 subjects there were 619 valid cases; 62.5% were female and 37.5% were male; 22% of the 1994 sample were smokers which increased to 33% in 1996. However, over the two year period, there was not a noticeable change in the proportion of smokers by gender. Over this period there were movements in the smoking status as follows; 61% remained non-smoker, 17% remained smoker, 17% were non-smoker in 1994 but smoker in 1996, and 5% were smoker in 1994 but non-smoker in 1996.

Table 6. Smoking status over the time points

1994		*Sex*		*Total*
Freqs (Col %s)		*Male*	*Female*	
Smoker	No	188 (81.0%)	296 (76.5%)	484 (78.2%)
	Yes	44 (19.0%)	91 (23.5%)	135 (21.8%)
Total		232 (100%)	387 (100%)	619 (100%)

1996		*Sex*		*Total*
Freqs Col %s)		*Male*	*Female*	
Smoker	No	164 (70.4%)	248 (64.2%)	412 (66.6%)
	Yes	69 (29.6%)	138 (35.8%)	207 (33.4%)
Total		233 (100%)	386 (100%)	619 (100%)

		Smoker 1996		*Total*
Freqs (Row %s)		No	Yes	
Smoker 1994	No	380 (78.5%)	104 (21.5%)	484 (100 %)
	Yes	32 (23.7%)	103 (76.3%)	135 (100%)
Total		412 (66.6%)	207 (33.4%)	619 (100%)

This data set provides only two time observations on a young adult's health related behaviour. More linked observations on the individuals prior to 1994 and post 1996 are essential to enable us to unravel some of the complexities of interactions between life processes and what ever impact they may have on smoking status over time. However, even with two time observations per individual, we can illustrate how the move from cross-sectional to longitudinal observational data can provide added value from a statistical modelling perspective.

Table 7. Result of bivariate logistic model of smoking (one explanatory variable at a time);N=1238

Explanatory Variables	Chi-sq	p
Gender	4.16	0.0244
Age	26.92	0.0000
At least one family member smokes	40.10	0.0000
Drinks	91.16	0.0000
Best friend smokes	172.42	0.0000
Consider health when choosing food	9.15	0.0124
Happy with weight	10.76	0.0006
Have a partner	29.85	0.0000
At ease with opposite sex	13.56	0.0001
Worry about money	55.40	0.0000
Worry about family problems	14.81	0.0003

Statistical Analysis of Longitudinal Data

The outcome variable is a binary ('0' non-smoker; '1' smoker) variable. With a binary dependent variable and many independent variables, the common statistical approach is to fit a logistic regression model to the data. It can be noticed, table 7, that all the variables are statistically significant when entered into the model on their own. Once again it is worth remembering the high multicollinearity in data as suggested by table 3. The adopted statistical modelling approach allows control for other variables when testing a variable of interest in the model. For example to get an idea of the effect of "worry about money" on smoking, variables such as age, sex, happy with weight, whether drinks, and so on, are controlled for in the model. However, of particular concern is the longitudinal nature of the data set. The logistic regression is essentially a cross-sectional model and fitting such a model to longitudinal data will lead to a well known specification error and misleading result[56]. Furthermore, the model must allow for the possibility that substantial variation between respondents will be due to the heterogeneity which was discussed in the introduction. The model applied in this section is the logistic-normal random effects model[46-48]. This model incorporates a normal mixing distribution to account for the possibility of residual heterogeneity (scale parameter ω) in the data (see appendix III). The model can be fitted using the package SABRE (Software for the Analysis of Binary Recurrent Events)[49,50]. Some individuals will never (or have a very low probability of) change, i.e. will always be a smoker or will never smoke. These individuals are referred to as 'stayers'. SABRE provides the additional flexibility of incorporating "stayers" into the model by supplementing the normal mixing distribution with mass-points at $+/- \infty$ (see appendix III). Three models were fitted in SABRE: ordinary logistic regression model (table 8), a logistic-normal random effects model assuming no stayers (table 9), and a logistic-normal random effects model with stayers (table 10). With having only two time observations, it is impractical for us to control for past behaviour in this case, though it is possible to do in SABRE.

To demonstrate the consequences of fitting inappropriate models to data a standard longitudinal model, Generalised Estimating Equations (GEE), was also fitted to the data. The results from this model fitting exercise (table 11) may then be compared with those from SABRE that uses a methodology which allows control for heterogeneity.

Table 8. Results from pooled cross-sectional analysis; N=1238, (Deviance=1162.9; >> much greater than, << much less than)

Explanatory Variables	Parameter	Estimate	S. Error	χ^2	P
Gender	Male	0.00		2.4	>0.1
	female	0.25	0.17		
Age				5.6	>0.05
	15 and under	0.00			
	16 years	0.50	0.23		
	17 years	0.29	0.19		
	18 and over	0.34	0.23		
At least one family member smokes				10.4	<0.005
	yes	0.00			
	no	-0.48	0.15		
Drinks				42.9	<<0.0001
	yes	0.00			
	no	-1.26	0.21		
Best friend smokes				88	<<0.0001
	yes	0.00			
	no	-1.49	0.17		
Consider health when choosing food				11.2	<0.005
	never	0.00			
	sometimes	-0.66	0.23		
	always	-0.93	0.28		
Happy with weight				9	<0.005
	put on/lose	0.00			
	happy	-0.38	0.15		
Have a partner				2.9	>0.05
	yes	0.00			
	no	-0.26	0.15		

Table 8. (Continued).

Explanatory Variables	Parameter	Estimate	S. Error	χ^2	P
Gender	Male	0.00		2.4	>0.1
	female	0.25	0.17		
At ease with opposite sex				3.2	>0.05
	yes	0.00			
	no	-0.45	0.25		
Worry about money				11.2	<0.005
	never	0.00			
	a little	0.19	0.19		
	a lot	0.62	0.19		
Worry about family problems				1.5	>0.1
	never	0.00			
	a little	0.16	0.19		
	a lot	0.21	0.18		

Table 9. Results from longitudinal analysis using Sabre without Stayers; N=619, (Deviance=1091.26; >> much greater than, << much less than)

Explanatory Variables	Parameter	Estimate	S. Error	χ^2	P
Gender	Male	0.00		1.8	>>0.1
	female	0.43	0.32		
Age				10.5	<0.025
	15 and under	0.00			
	16 years	0.99	0.39		
	17 years	0.74	0.28		
	18 and over	0.86	0.41		
At least one family member smokes				7.4	<0.01
	yes	0.00			
	no	-0.76	0.28		
Drinks				39	<<0.0001
	yes	0.00			
	no	-1.99	0.37		
Best friend smokes				76	<<0.0001
	yes	0.00			
	no	-2.29	0.31		

Table 9. (Continued).

Explanatory Variables	Parameter	Estimate	S. Error	χ^2	P
Gender	Male	0.00		1.8	>>0.1
	female	0.43	0.32		
Consider health when choosing food				6.9	<0.05
	never	0.00			
	sometimes	-0.72	0.41		
	always	-1.28	0.49		
Happy with weight				5.7	<0.025
	put on/lose	0.00			
	happy	-0.63	0.27		
Have a partner				1.3	>>0.1
	yes	0.00			
	no	-0.29	0.26		
At ease with opposite sex				2.1	>>0.1
	yes	0.00			
	no	-0.59	0.41		
Worry about money				5.7	0.05
	never	0.00			
	a little	0.12	0.31		
	a lot	0.72	0.33		
Worry about family problems				2.82	>>0.1
	never	0.00			
	a little	0.42	0.32		
	a lot	0.47	0.31		
Scale (ω)		2.38	0.31		

Table 10. Results from longitudinal analysis with stayers using Sabre; N=619, (Deviance=1084.72; >> much greater than, << much less than)

Explanatory Variables	Parameter	Estimate	S. Error	χ^2	P
Gender	Male	0.00		0.6	>>0.1
	female	0.25	0.32		
Age				12	<0.01
	15 and under	0.00			
	16 years	1.00	0.36		
	17 years	0.75	0.27		
	18 and over	0.85	0.39		
At least one family member smokes				7.2	<0.01
	yes	0.00			
	no	-0.71	0.27		
Drinks				39	<<0.0001
	yes	0.00			
	no	-1.86	0.33		
Best friend smokes				80.5	<<0.0001
	yes	0.00			
	no	-2.19	0.28		
Consider health when choosing food				10.1	<0.01
	never	0.00			
	sometimes	-0.75	0.39		
	always	-1.45	0.47		
Happy with weight				6.2	<0.025
	put on/lose	0.00			
	happy	-0.63	0.26		
Have a partner				0.4	>>0.1
	yes	0.00			
	no	-0.16	0.26		
At ease with opposite sex				1.7	>>0.1
	yes	0.00			
	no	-0.54	0.41		

Table 10. (Continued).

Explanatory Variables	Parameter	Estimate	S. Error	χ^2	P
Gender	Male	0.00		0.6	>>0.1
	female	0.25	0.32		
Worry about money				5.8	0.05
	never	0.00			
	a little	0.13	0.29		
	a lot	0.71	0.31		
Worry about family problems				3.4	>0.1
	never	0.00			
	a little	0.52	0.32		
	a lot	0.44	0.29		
Scale (ω)		0.69	0.69		
				PROBABILITY	
	ψ_0 (end-point0)	0.58	0.16	0.36	
	ψ_1 (end-point1)	0.02	0.02	0.01	

Table 11. Results from fitting a GEE model to the data using GENSTAT

Explanatory Variables	Parameter	Estimate	S. Error
Gender	Male	0	
	female	0.254	0.165
Age			
	15 and under	0	
	16 years	0.504	0.229
	17 years	0.294	0.186
	18 and over	0.342	0.235
At least one family member smokes			
	yes	0	
	no	-0.483	0.15
Drinks			
	yes	0	
	no	-1.259	0.208
Best friend smokes			
	yes	0	
	no	-1.497	0.17

Table 11. (Continued).

Explanatory Variables	Parameter	Estimate	S. Error
Gender	Male	0	
	female	0.254	0.165
Age			
Consider health when choosing food			
	never	0	
	sometimes	-0.655	0.234
	always	-0.927	0.28
Happy with weight			
	put on/lose	0	
	happy	-0.379	0.154
Have a partner			
	yes	0	
	no	-0.257	0.15
At ease with opposite sex			
	yes	0	
	no	-0.45	0.259
Worry about money			
	never	0	
	a little	0.192	0.19
	a lot	0.622	0.196
Worry about family problems			
	never	0	
	a little	0.155	0.187
	a lot	0.213	0.182

Results from Lngitudinal Study

Tables 8-10 show the results from fitting the three models: a standard conventional logistic model to the pooled data from 1994 and 1996 (table 8), a logistic-normal random effects model assuming no stayers (table 9) and a logistic-normal random effects model with stayers (table 10). The tables provide the list of variables and their categories (parameters), their estimates and standard errors, chi-squared (χ^2) goodness of fit tests and their associated p-values. The statistical significance of a variable in the model is indicated by the χ^2 and its associated p-value. For this analysis the significance level was set to 5% (α=0.05). Thus, a χ^2 showing a p-value of less than or equal to 0.05 (e.g. <0.005, <0.0001) would indicate a statistically significant variable in the model. Positive estimates indicate likelihood of being a smoker compared with a reference category (usually the first category) e.g. 16 year old pupils are more likely to be smokers than those 15 and under. Similarly, negative estimates indicate likelihood of being a non-smoker e.g. those who claimed that their best friend did not smoke are less likely to be smoker (or more likely to be non-smoker) than those whose best friend was a smoker. As demonstrated in the cross-sectional analyses section the parameter estimates can easily be translated into odds ratios (OR) and interpreted appropriately. However, in this section our main concern is the comparison of the different models.

With the standard logistic regression model, the variables gender and 'worry about family problems' appear non-significant after controlling for other variables. Both variables were significant on their own without any control (gender at the 5% and 'worry about family problems' at the 0.5% significance levels). Similarly, age, highly significant on its own, is only marginally significant after controlling for other variables. Out of the remaining variables 'at ease with opposite sex' and 'have a partner' are also marginally significant (at the 10% level). All the other variables in the model appear significant at the 0.5% level.

In general the results suggest that having non-smoking family members, not drinking, considering health when choosing food and not worrying about money problems appear to reduce the likelihood of being a smoker. Furthermore, for each parameter estimate, an odds ratio and 95% confidence interval could easily be calculated, as in table 12.

Table 12. ORs and 95% C.I. for the variable 'best friend smokes'

Parameter		Estimate	S. Error	OR	Lower	Upper
From table 8 –	No	0.00		1.00		
	Yes	1.50	0.17	4.47	3.20	6.23
From table 9 –	No	0.00		1.00		
	Yes	2.29	0.31	9.88	5.42	18.04
From table 10 –	No	0.00		1.00		
	Yes	2.19	0.28	8.90	5.11	15.50

Our interest in this study is to explore how the parameter estimates change with increasing complexity in the modelling. A comparison of the standard logistic regression model (table 8) with the logistic-normal random effects models (tables 9 and 10) reveals that, after controlling for residual heterogeneity (omitted variables), apart from age, all the variables that were marginally significant in the standard model have ceased to be so in the random effects models. All the significant variables in table 8 remain significant in the random effects models of tables 9 and 10. However, it can be noticed that apart from age, the only objective variable remaining in the models, the effects of the rest are diminished. Furthermore, an examination of the parameter estimates and their standard errors suggests that the standard logistic model has overestimated the effects of these variables. For example, table 12 shows that the effect of 'best friend', though statistically significant in all the models, has been estimated with less precision given the wider confidence intervals compared to those derived from the standard model. This suggests that the cross-sectional model may be providing a false sense of accuracy leading to erroneous conclusions.

The change in the age effect from standard logistic model to logistic-normal model serves to demonstrate the complex inter-relationships in data due to the presence of the subjective variables. The effects of the subjective variables are inflated, very likely due to their relationship with the outcome variable, smoking, through the omitted variables. The inflated effect of some of the subjective variables which may be age-related (e.g. drink, have a partner) is to artificially control for the effect of age. Thus, the age effect may appear marginally significant in table 8. However, controlling for the residual heterogeneity, in tables 9 and 10, the age effect appears statistically significant.

The change in deviance from the standard logistic model to the logistic-normal random effects model without stayers is highly significant (1162.9 – 1091.3 = 71.6 on 1 d.f.), as is the estimate of the scale parameter (ω), table 9, indicating that there is substantial residual heterogeneity due to omitted variables. The results suggest that ignoring heterogeneity may lead to underestimation. The change in deviance from the random effects model without stayers to the random effects model with stayers is significant at the 5% level (1091.3 – 1084.7 = 6.6 on 2 d.f.), indicating that there is a significant proportion of stayers in the sample. Indeed, inspection of the estimate of endpoint 0 (ψ_0), table 10, reveals a highly significant proportion of stayers in state 0; in other words, 36% of the pupils claimed in both 1994 and 1996 that they had never smoked or had given up smoking (be it prior to 1994 or within the 1994-1996 project window). Endpoint 1 (ψ_1) is not significant at the 5% level: only 1% of the pupils claimed that they had smoked either regularly or occasionally in both 1994 and 1996. The scale parameter (ω) is no longer significant; in other words, the residual heterogeneity revealed by the previous model has been explained by the high proportion of non-smoking stayers in the current model.

As mentioned earlier (see table 11), another standard random effect model, GEE (Generalised Estimating Equations), that the literature recommends for longitudinal data analysis using GenStat statistical software package was also fitted to the model. It is interesting to note that a comparison of results from applying GEE, table 11, produced estimates that were similar to the estimates provided by the ordinary logistic model (table 8). That is, no real gains over and above the standard cross-sectional model were achieved. It is therefore prudent to adopt methodologies that control for residual heterogeneity.

The results, based on our sample, can be interpreted as: the likelihood of being a smoker appears to increase with age; with exposure to smoking and drinking as measured by the variables "at least one family member smokes", "best friend smokes" and "drinks"; with emotional dependence as measured by the variables "happy with weight" and "worry about money" and decreases with having a healthy attitude as measured by the variable "consider health when choosing food". The variable "worry about money" is only marginally significant and the remaining variables are non-significant even at the 20% level. Perhaps the most important aspect of these results is the statistically significant "omitted variables" effects.

Conclusion

As noted in the introduction, when using survey type data to investigate the relationship between smoking and explanatory variables a number of analytical issues must be addressed. Also noted in the introduction was the large number of variables that have been associated with teenage smoking. Certainly, for this study, all the variables included in the analysis appeared highly significant on their own (see table 2). How the explanatory variables are related with each other will have an impact on the final results. This is referred to as multicollinearity (e.g. see[57]. page 105). For the analyses in this chapter the issue of multicollinearity was addressed within the adopted statistical modelling framework (see statistical analysis section). Consequently, it is noticeable that half of the variables have ceased to be significant (see tables 4 and 5). This approach controls only for the observed multicollinearity.

We know that there are variables that may not, or cannot be observed in a survey and therefore omitted from the study such as personality, the feel good factor. The effect of omitted variables, if they exist, is to inflate the relationship between the response (smoking) and the explanatory variables [22,40]. It is also important to have measures of past behaviour on smoking and explanatory variables in order to gain some insight into the direction of causality e.g. the confidence and smoking relationship. Although, multicollinearity can be addressed within the statistical modelling framework, to address the omitted variables and past behaviour effects longitudinal data is required. In the absence of longitudinal data, the simple and pragmatic approach presented in table 5, using an awareness of substantives issues (omitted variables effect, past behaviour and multicollinearity), will assist in gaining insight into the process to guide and inform interpretation of the results from cross-sectional studies. Perhaps the most obvious example from tables 4 and 5 is the effect of the variables "which parent live with". The result for this variable suggests that those with foster parents have a much higher likelihood of being a smoker. Does this imply ruling out foster parenting as part of the social care services? As suggested in the results section, this result may well be due to the past behaviour effect not included in the cross sectional study.

The results from this study suggest that subjective variables play an intervening role. For example, the peer pressure effect (the variable "best friend smokes") in itself may not be a direct and independent effect on smoking. In fact this variable may owe its significance, at least in part, to an unobserved phenomenon or a latent variable such as a resilience factor [58] that influences teenage decision making. Resilience in turn may be governed by other social and environmental variables. For example, there is some evidence to suggest that parental influence indirectly predicts lower levels of smoking[36-38]. On the other hand there is a large body of literature on the important role the media plays and its effect on society (e.g. [59]). Norton et al [35] also make a similar conclusion that peer behaviour as a measure of peer effect is a complex subjective variable. They further conclude that including peer behaviour in the analysis rather than actual peer tobacco use could lead to inconsistencies in results. Inconsistencies in results may lead to inconsistencies in the interpretation of results and misleading conclusions.

Therefore, inconsistencies have been noted in the literature[8, 35] but have not been fully explained. For example, based on the review of the literature, Tyas [8] suggested that smoking is often used as a mechanism to cope with stress. Table 4 also suggests that those pupils who worry are more likely to be smokers. The simple analysis of table 5, and the results from the random effects models, tables 9 and 10, suggests that worrying about family problems and being at ease with the opposite sex are no longer significant, and worrying about money is significant at 10%. The calming effect of smoking as a reason for smoking is not fully justified even when it is reported by the respondents themselves. Such a conclusion projects the assumption that the majority of adolescents do not feel stressed or worry. At the same time, most of the studies reviewed by Tyas are cross-sectional and do not provide historical information on smoking. The calming effect of smoking could well be a feed-back effect as a cessation will often be accompanied by feelings of unease and anxiety [21,26]. Non-smokers who do not know the effect of smoking on their stress levels may therefore distinguish between the reasons for their anxiety/stress and try to deal with it whilst others may take up dangerous sports and so on. This ambiguity in interpreting the results is further exacerbated by the subjective effect of smoking, e.g. feelings of higher self-esteem and being in control[15,21]; a perceived 'benefit' effect as utilised in the risk models [16,17].

The reported relationship between high self-esteem and smoking serves to demonstrate these difficulties. Quite apart from the problems associated with measurement of self-esteem and multicollinearity, the main issue with such variables is change over time. To infer from cross-sectional data a relationship between smoking and high self-esteem without the knowledge of levels of self-esteem prior to smoking is unwise, and, may lead to erroneous conclusions. For example, Murphy et al[15] reported low self-esteem among the female group who indicated an intention to smoke. This means that the association between higher self-esteem and smoking[23] may become untenable, as it is likely that the individuals had lower self-esteem prior to taking up smoking. Yet, survey studies often treat a mix of observations (e.g. parental smoking behaviour and self-esteem, or psychological and environmental measures) as independent correlates (i.e. that no other effects are present) of smoking. Such an approach ignores the consequences of, both observed and unobserved multicollinearity and residual heterogeneity in data.

As discussed earlier, in behavioural studies, the possibility of a past behaviour effect should not be discounted (e.g. state dependence and duration dependence). It would have been preferable to follow up pupils from an earlier age before the uptake of smoking, and to collect observations on more than two time points, thereby allowing us to incorporate past behaviour, pathways to smoking/giving up/smoking, and other dynamics of behaviour into the analysis. Currently, with the Sabre methodology, we are also limited to a binary outcome, although theoretically the methodology applies to a multinomial outcome (e.g. regular smoker, party smoker, non-smoker). How the Sabre methodology may be extended in order to handle other features of longitudinal data, such as dropout/attrition, is a topic of current research. Furthermore, the individual specific error term accounting for heterogeneity is time-constant. Thus, the model does not account for time-varying heterogeneity (such as the feel good factor). Some of these limitations, such as accounting for time-varying heterogeneity, may be overcome by adopting a pragmatic multi-method approach e.g. the Shahtahmasebi-Davies approach[3,60].

One of the major difficulties with survey type studies is addressing residual heterogeneity (inherent variation due to omitted variables). The effects of omitted variables, if they exist, are to inflate the relationship between the outcome variable (smoking) and the explanatory variables by underestimating the standard errors[22,40]. Indeed, the comparison of the results from the standard and random effects models suggests such underestimation due to the omitted variables. Almost half the variables that were reported as significant in the standard logistic regression model (tables 4 and 8) ceased to be significant in the random effects models. Furthermore, the standard model appeared to underestimate the model parameters. For example, the peer pressure effect (the variable "best friend smokes") in itself may not be a direct and independent effect on smoking. In fact this variable may owe its significance, at least in part, to an unobserved phenomenon or a latent variable such as a resilience factor[58] that influences teenage decision making. Resilience in turn may be governed by personal characteristics and other social and environmental variables e.g. parental influence[36-38], the important role of the media and its effect on society (e.g. see [59]). This means that the act of being "happy with weight" or "worrying" may not directly increase the likelihood of being a smoker. Such variables appear to be highly correlated with the omitted variables, thereby acting as proxies for individual characteristics which had not been measured. Failure to address the substantive and analytical issues may lead to inconsistencies in results[8,35] and misleading conclusions.

One of the main challenges facing researchers, practitioners and policy makers must surely be how to inform the process of decision/policy making. Health promotion programmes must be based on reliable evidence from appropriate longitudinal research designs. Complexities arise usually as a result of ignoring substantive issues (e.g. subjectivity, objectivity and residual heterogeneity) of the study leading to mis-specification, mis-interpretation and misleading conclusions. Preventional policies that are based on cross-sectional surveys or focus on certain variables such as peer pressure often fail to take the complex dynamic behaviour of the young individuals into account. Such policies focus on influencing the "action" indicated by a variable rather than the underlying effect that the variables represent. Furthermore, health promotion (interventional and preventional) policies very rarely integrate an evaluation programme.

In studying a dynamic social behaviour such as smoking it is absolutely essential to adopt appropriate analytical methodologies of appropriate data collected using appropriate study design. An appropriate study design would incorporate substantive issues related to the dynamics of the process under investigation. For example, standard statistical methods such as logistic regression may be applied effectively to cross-sectional data, but cannot be utilised to exploit fully the richness of longitudinal data. With survey or observational studies it is possible to measure a wide range and mix of individual, social and environmental variables. On the other hand, some other variables such as personality and social attrition are un-observed, leading to complex inter-relationships and interactions in data requiring additional complexities in the methodology. Caution must be exercised when interpreting the results from survey or observational studies even when they are based on multivariate analyses. In this chapter, I demonstrated methods of examining and re-assessing evidence derived from appropriate cross-sectional and longitudinal studies. For example, Flay et al [60] using structural equation modelling suggested that the "best friend" effect on adolescent initiation into smoking is a direct effect, whilst the analysis presented in this chapter suggests otherwise. Such a result has important implications for policy as well as theory. Smoking is not an event that occurs on its own, it is the outcome of a dynamic decision making process. We need to understand the whole process.

Teenage smoking was used to illustrate some important issues of what may constitute evidence in developing interventional and preventional policy/programmes in any behavioural outcome (e.g. youth suicide, obesity, health, mental health). The relationship between evidence, researchers and other actors who play a role in informing policy formation must surely be re-examined.

Acknowledgements

The data for this study was provided with the kind permission of the Public Health Directorate, Northern and Yorkshire NHS Executive, John Snow House, Durham University Science Park, Durham DH1 3YG. Tony Goodall was the coordinator of Yorkshire Heartbeat (Public Health Department) who initiated the Health Behaviour Related survey, which was carried out by the Schools Health Education Unit, Exeter University.

References

[1] National Institute of Health. Interventions to prevent HIV risk behaviour. Washington, DC. 1997.

[2] World Health Organisation. Coming of Age: from facts to action for adolescent sexual and reproductive health. WHO/FRH/ADH/97.1. Geneva. 1997.

[3] Shahtahmasebi S. Statistical modelling of dependency in old age (PhD thesis). Bangor, North Wales: University of Wales, 1995.

[4] Short, Stephanie. Elective Affinities: Research and Health Policy Development. Heather Gardner (Ed.) Health Policy in Australia. Oxford University Press. Melbourne. 1996.

[5] Maxim Institute: http://www.scoop.co.nz/stories/PO0611/S00149.htm – see also New Zealand Herald http://www.nzherald.co.nz/section/1/story.cfm?c_id=1 and objectid=10409902.

[6] Cassidy B. The role of ICT on the literacy levels of young people with learning difficulties and/or disabilities. PhD Thesis. School of Information Management, Leeds Metropolitan University, Leeds, UK. 2007.

[7] Pletcher JR, Schwarz DF. Current concepts in adolescent smoking. *Current Opinion in Pediatrics*. 2000;12(5):444-9.

[8] Tyas SL, Pederson LL. Psychosocial factors related to adolescent smoking: a critical review of the literature. *Tobacco Control*. 1998;7(4):409-20.

[9] Jensen EJ, Overgaard E. Investigation of smoking habits among 14-17-year-old boarding school pupils: Factors which influence Smoking Status. *Public Health*. 1993; 107:117-23.

[10] Hine C. Report on stopping or reducing smoking: issues for Health Authorities. Bristol: University of Bristol, Health Care Evaluation Unit. Department of Epidemiology and Public Health Medicine, 1992.

[11] Lader D, Matheson J. Smoking among secondary school children in 1990. An enquiry carried out by Social Survey Division of OPCS on behalf of the Department of Health, the Welsh Office and the Scottish Office Home and Health Department: OPCS, Social Survey Division. London: HMSO, 1991.

[12] Goddard E. Why children start smoking. An enquiry carried out by the Social Survey Division of OPCS on behalf of the Department of Health: OPCS, Social Survey Division London: HMSO, 1990.

[13] Bolling K. Smoking among secondary school children in England in 1993. An enquiry carried out by Social Survey Division of OPCS on behalf of the Department of Health: OPCS. Social Survey Division London: *HMSO,* 1994.

[14] Sussman SC, Dent W. Group self-identification and adolescent cigarette smoking: a 1-year prospective study. J Abn Psychol 1994;103(3):576-80.

[15] Murphy NT, Price CJ. The influence of self-esteem, parental smoking and living in tobacco production region on adolescent smoking behaviour. *J. School Health.* 1988;58(10):401-5.

[16] Parsons JT, Siegel AW, Cousins JH. Late adolescent risk-taking: effect of perceived benefits and perceived risks on behavioural intentions and behavioural change. *J. Adolescence.* 1997;20:381-92.

[17] Moore S, Gullone E. Predicting adolescent risk behaviour using a personalized cost-benefit analysis. *J. Youth Adolescence.* 1996;25(3):343-59.

[18] Smith AMA, Rosenthal DA. Adolescents' perceptions of their risk environment. *J. Adolescence.* 1995; 18:229-245.

[19] Upadhyaya HP, Deas D, Brady KT, Kruesi M. Cigarette smoking and psychiatric comorbidity in children and adolescents. *J. Am. Acad. Child Adolesc. Psychiatr.* 2002;41(11):1294-305.

[20] Shek DT. Family environment and adolescent psychological well-being, school adjustment, and problem behaviour: a pioneer study in a Chinese context. *J. Genetic Psychol.* 1997; 158(1):113-28.

[21] McNeill AD, Jarvis M, West R. Subjective effects of cigarette smoking in adolescents. *Psychopharmacology.*-(Berl) 1987;92(1):115-7.

[22] Davies RB. From cross-sectional to longitudinal analysis. In: Dale A, Davies RB, editors. Analysing social and political change: A casebook of methods. London: Sage, 1994:20-40.

[23] Clayton S. Gender differences in psychosocial determinants of adolescent smoking. *J. School Health.* 1991;61(3):115-20.

[24] Paavola M, Vartianian E, Puska P. Predicting adult smoking: the influence of smoking during adolescence and smoking among friends and family. *Health Edu. Res.* 1996;11(3):309-15.

[25] Soldz S, Cui X. Pathways through adolescent smoking: a 7-year longitudinal grouping analysis. *Health Psychol.* 2002;21(5):495-504.

[26] McNeill AD. The development of dependence on smoking in children. *Psychopharmacology.*-(Berl) 1991; 92 (1):115-7.

[27] Stead M, Hastings G, Tudor-Smith C. Preventive adolescent smoking: a review of options. *Health Edu. J.* 1996;55:31-54.

[28] Moolchan ET, Ernst M, Henningfield JE. A review of tobacco smoking in adolescents: treatment implications. *J. Am. Acad. Child Adolesc. Psychiatr.* 2000;39(6):682-93.

[29] Giovannucci E. An updated review of the epidemiological evidence that cigarette smoking increases risk of colorectal cancer. *Cancer Epidemiol. Biomarkers Prev.* 2001;10(7):725-31.

[30] Balding J. Young People in 1991. Exeter: University of Exeter, Schools Health Education Unit, 1992.

[31] GLIM. Generalised Linear Interactive Modelling. 4 ed. Oxford, UK: NAG, 1993.

[32] Shahtahmasebi S, Davies R, Wenger C. A longitudinal analysis of factors related to survival in old age. *Gerontologist.* 1992;333:404-13.

[33] Wenger GC, Davies R, Shahtahmasebi S. Morale in Old Age: Refining the Model. *Int. J. Geriatric Psychiatr.* 1995; 10:933-43.

[34] Royal College of Physicians. Smoking and the Young. London, 1992.

[35] Norton EC, Lindrooth RC, Ennett ST. How measures of perception from survey data lead to inconsistent regression results: evidence from adolescent and peer substance use. *Health Econ.* 2003;12(2):139-48.

[36] Charlton A. The Brigantia Smoking Survey: a general review. Public Education About Cancer. *UICC Technical Report Series.* 1984;77:92-102.

[37] U.S. Department of Health and Human Services. Preventing Tobacco Use Among Young People. A Report of the Surgeon General: Public Health Service, Centers for Disease Control and Prevention, National Center for Chronic Disease Prevention and Health Promotion, Office on Smoking and Health, 1994.

[38] Eiser J, Morgan M, Gammage P, Gray E. Adolescent smoking: attitudes, norms and parental influences. *Br. J. Soc. Physio.* 1989;28:193-202.

[39] Stuart A. The idea of sampling. High Wycombe: Charles Griffin Ltd, 1984.

[40] Davies RB. The limitation of cross-sectional analysis. In: Crouchley R, ed. Longitudinal Data Analysis. London: Sage, 1987.

[41] Conrad KM, Flay BR, Hill D. Why children start smoking cigarettes: predictors of onset. *Br. J. Addiction.* 1992;87:1711-24.

[42] Glendinning A, Shucksmith J, Hendry L. Social class and adolescent smoking behaviour. *Soc. Sci. Medicine.* 1994;38(10):1149-60.

[43] Oakley A, Brannen J, Dodd K. Young people, gender and smoking in the United Kingdom. *Health Promotion Int.* 1992;7(2):75-88.

[44] Gibbons RD, Hedeker DR, Elkin I, Waternaux C, et al. Some conceptual and statisticalal issues in analysis of longitudinal psychiatric data: Application to the NIMH Treatment of Depression Collaborative Research Program dataset. *Archives of General Psychiatry.* 1993;50(9):739-750.

[45] Everitt BS. Analysis of longitudinal data: beyond MANOVA. *British Journal of Psychiatry.* 1998;172:7-10.

[46] Davies R, Pickles A. Accounting for omitted variables in a discrete time panel data of residual mobility. *Quality and Quantity.* 1986;20:219-233.

[47] Davies RB, Pickles AR. Robustness in modelling dynamics of choice. InHauer J, Timmermans H, Wrigley N. (Eds.) Contemporary Developments in Quantitative Geography. Dordrecht, the Netherlands: D Reidel; 1987.

[48] Davies R, Flowerdew R. Modelling Migration Careers Using Data from a British Survey. *Geographical Analysis.* 1992;24:35-57.

[49] Barry J, Francis B, Davies R. Software for Analysis of Binary Recurrent Events (SABRE): A guide for users. In. Lancaster: Centre for Applied Statistics, Lancaster University; 1990.

[50] Berridge D, dos Santos D. Modelling ordinal recurrent events. In: Banks R et al. (Eds.) *Survey and Statistical Computing.* 1996; 233-340.

[51] Bell R, Pavis S, Amos A, Cunningham-Burley S. Continuities and changes: teenage smoking and occupational transition. *J. Adolesc.* 1999; 22(5):683-94.

[52] Carlin JB, Wolfe R, Coffey C, Patton GC. Analysis of binary outcomes in longitudinal studies using weighted estimating equations and discrete-time survival methods: prevalence and incidence of smoking in an adolescent cohort. *Stat. Med.* 1999;18(19):2655-79.

[53] Sashegyi AI, Brown KS, Farrell PJ. Application of a generalized random effects regression model for cluster-correlated longitudinal data to a school-based smoking prevention trial. *Am. J. Epidemiol.* 2000;152(12):1192-200.

[54] Lawlor DA., O'Callaghan J., Mamun AA., et al. Early life predictors of adolescent smoking: findings from the Mater-University study of pregnancy and its outcomes. *Paediatric and Perinatal Epidemiology.* 2005;19, 377-387.

[55] Higgins A. and Conner M. Understanding adolescent smoking: the role of the Theory of Planned Behaviour and implementation intentions. *Psychology, Health and Medicine.* 2003;8(2),173-186.

[56] Davies R, Martin AM, Penn R. Linear modelling with clustered observations an illustrative example of earnings in the engineering industry. *Environment and Planning.* A 1988;20:1069-1084.

[57] Wallace D, Silver JL. Econometrics - An introduction. New York: Addison-Wesley, 1988.

[58] Braverman MT. Research on resilience and its implications for tobacco prevention. *Nicotine Tob. Res.* 1999(1 Suppl 1):S67-72.

[59] MacFadyen L, Hastings G, Mackintosh A. Cross sectional study of young people's awareness of and involvement with tobacco marketing. *BMJ.* 2001;3(322):513-7.

[60] Flay BR, Hu FB, Siddiqui O, Day LE, Hedeker D, Petraitis J, et al. Differential influence of parental smoking and friends' smoking on adolescent initiation and escalation of smoking. *J. Health Socl. Behavior.* 1994;35(3):248-65.

Appendix I: Additional Information on Some Variables

Definitions

Smokers: are those who claimed to smoke either regularly or occasionally; non-smokers are those who either never smoked or had given up smoking.

Missing Values Category: this category was created if the proportion of non-response (missing values) for any question was greater than 1%, otherwise, missing values re-category was assigned to the category with the highest cell frequency.

The following variables are created from the data set (25):

Social class - the only measure of class available from the survey is crudely based on the type of newspaper read by the household of the respondent: High = Quality Broadsheet newspapers (e.g. Times, Guardian, Telegraph, Independent, Scotsman, Observer); Medium = quality tabloid newspapers (e.g. Mail, Express, Today, Scottish Daily Express); Low = popular tabloid newspapers (e.g. Star, Mirror, Sun, Scottish Daily Record, Sunday Sport, Sunday People).

Self-esteem - this variable is based on 9 statements each allowing a score of 0-2; "0" agree, "1" not sure and "2" disagree. The total will take a value of 0-18, of which a score of 0-4 is low, 5-9, and 10-14 are "lower middle" and "upper middle" respectively, and 15-18 is high self-esteem. The statements are:

"There is lots of things about myself that I would like to change."
"When I have something to say in front of teachers, I usually feel uneasy."
"I often fall out with other pupils at school."
"I often feel lonely at school."
"I think other pupils usually say nasty things about me."
"When I want to tell a teacher something I usually feel shy."
"I often have to find new friends because my old ones are with somebody else."
"I usually feel foolish when I have to talk to my parents."
"I feel comfortable talking to other pupils at school."

Appendix II: The Logistic Model

To fit a normal regression to a binary variable (1/0 indicating yes/no, or, success/failure) data needs to be transformed. Generally a suitable transformation is the *logit* often referred to as logistic regression with the probability density function given by:

$$p(y_i = 1) = \frac{\exp(\beta x_i)}{1 + \exp(\beta x_i)}$$

One of the advantages of the logit model is that we can estimate the probability of a "smoker" using the prevalence rate in the sample. Alternatively, the **odds** of being a smoker can be derived as follows:

let x_{1i} represent sex; x_{1i}=0=male, x_{1i}=1=female and let β_1 be the logistic coefficient of x_{1i}:

logit (p_1; y=smoker|female)
$= \alpha + \beta_1 (x_{1i}=1) + \beta_2 x_{2i} + \ldots$

i.e the **log odds** of being a smoker given a female respondent, while the **log odds** for a male respondent is given by

logit (p_2; y=smoker|male)
$= \alpha + \beta_1 (x_{1i}=0) + \beta_2 x_{2i} + \ldots$

because β_1 is the difference between the two logs, i.e.

logit (p_1) - *logit* (p_2)
$= \beta_1 \Rightarrow \log (p_1/p_2) = \beta_1$
$\Rightarrow$ log (Odds Ratio)
$= \beta_1 \Rightarrow OR = \exp(\beta_1)$

The confidence limits (CLs) for the *OR* can easily be obtained from the standard errors of the logistic coefficients.

Appendix III: The Longitudinal Model

Consider the conventional logistic model, where each observation is assumed to be independent, the contribution by the ith case and tth event is given by

$$L_{it}(\underline{\beta}) = \frac{\exp(\beta' x_{it})^{y_{it}}}{1 + \exp(\beta' x_{it})}$$

where y_{it} is the response variable (0=non-smoker; 1=smoker), x_{it} is a vector of explanatory variables and $\underline{\beta}$ is a vector of parameter estimates. For the longitudinal application the logistic model is modified to include an individual-specific random error term ε_i in the linear predictor to account for omitted variables. For the sequence of outcomes for the ith individual, this random effects model has the integrated (or marginal) likelihood

$$L_i(\underline{\beta}) = \int \prod_{t=1}^{T_i} [g(y_{it} \mid \beta; x_{it}; \varepsilon_i)] \bullet f(\varepsilon_i) d\varepsilon_i$$

where

$$g(y_{it} \mid .) = \frac{\exp(\beta' x_{it} + \varepsilon_i)^{y_{it}}}{1 + \exp(\beta' x_{it} + \varepsilon_i)}$$

$f(\varepsilon)$ is the probability density function (mixing distribution) of the error term and T_i is the length of the sequence. SABRE uses Gaussian quadrature for the numerical evaluation of each likelihood integral, assuming a normal parameter form for f(.) then the integrated likelihood becomes

$$L_i(\theta,\beta,\omega,x_{it},z)=\sum_{q=1}^{Q}\left[\prod_{t=1}^{T_i}L_{ij(i,t)t}(\theta,\beta,\omega,x_{it},z_q)\right]p_q$$

$$L_i(\underline{\beta})=\int\prod_{t=1}^{T_i}[g(y_{it}\mid\beta;x_{it};\varepsilon_i)]\bullet f(\varepsilon_i)d\varepsilon_i$$

where z_q and p_q, q=1,...,Q are the Q fixed quadrature locations and probabilities respectively, and the scale parameter ω is the unknown standard deviation of the mixing distribution.

SABRE also includes a facility which allows for stayers, with the quadrature points supplemented by empirically determined masses at extremes (plus and minus infinity) of the mixing distribution, giving the sequence likelihood

$$L_i^*=\frac{\psi_0\prod_{t=1}^{T_i}(1-y_{it})+\psi_1\prod_{t=1}^{T_i}(y_{it})+L_i}{1+\psi_0+\psi_1}$$

where ψ_0 and ψ_1 are the unknown but estimable end-point parameters and L_i is the sequence likelihood given above. The estimated proportions of the population which are stayers in state 0 and state 1 are given by

$$\rho_0=\frac{\psi_0}{1+\psi_0+\psi_1}\text{ and }\rho_1=\frac{\psi_1}{1+\psi_0+\psi_1}.$$

SEE (25,26) FOR MORE DETAILS ON SABRE AND TO OBTAIN A FREE COPY SEE http://www.cas.lancs.ac.uk/software/sabre/sabre.html.

Index

A

B

C

D

E

F

G

H

I

N

O

P

Q

R

S

T

U

V

W

X

Y

Z